Pharmacologia

Or, The History of Medicinal Substances

John Ayrton Paris

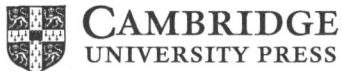

CAMBRIDGE
UNIVERSITY PRESS

CAMBRIDGE
UNIVERSITY PRESS

University Printing House, Cambridge, CB2 8BS, United Kingdom

Cambridge University Press is part of the University of Cambridge.

It furthers the University's mission by disseminating knowledge in the pursuit of
education, learning and research at the highest international levels of excellence.

www.cambridge.org
Information on this title: www.cambridge.org/9781108069847

© in this compilation Cambridge University Press 2015

This edition first published 1820
This digitally printed version 2015

ISBN 978-1-108-06984-7 Paperback

CAMBRIDGE LIBRARY COLLECTION

Books of enduring scholarly value

History of Medicine

It is sobering to realise that as recently as the year in which On the Origin of Species was published, learned opinion was that diseases such as typhus and cholera were spread by a 'miasma', and suggestions that doctors should wash their hands before examining patients were greeted with mockery by the profession. The Cambridge Library Collection reissues milestone publications in the history of Western medicine as well as studies of other medical traditions. Its coverage ranges from Galen on anatomical procedures to Florence Nightingale's common-sense advice to nurses, and includes early research into genetics and mental health, colonial reports on tropical diseases, documents on public health and military medicine, and publications on spa culture and medicinal plants.

Pharmacologia

The physician and author John Ayrton Paris (1785–1856), several of whose other medical and popular works have been reissued in the Cambridge Library Collection, published the first edition of this book in 1812. It was immediately successful, and went into eight further editions until 1843: this reissue is of the 1820 third edition. Many volumes on materia medica existed at the time, and Paris claims in his preface that he is not disparaging these competitor works, but that they presume too much prior knowledge on the part of the reader. His own work is designed to inform the student of the properties and effects of each medicinal substance, and how they function, both alone and in combinations. This will lead to greater understanding of the efficacy of medicines, and also help to prevent their adulteration. The qualities of each ingredient are discussed, and formulae and doses provided.

Cambridge University Press has long been a pioneer in the reissuing of out-of-print titles from its own backlist, producing digital reprints of books that are still sought after by scholars and students but could not be reprinted economically using traditional technology. The Cambridge Library Collection extends this activity to a wider range of books which are still of importance to researchers and professionals, either for the source material they contain, or as landmarks in the history of their academic discipline.

Drawing from the world-renowned collections in the Cambridge University Library and other partner libraries, and guided by the advice of experts in each subject area, Cambridge University Press is using state-of-the-art scanning machines in its own Printing House to capture the content of each book selected for inclusion. The files are processed to give a consistently clear, crisp image, and the books finished to the high quality standard for which the Press is recognised around the world. The latest print-on-demand technology ensures that the books will remain available indefinitely, and that orders for single or multiple copies can quickly be supplied.

The Cambridge Library Collection brings back to life books of enduring scholarly value (including out-of-copyright works originally issued by other publishers) across a wide range of disciplines in the humanities and social sciences and in science and technology.

PHARMACOLOGIA;

OR

THE HISTORY

OF

Medicinal Substances,

WITH A VIEW TO ESTABLISH

THE ART OF PRESCRIBING

AND OF

COMPOSING EXTEMPORANEOUS FORMULÆ

UPON

FIXED AND SCIENTIFIC PRINCIPLES;

ILLUSTRATED BY FORMULÆ,
IN WHICH THE INTENTION OF EACH ELEMENT
IS DESIGNATED BY KEY LETTERS.

BY

JOHN AYRTON PARIS, M.D. F.L.S.

Fellow of the Royal College of Physicians of London,

Member of the Royal Medical Society of Edinburgh, and late Senior
Physician to the Westminster Hospital.
&c. &c.

Quis Pharmacopœo dabit leges, ignarus ipse agendorum?----Vix profecto dici potest,
quantum hæc ignorantia rei medicæ inferat detrimentum.

GAUB: METHOD: CONCINN: FORMUL.

Third Edition, very considerably enlarged.

LONDON:

PRINTED AND PUBLISHED BY W. PHILLIPS,
George Yard, Lombard Street.
SOLD ALSO BY BURGESS & HILL, GREAT WINDMILL STREET,
AND OTHER BOOKSELLERS.

1820.

PREFACE TO THE THIRD EDITION.

THE Public are already in possession of many pharmaceutical compendiums and epitomes of plausible pretensions, composed with a view of directing the practice of the junior, and of relieving the occasional embarrassments of the more experienced practitioner. Nothing is farther from my intention than to disparage their several merits, or to question their claims to professional utility; but, in truth and justice it must be confessed that, as far as these works relate to the art of composing scientific prescriptions, their authors have not escaped the too common error of supposing, that the reader is already grounded in the first principles of the science; or, to borrow the figurative illustration of a popular writer, *that while they are in the ship of science, they forget the disciple cannot arrive without a boat.* I am not acquainted with any book that is calculated to furnish such assistance, or which professes to teach the GRAMMAR, and ground work of this important branch of medical knowledge. Numerous are the works which present us with the detail, but no one with the philosophy of the subject. We have copious catalogues of formal recipes, and many of unexceptionable propriety, but the compilers do not discuss the principles upon which they were constructed, nor do they explain the part which each ingredient is supposed to perform in the general scheme of the formula; they cannot therefore lead to any useful generalization, and the young practitioner, without a beacon that can direct his

course in safety, is abandoned to the alternative of
two great evils—a feeble and servile routine, on one
hand, or, a wild and lawless empiricism, on the other.
The present volume is an attempt to supply this
deficiency : and while I am anxious to ' catch the
ideas which lead from ignorance to knowledge,' it is
not without hope, that I may also be able to suggest the means by which our already acquired knowledge may be more widely and usefully extended;
and, by offering a collective and arranged view of the
objects and resources of medicinal combination, to
establish its practice upon the basis of science, and,
thereby, to render its future career of improvement,
progressive with that of the other branches of medicine;
or, to follow up the figurative illustration already
introduced, *to furnish a boat, which may not only convey the disciple to the ship, but which may also assist
in piloting the ship herself from her shallow and trea-
cherous moorings.* That the design however of the
present work may not be mistaken, it is essential to
remark, that it is elementary only in reference to the
art of prescribing, for it is presumed that the student is already acquainted with the common manipulations of pharmacy, and with the first principles of
chemistry. When any allusions are made to the processes of the Pharmacopœia, they are to be understood as being only supplementary, or as explanatory
of their nature, in reference to the application or
medicinal powers of the substance in question. The
term *Pharmacologia*, as applied to the present work,
may therefore be considered as contradistinctive to
that of *Pharmacopœia;* for while the latter denotes
the processes for preparing, the former comprehends
the scientific methods of administering medicinal bodies, and explains the objects and theory of their

operation. The articles of the Materia Medica have been arranged in alphabetical order, not only as being that best calculated for reference, but one, which, in an elementary work at least, is less likely to mislead, than any arrangement founded on their medicinal powers; for in consequence of the difficulty of discriminating, in every case, between the primary and secondary effects of a medicine, substances, very dissimilar in their nature, have been enlisted into the same artificial group, and, when several of such bodies have, from a reliance upon their unity of action, been associated together in a medicinal mixture, it has too often happened, that, like the armed men of Cadmus, they have opposed and destroyed each other. The object and application of the red marginal letters, to which the name of *Key Letters* has been given, are fully explained in the introductory essay, and it is hoped, that the scheme possesses a more substantial claim to notice than that of mere novelty : it will be perceived, that in the enumeration of the officinal formulæ, these letters are also occasionally used, to express the manner in which the particular substance, under the head of which it stands, operates in the combination. If any apology be necessary for the introduction of the medicinal formulæ, it may be offered in the words of Quintillian, who very justly observes, " *In omnibus fere minus valent præcepta quam exempla;* or in the language of Seneca, " *Longum est iter per præcepta, breve et efficax per exempla.*" Under the history of each article, I have endeavoured to concentrate all that is required to be known for its efficacious administration, such as, 1. *Its sensible qualities.* 2. *Its chemical composition,* or the constituents in which its medicinal activity resides. 3. *Its relative solubility in different menstrua, and the*

*proportions in which it should be mixed, or combined
with different bodies, in order to produce suspension, or
saturation.* 4. *The Incompatible Substances,* that is
to say, those substances which are capable of destroying its properties, or of rendering its flavour, or
aspect, unpleasant, or disgusting. 5. *The most eligible forms in which it can be exhibited.* 6. *Its specific
doses.* 7. *Its Medicinal Uses, and Effects.* 8. *Its
Officinal Preparations.* 9. *Its Adulterations.* That
such information is indispensable, for the elegant and
successful exhibition of a remedy, must be sufficiently
apparent ; the injurious changes, and modifications
which substances undergo, when they are improperly
combined by the ignorant practitioner, are not as
some have supposed imaginary, the mere *deliramenta
doctrinæ,* or the whimsical suggestions of theoretical
refinement, but they are really such as to render
their powers unavailing, or to impart a dangerous
violence to their operation. " *Unda dabit flammas et
dabit ignis aquas.*"

In the history of the different medicinal preparations, the pharmacopœia of the London College is the
standard to which I have always referred, although
it will be perceived that I have frequently availed
myself of the resources with which the pharmacopœiæ
of Edinburgh and Dublin abound. To a knowledge
of the numerous adulterations to which each article
is so shamefully exposed, too much importance can
be scarcely attached; and under this palpable source
of medicinal fallacy and failure, may be very fairly
included those secret and illegitimate deviations from
the acknowledged modes of preparation, as laid down
in the pharmacopœia, whether practised, as an expedient to obtain a lucrative notoriety, or from a
conceit of their being improvements upon the ordinary

processes; for instance, we have lately heard of a wholesale chemist who professes to supply a syrup of roses of very superior beauty, and for this purpose, he substitutes the petals of the *red* (rosa gallica) for those of the *damask* rose (rosa centifolia); we need not be told, that a preparation of more exquisite colour may be thus afforded, but allow me to ask if this *underhanded* substitution be not a manifest act of injustice to the medical practitioner, who instead of a laxative syrup, receives one which is marked by the opposite character of astringency. These observations will, of course, not apply to those articles, which are *avowedly* prepared by a new process, for in that case, the practitioner is enabled to make his election, and either to adopt, or refuse them, at his discretion. Thus, since the article *Extracta* in this work has been printed off, Mr. Barry has taken out a patent for making certain extracts, by evaporation *in vacuo;* we might almost say *a priori*, that the results must be more active than those obtained in the ordinary way, but they must pass the ordeal of experience, before they can be admitted into practice. As a brief notice of the more notorious *Quack Medicines* may be acceptable, the formulæ for their preparation have been appended in notes, each being placed at the foot of the particular article which constitutes its prominent ingredient; indeed, it is essential that the practitioner should be acquainted with their composition, for although he would refuse to superintend the operation of a boasted *panacea*, it is but too probable that he may be called upon to counteract its baneful influence.

From what has been thus stated, it will appear, that the volume now presented to the public has been so enlarged in its bulk, and extended in its views, that it rather merits the appellation of a new work, than that of a renewed edition of a former one.

The *Historical Introduction*, comprehending the substance of two of the lectures, which were delivered in the last year, before the Royal College of Physicians of London, from the recently established chair of Materia Medica, has been prefixed to the work, at the desire of several of the auditors; and I confess my readiness to comply with this request, as it enabled me at once to obviate any misconception, or unjust representation, of those remarks, which I felt it my bounden duty to offer to the College.

It will be observed, that the work itself is divided into two separate and very distinct parts, the *first* comprehending the principles of the art of combination,— the *second*, the medicinal history, and chemical habitudes of the bodies which are the subjects of such combination. These comprise every legitimate source of instruction, and to the young and industrious student, they are at once the Loom and the Raw Material. Let him therefore abandon those flimsy and ill adapted textures, that are kept ready fabricated for the service of ignorance and indolence, and by actuating the machinery himself, weave the materials with which he is here presented, into the forms and objects that may best fulfil his intentions, and meet the various exigencies of each particular occasion.

J. A. P.

Dover Street, January, 1820.

HISTORICAL INTRODUCTION.

AN INVESTIGATION OF THE MORE REMARKABLE
CAUSES WHICH HAVE, IN DIFFERENT AGES, OPE-
RATED IN PRODUCING THE REVOLUTIONS THAT
CHARACTERISE THE HISTORY OF MEDICINAL
SUBSTANCES.

[*This, and the succeeding Essay, on the subject of Medicinal Combinations, comprehend the substance of
Four Lectures, delivered by the Author before the
Royal College of Physicians, on the Philosophy of
the Materia Medica, in June,* 1819.]

BEFORE I proceed to discuss the particular views
which I am prepared to submit to the College, on the
important but obscure subject of medicinal combination, I propose to take a sweeping and rapid sketch
of the different moral and physical causes which have
operated in producing the extraordinary vicissitudes,
which so eminently characterise the history of Materia
Medica. Such an introduction is naturally suggested
by the first glance at the extensive and motley as-

a

semblage of substances, with which our cabinets* are
overwhelmed. It is impossible to cast our eyes over
such multiplied groups, without being forcibly struck
with the palpable absurdity of some—the disgusting
and loathsome nature of others—the total want of
activity in many—and the uncertain and precarious
reputation of all—or, without feeling an eager curio-
sity to enquire, from the combination of what causes
it can have happened, that substances, at one period
in the highest esteem, and of generally acknowledged
utility, could have fallen into total neglect and disrepute ;—why others, of humble pretensions, and little
significance, could have maintained their ground for
so many centuries; and on what account, materials of
no energy whatever, could have received the indis-
putable sanction, and unqualified support, of the best
and wisest practitioners of the age. That such fluc-
tuations in opinion, and versatility in practice, should
have produced, even in the most candid and learned
observers, an unfavourable impression, with regard
to the general efficacy of medicines, can hardly excite
our astonishment, much less our indignation ; nor can
we be surprised to find, that another portion of mankind has at once arraigned Physic as a fallacious art,
or derided it as a composition of error and fraud.
They ask—and it must be confessed that they ask

---

* The College of Physicians may now be said to possess one of the
most complete collections of Materia Medica in Europe. That, collected by Dr. Burges, and presented to the College after his death by
Mr. Brande, to whom it was bequeathed, has lately been collated with
the cabinet of Dr. Coombe, purchased for that purpose. Its arrangement has been directed by a feeling of convenience for reference,
rather than by any theoretical views relative to the natural, chemical,
and medicinal histories of its constituent parts. Under proper regula-
tions, it is accessible to the studious and respectable members of the
profession.

with reason—what pledge can be afforded them, that the boasted remedies of the present day will not, like their predecessors, fall into disrepute, and, in their turn, serve only as humiliating memorials of the credulity and infatuation of the physicians who commended, and prescribed them? There is surely no question, connected with our subject, which can be more interesting and important, no one which requires a more cool and dispassionate enquiry, and certainly not any which can be more appropriate for a lecture, introductory to the history of Materia Medica. I shall therefore proceed to examine with some attention the revolutions which have thus taken place in the opinions and belief of mankind, with regard to the efficacy and powers of different medicinal agents ; such an enquiry, by referring them to causes, capable of a philosophical investigation, is calculated to remove many of the unjust prejudices which have been excited, to quiet the doubts and alarms which have been so industriously propagated, and, at the same time, to obviate the recurrence of several sources of error and disappointment.

This moral view of events, without any regard to chronological minutiæ, way be denominated the PHILOSOPHY OF HISTORY, and should be carefully distinguished from that technical and barren erudition, which consists in a mere knowledge of *names* and *dates*. It has been very justly observed, that there is a certain maturity of the human mind, acquired from generation to generation, in the *mass*, as there is in the different stages of life, in the *individual* man ; what is history, when thus philosophically studied, but the faithful record of this progress? pointing out for our instruction the various causes

a 2

which have retarded or accelerated its progress in different ages and countries.

In tracing the history of the Materia Medica to its earliest periods, we shall find that its progress towards its present advanced state, has been very slow and unequal, very unlike the steady, and successive improvement, which has attended other branches of natural knowledge; we shall perceive even that its advancement has been continually arrested, and often entirely subverted, by the caprices, prejudices, superstitions, and knavery of mankind; unlike too the other branches of science, it is incapable of successful generalization; in the progress of the history of remedies, when are we able to produce a discovery or improvement, which has been the result of that happy combination of Observation, Analogy, and Experiment, which has so eminently rewarded the labours of modern science? Thus, OBSERVATION led Newton to discover, that the refractive power of transparent substances was, in general, in the ratio of their density, but, that of substances of equal density, those which possessed the refractive power in a higher degree were inflammable. ANALOGY enabled him to conclude that, on this account, water even must contain an inflammable principle, and EXPERIMENT enabled Cavendish and Lavoisier to demonstrate the surprising truth of Newton's induction, in their immortal discovery of the chemical composition of this fluid; but it is clear that such principles of research, and combination of methods, can rarely be applied in the investigation of remedies, for every problem which involves the phenomena of life is unavoidably embarrassed by circumstances, so complicated in their nature, and fluctuating in their operation, as to set at defiance every attempt to appreciate their influence; thus an observation, or experiment, upon the effects of a medicine, is liable to a thousand fallacies, unless it be carefully repeated under the various circumstances of health and disease, in different climates, and on different constitutions. We all know how very differently opium, or mercury, will act upon different individuals, or even upon the same individual, at different times, or under different circumstances; the effect of a stimulant upon the living body is not in the ratio of the intensity of its impulse, but in proportion to the degree of excitement, or vital susceptibility of the individual, to whom it is applied: this is illustrated in a clear and familiar manner, by the very different sensations of heat which the same temperature will produce under different circumstances: in the road over the Andes, at about half way, between the foot and the summit, there is a cottage, in which the ascending and descending travellers meet; the former, who have just quitted the sultry vallies at the base, are so relaxed, that the sudden diminution of temperature produces in them the feeling of intense cold, whilst the latter, who have left the frozen summits of the mountain, are overcome by the distressing sensation of extreme heat. But we need not climb the Andes for an illustration; if we plunge one hand into a basin of hot, and the other into one of cold water, and then mix the contents of each vessel, and replace both hands in the mixture, we shall experience the sensation of heat and cold, from one and the same medium; the hand, that had been previously in the hot, will feel cold, whilst that which had been immersed in the cold water, will experience a sensation of heat. Upon the same principle, ardent spirits will produce very opposite effects upon different constitutions, and temperaments.

To such causes we must attribute the barren labours of the ancient empirics, who saw without discerning, and concluded without reasoning; nor should we be surprised at the very imperfect state of the materia medica, as far as it depends upon what is commonly called experience. John Ray attempted to enumerate the virtues of plants from *experience*, and the system serves only to commemorate his failure : Vogel likewise professed to assign to substances, those powers which had been learnt from accumulated experience; and he speaks of *roasted toad*, as a specific for the pains of gout, and asserts that a person may secure himself for the whole year, from angina, by eating a roasted swallow! Such must ever be the case, when medicines derive their origin from false experience, and their reputation from blind credulity.

ANALOGY has undoubtedly been a powerful instrument in the improvement, extension, and correction of the materia medica, but it has been chiefly confined to modern times, for in the earlier ages, Chemistry had not so far unfolded the composition of bodies, as to furnish any just idea of their relations to each other, nor had the science of Botany taught us the value and importance of the natural affinities which exist in the vegetable kingdom.

With respect to the fallacies to which such analogies are exposed, I shall hereafter speak at some length, and examine the pretensions of those *ultra* chemists of the present day, who have, upon every occasion, arraigned, at their self constituted tribunal, the propriety of our medicinal combinations, and the validity of our pharmacopœias.

In addition to the obstacles, already enumerated,

the progress of our knowledge, respecting the virtues
of medicines, has met with others of a moral character,
which have deprived us, in a great degree, of another
obvious method of research, and rendered our depen-
dance upon testimony uncertain, and often entirely
fallacious. The human understanding, as Lord Bacon
justly remarks, is not a mere faculty of apprehension,
but is affected, more or less, by the will and the
passions; what man wishes to be true, that he too
easily believes to be so, and I conceive that physic
has, of all the sciences, the least pretensions to proclaim
itself independent of the empire of the passions.

In our researches to discover, and fix the period when
remedies were first employed for the alleviation of
bodily suffering, we are soon lost in conjecture, or
involved in fable; we are however unable to reach
the period in any country, when the inhabitants were
destitute of medical resources; the personal feelings
of the sufferer, and the anxiety of those about him,
must, in the rudest state of society, have incited a
spirit of industry and research, to procure alleviation,
the modification of heat and cold, of moisture and
dryness, and the regulation and change of diet, and
habits, must have intuitively suggested themselves for
the relief of pain, and when these resources failed,
charms and amulets were the natural expedients of
the barbarian ever more inclined to indulge the delusive hope of superstition, than to listen to the voice
of sober reason. Traces of amulets may be discovered
in very early history; Galen affirms that king Nechep-
sus, 630 years before the christian era, had written,
that a green jasper, cut into the form of a dragon
surrounded with rays, if applied externally, would
strengthen the stomach, and organs of digestion. In
the progress of civilization, various fortuitous incidents,

and even errors in the choice, and preparation of aliments, must have gradually unfolded the remedial
powers of many natural substances; these were recorded, and the authentic history of medicine may
date its commencement from the period when such
records began. The Chaldeans and Babylonians, we
are told by Herodotus, carried their sick to the public
roads and markets, that travellers might converse
with, and communicate to them, any remedies, which
had been successfully used in similar cases : this custom
continued during many ages in Assyria; and Strabo
states that it prevailed also amongst the ancient
Lusitanians, or Portuguese: in this manner however
the results of experience descended only by oral tradition; it was in the temple of Esculapius in Greece,
that medical information was first recorded; diseases
and cures were there registered on durable tablets of
marble; the priest and priestesses, who were the
guardians of the temple, prepared the remedies, and
directed their application, and thus commenced the
profession of physic. With respect to the actual nature
of these remedies, it is useless to enquire; the lapse of
ages, loss of records, change of language, and ambiguity of description, have rendered every learned research unsatisfactory; indeed we are in doubt with
regard to many of the medicines which even Hippocrates employed. It is however clearly shewn by
the earliest records, that the ancients were in the
possession of many powerful remedies; thus Melampus
of Argos, the most ancient Greek physician with whom
we are acquainted, is said to have cured one of the
Argonauts of sterility, by administering the rust of
iron in wine for ten days; and the same physician
used hellebore, as a purge, on the daughters of king
Prætus, who were afflicted with melancholy. Vene-

section was also a remedy of very early origin, for
Podalirius, on his return from the Trojan war, cured
the daughter of Damethus, who had fallen from a
height, by bleeding her in both arms. Opium, or a
preparation of the poppy, was certainly known in the
earliest ages; it was probably opium that Helen
mixed with wine, and gave to the guests of Menelaus,
under the expressive name of *nepenthe*, to drive away
their cares, and encrease their hilarity ; and this conjecture receives much support from the fact, that the
nepenthe of Homer was obtained from Egypt.

The revolutions and vicissitudes which remedies
have undergone, in medical, as well as popular opinion,
from the ignorance of some ages, the learning of others,
the superstitions of the weak, and the designs of the
crafty, afford an ample subject for philosophical reflection ; some of these revolutions, I shall proceed to
investigate, classing them under the prominent causes
which have produced them, viz.   Superstition—Credulity—Scepticism—False Theory—Devotion to Authority, and Established Routine—The assigning to
Art that which was the effect of unassisted Nature—
Ambiguity of Nomenclature—The progress of Botanical Science—The application, and misapplication
of Chemical Philosophy—The Influence of Climate
and Season on Diseases, as well as on the properties,
and operations of their Remedies—The ignorant Preparation, or fraudulent Adulteration of Medicines.
—The unseasonable collection of those remedies
which are of vegetable origin.—The obscurity which
has attended the operation of compound medicines.

SUPERSTITION.

A belief in the interposition of supernatural powers,
in the direction of earthly events, has prevailed in
every age and country, in an inverse ratio with its
state of civilization, or, in the exact proportion to its
want of knowledge. "In the opinion of the ignorant
multitude," says Lord Bacon, " witches and impostors
have always held a competition with physicians."
Galen also complains of this circumstance, and observes, that his patients were more obedient to the
oracle, in the temple of Esculapius, or to their own
dreams, than they were to his prescriptions. The
same popular imbecility is evidently allegorized in
the mythology of the ancient poets, when they made
both ESCULAPIUS and CIRCE the children of APOLLO;
in truth, there is an unaccountable propensity in the
human mind, unless subjected to a very long course
of discipline, to indulge in the belief of what is im-
probable and supernatural; and this is perhaps more
conspicuous with respect to physic, than to any other
affair of common life, both because the nature of
diseases and the art of curing them, are more obscure,
and because disease necessarily awakens fear, and fear
and ignorance are the natural parents of superstition;
every disease therefore, the origin and cause of which
did not immediately strike the senses, have in all ages,
been attributed, by the ignorant, to the wrath of
heaven, to the resentment of some invisible demon,
or to some malignant aspect of the stars; and hence
the introduction of a rabble of superstitious remedies,
not a few of which were rather intended as expiations
at the shrines of these offended spirits, than as natural
agents possessing medicinal powers. The introduction
of precious stones into the materia medica, arose from

an Arabian superstition of this kind; indeed De Boot, who has written extensively upon the subject, does not pretend to account for the virtues of gems, upon any philosophical principle, but from their being the residence of spirits, and he adds that such substances, from their beauty, splendour, and value, are well adapted as receptacles for *good* spirits!

Every substance whose origin is involved in mystery, has at different times, been eagerly applied to the purposes of medicine; not long since, one of those showers, which are now known to consist of the excrement of insects, fell in the north of Italy, the inhabitants regarded it as Manna, or some supernatural panacea, and they swallowed it with such avidity, that it was only by extreme address, that a small quantity was obtained for a chemical examination. A propensity to attribute every ordinary and natural effect to some extraordinary, and unnatural cause, is one of the striking peculiarities of medical superstition; it seeks also explanations from the most preposterous agents, when obvious and natural ones are in readiness to solve the problem. Soranus, for instance, who was cotemporary with Galen, and wrote the life of Hippocrates, tells us that honey proved an easy remedy for the aphthæ of children, but, instead of at once referring the fact to the medical qualities of the honey, he very gravely explains it, from its having been taken from bees that hived near the tomb of Hippocrates! And even those salutary virtues, which many herbs possess, were, in these times of superstitious delusion, attributed rather to the planet, under whose ascendency they were collected, or prepared, than to any natural and intrinsic properties in the plants themselves; indeed such was the supposed importance of planetary influence, that it was usual to prefix to

receipts a symbol of the planet, under whose reign the
ingredients were to be collected, and it is not perhaps
generally known, that the character which we at this
day place at the head of our prescriptions, and which
is understood, and supposed to mean *recipe*, is a relict
of the astrological symbol of Jupiter, as may be seen
in many of the older works on pharmacy, although it
is at present so disguised by the addition of the down
stroke, which converts it into the letter ℞, that were
it not for its *cloven* foot, we might be led to question
the fact of its superstitious origin.

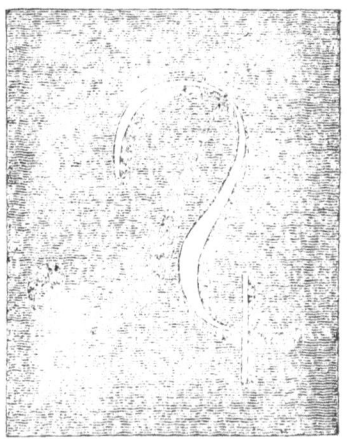

A knowledge of this ancient and popular belief in
sideral influence, will enable us to explain many
superstitions in physic; it was for this reason, that
the metals were first distinguished by the names and
signs of the planets, and as the latter were supposed
to hold dominion over time, so were astrologers led
to believe that some, more than others, had an influence on certain days of the week; and moreover, that
they could impart to the corresponding metals, con-

siderable efficacy upon the particular days which were devoted to them; from the same belief, some bodies were only prepared on certain days in the year; the celebrated earth of Lemnos, was, as Galen describes, periodically dug, with great ceremony, and it continued for many ages to be highly esteemed for its virtues; even at this day, the pit in which the clay is found is annually opened, with solemn rites, by the priests, on the sixth day of August, six hours after sun rising, when a quantity is taken out, washed, dried, and then sealed with the grand Signior's seal, and sent to Constantinople. Formerly it was death to open the pit, or to seal the earth, on any other day in the year.

It is not the least extraordinary feature in the history of medical superstition, that it should so frequently involve in its trammels, persons, who on every other occasion, would resent with indignation any attempt to talk them out of their reason, and still more so, to persuade them out of their senses; and yet, we have continual proofs of its extensive influence over powerful and cultivated minds: we need only recal to our recollection the number of persons, of superior rank, and intelligence, who were actually persuaded to submit to the magnetising operations of Miss Prescott, and even some of them were induced to believe, that a beneficial influence had been produced from the spells of this modern Circe.

Lord Bacon, with all his philosophy, betrayed a disposition to believe in the virtues of charms and amulets; and Boyle seriously recommends the thigh bone of an executed criminal, as a very powerful remedy. Amongst the remedies of Sir Theodore Mayerne, known to commentators as the Doctor Caius of Shakespeare, who was physician to three English Sovereigns, and who, by his personal authority, put an end to the distinctions of chemical and galenical practitioners in England, we shall find the secundines of a woman in her first labour with a male child; the bowels of a mole, cut open alive; mummy made of the lungs of a man who had died a violent death; with a variety of remedies, equally absurd and disgusting.

It deserves to be particularly noticed, that many of the practices which superstition has, at different times suggested, have not been alike absurd, nay, some of them have even possessed, by accident, natural powers of considerable efficacy, whilst others, although ridiculous in themselves, have actually led to results and discoveries of great practical importance. The most remarkable instance of this kind upon record, is that of the *Sympathetic* powder of Sir Kenelm Digby,* Knight of Montpellier. Whenever any wound had been inflicted, this powder was applied to the weapon that had inflicted it, which was, moreover, covered with ointment, and dressed two or three times a day.† The wound itself in the mean time

* See "Sir Kenelm Digby's Discourse upon the Cure by Sympathy, pronounced at Montpellier, before an assembly of Nobles, and learned men. Translated into English, by R. White, Gentleman, and published in 1658." King James VI. obtained from Sir Kenelm the discovery of his secret, which he pretended had been taught him by a Carmelite Friar, who had learned it in Armenia, or Persia.

† This superstitious practice is repeatedly alluded to by the poets: thus Walter Scott, in the Lay of the Last Minstrel.

> "*But she has ta'en the broken lance,*
> "*And washed it from the clotted gore,*
> "*And salved the splinter o'er and o'er.*
> "*William of Deloraine, in trance,*
> "*Whene'er she turned it round and round,*
> "*Twisted, as if she galled his wound.*
> "*Then to her maidens she did say,*
> "*That he should be whole man and sound.*"

Canto iii. St. xxiii.

was directed to be brought together, and carefully bound up with clean linen rags, but, ABOVE ALL, TO BE LET ALONE for seven days; at the end of which period, the bandages were removed, when the wound was generally found perfectly united; the triumph of the cure was decreed to the mysterious agency of the sympathetic powder, which had been so assiduously applied to the weapon, whereas, it is hardly necessary to observe, that the promptness of the cure depended upon the total exclusion of air from the wound, and upon the sanative operations of nature not having received any disturbance from the officious interference of art; the result, beyond all doubt, furnished the first hint, which led surgeons to the improved practice of healing wounds, by what is technically call the *first intention*.

The rust of the spear of Telephus, mentioned in Homer as a cure for the wounds, which that weapon

Dryden has also introduced the same superstition in his Enchanted Island. Act v. Scene ii.

Ariel. *Anoint the sword which pierced him with this*
       Weapon salve, and wrap it close from air
       Till I have time to visit it again.—

Again, in scene 4th, Miranda enters with Hippolito's sword, wrapt up.

Hip. *O my wounds pain me,*
                              (she unwraps the sword)
Mir. *I am come to ease you.*
Hip. *Alas I feel the cold air come to me;*
     My wound shoots worse than ever,
Mir. *Does it still grieve you?*
                              (She wipes and anoints the sword)
Hip. *Now, methinks, there's something laid just upon it,*
Mir. *Do you find, no ease?*
Hip. *Yes, yes; upon the sudden all this pain*
     Is leaving me—Sweet heaven, how I am eased!

inflicted, was probably *Verdegris*, and led to the discovery of its use as a surgical application.

The inoculation of the small pox in India, Turkey, and Wales, observes Sir Gilbert Blane, was practised on a superstitious principle, long before it was introduced as a rational practice into this country. The superstition consisted in buying it—for the efficacy of the operation, in giving safety, was supposed to depend upon a piece of money being left by the person who took it for insertion. The members of the National Vaccine Establishment, during the period I had a seat at the board, received from Mr. Dubois, a Missionary in India, a very interesting account of the services, derived from superstitious influence, in propagating the practice of vaccination through that uncivilized part of the globe. It appears from this document, that the greatest obstacle which vaccination encountered, was a belief that the natural small pox was a dispensation of a mischievous deity among them, whom they called MAH-RY UMMA, or rather, that this disease was an incarnation of the dire Goddess herself, into the person who was infected with it; the fear of irritating her, and of exposing themselves to her resentment, necessarily rendered the natives of the East decidedly averse to vaccination, until a superstitious impression, equally powerful, with respect to the new practice, was happily effected, this was no other than a belief, that the Goddess MAH-RY UMMA, had spontaneously chosen this new, and milder mode of manifesting herself to her votaries, and that she might be worshipped, with equal respect, under this new shape.

HYDROMANCY is another superstition, which has incidentally led to the discovery of the medicinal virtues of many mineral waters; a belief in the divining nature of certain springs and fountains, is, perhaps, the most ancient and universal of all superstitions. The Castalian fountain, and many others amongst the Græcians, were supposed to be of a prophetic nature; by dipping a fair mirror into a well, the Patræans of Greece received, as they imagined, some notice of ensuing sickness, or health; at this very day, the sick and lame are attracted to various hallowed springs, and to this practice, which has been observed for so many ages, and in such different countries, we are, no doubt, indebted for a knowledge of the sana-tive powers of many mineral waters. There can, moreover, be no doubt, but that in many cases, by affording encouragement and confidence to a dejected patient, and serenity to his mind, whether by the aid of reason, or the influence of superstition, much benefit may arise, for the salutary and curative efforts of nature, in such a state of mind, must be much more likely to succeed. Amongst the numerous instances which have been cited to shew the power of faith over disease, or of the mind over the body, the *cures per-formed by Royal Touch* have been generally selected; but it would appear, upon the authority of Wiseman, that the cures, which were thus effected, were in reality produced by a very different cause, for he states that part of the duty of the Royal Physicians and Serjeant Surgeons, was to select such patients afflicted with scrophula as evinced a tendency towards reco-very, and that they took especial care to choose those who approached the age of puberty; in short, those only were produced, whom nature had shewn a dispo-sition to cure; and as the touch of the king, like the sympathetic powder of Digby, secured the patient from the mischievous importunities of art, so were the efforts of nature left free and uncontrolled, and

b

the cure of the disease was not retarded, or opposed
by the operation of adverse remedies. The wonderful
cures of Valentine Greatracks, performed in 1666,
which were witnessed by cotemporary prelates, members of parliament, and fellows of the royal society,
amongst whom was the celebrated Mr. Boyle, would
probably, upon investigation, admit of a similar
explanation; it deserves, however, to be noticed,
that in all records of extraordinary cures, performed
by mysterious agents, there is a great desire to con-
ceal the remedies, and other curative means, which
were simultaneously administered with them; thus
Oribasius commends in high terms, a necklace of
Pæony root, for the cure of Epilepsy; but we learn
that he always took care to accompany its use with
copious evacuations, although he assigns to them no
share of credit in the cure.

The advantages which I have stated to have occasionally arisen from superstitious influence, must be
understood as being purely accidental; indeed, in the
general history of superstitious practices, we do not
find that their application was generally commended
in cases likely to be influenced by the powers of faith,
or of the imagination, but that, on the contrary, they
were as frequently directed in affections that were
entirely placed beyond the control of the mind.
Homer tells us, for instance, that the bleeding of
Ulysses was stopped by a charm; and Cato, the censor,
has favoured us with an incantation, for the reduction
of a dislocated limb.

CREDULITY;

Although it is nearly allied to Superstition, yet it differs very widely from it. Credulity is an unbounded belief in what is possible, although destitute of proof, and perhaps of probability, but Superstition is a belief in what is wholly repugnant to the laws of the physical and moral world; thus, if we believe that an inert plant possesses any remedial power, we are *credulous*, but if we were to fancy, that by carrying it about with us, we should become invulnerable, we should in that case be *superstitious*. Credulity is a far greater source of error than Superstition, for the latter must be always more limited in its influence, and can exist only, to any considerable extent, in the most ignorant portion of society, whereas the former diffuses itself through the minds of all classes, by which the rank and dignity of science are degraded, its valuable labours confounded with the vain pretensions of empiricism; and ignorance is enabled to claim for itself the prescriptive right of delivering oracles amidst all the triumphs of truth, and the progress of philosophy. Nor is this mental imbecility characteristic of any age or country. England has indeed, by a late continental writer,* been accused of possessing a larger share of credulity than its neighbours, and it has been emphatically called " *The Paradise of Quacks*," but with as little truth, as candour. If we refer to the works of Ætius, written more than 1300 years ago, we shall discover the existence of a similar infirmity with regard to physic; this author has collected a multitude of receipts, particularly those that had been celebrated, or used as *Nostrums*, many of which, he mentions, with no other view, than to expose their folly, and to inform us at what an extravagant price

* See a Tour through England by Dr. Nemnich of Hamburgh.

they were purchased ; we accordingly learn from him, that the collyrium of Danaus was sold at Constantinople for 120 numismata, and the cholical antidote of Nicostratus for two talents ; in short, we shall find an unbounded credulity with respect to the powers of inert medicines, from the elixir, and *alkahest* of Paracelsus, and Van-Helmont, to the tar water of bishop Berkley, the metallic tractors of Perkins, the animal magnetism of Miss Prescott, and may I not add with equal justice to the nitro-muriatic acid bath of Dr. Scott? The description of Thessalus, the Roman empiric in the reign of Nero, as drawn by Galen, applies, with equal fidelity and force, to the medical Charlatan of the present day ; and, if we examine the writings of Scribonius Largus, we shall obtain ample evidence that the same ungenerous selfishness,* of keeping medicines secret, prevailed in ancient, no less than in modern times.

SCEPTICISM.

Credulity has been just defined to be, *Belief without Reason*. Scepticism is its opposite, *Reason without Belief*, and is the natural, and invariable consequence of credulity, for it may be generally observed, that men, who believe without reason, are succeeded by others, whom no reasoning can convince ; a fact which has occasioned many extraordinary and violent revolutions in the *Materia Medica*, and a knowledge of it will enable us to explain the otherwise unaccountable rise and fall of many useless, as well as important articles. It will also suggest to the reflecting practitioner, a caution of great moment, to avoid the dangerous fault, imputed by Galen to Dioscorides, that of

---

* *Nostrum.* (our own.) This word, as its original meaning implies, is very significant of this characteristic attribute of quackery.

ascribing too many, and too great virtues, to one and
the same medicine; by bestowing unworthy and extravagant praise upon a remedy, we, in reality, do
but detract from its reputation, and run the risk of
banishing it from practice, for when the sober practitioner discovers by experience that a medicine falls
so far short of the efficacy ascribed to it, he abandons
its use in disgust, and is even unwilling to concede to
it that degree of merit, to which, in truth and justice,
it may be entitled; the inflated eulogiums bestowed
upon the operation of *digitalis,* in pulmonary diseases,
excited, for some time, a very unfair impression against
its use; and the injudicious manner in which the anti-
siphylitic powers of *Nitric Acid* have been aggrandised,
had very nearly exploded a valuable auxiliary from
modern practice.   It is well known with what avidity
the public embraced the expectations, given by Stoerck
of Vienna, with respect to the efficacy of *Hemlock;*
every body, says Dr. Fothergill, made the extract,
and every body prescribed it, but finding that it would
not perform the wonders ascribed to it, and that a
multitude of discordant diseases refused to yield, as
it was asserted they would, to its narcotic powers,
practitioners fell into the opposite extreme of absurdity, and declaring that it could do nothing at all,
dismissed it at once, as inert and useless.   May we
not then predict the fate of the *Cubebs,* which has been
lately restored to notice, with such extravagant praise,
and unqualified approbation?

FALSE THEORIES.

He who is governed by preconceived opinions, may
be compared to a spectator, who views the surround-
ing objects through coloured glasses, each assuming a
tinge similar to that of the glass employed; thus have

crouds of inert and insignificant drugs been indebted
to an ephemeral popularity, from the prevalence of a
false theory; the celebrated hypothesis of Galen, respecting the virtues and operation of medicines, may
serve as an example; it is a web of philosophical
fiction, which was never surpassed in absurdity. He
conceives that the properties of all medicines are derived from, what he calls, their elementary or *cardinal*
qualities, HEAT, COLD, MOISTURE, and DRYNESS.
Each of which qualities is again sub-divided into four
degrees, and a plant or medicine, according to his
notion, is cold, or hot, in the first, second, third, or
fourth gradation; if the disease is hot, or cold, in any
of these four stages, a medicine possessed of a contrary quality, and in the same proportionate degree of
elementary heat, or cold, must be prescribed. Salt-
ness, bitterness, and acridness depend, in his idea,
upon the relative degrees of heat and dryness in different bodies. It will be easily seen how a belief in
such an hypothesis must have multiplied the list of
inert articles in the materia medica, and have corrupted
the practice of physic. The variety of seeds derived
its origin from this source, and, until lately, medical
writers, in the true jargon of Galen, spoke of the
four greater and lesser hot and cold seeds; and in the
London Dispensatory of 1721, we find the powders of
hot and cold precious stones, and those of the hot and
cold compound powders of pearl.

THE METHODIC SECT, which was founded by the
Roman physician Themison, a disciple of Asclepiades,
as they conceived all diseases to depend upon *over-
bracing*, or *relaxation*, so did they class all medicines
under the head of *relaxing* and *bracing* remedies; and
although this theory has been long since banished from
the schools, yet it continues at this day to exert a

secret influence on medical practice, and to preserve from neglect some unimportant medicines.

THE STAHLIANS, under the impression of their ideal system, introduced *Archæal* remedies, and many of a superstitious and inert kind, whilst, as they on all occasions, trusted to the constant attention and wisdom of nature, so have they zealously opposed the use of some of the most efficacious instruments of art, as the Peruvian *bark*; and few physicians were so reserved in the use of general remedies, as bleeding, vomiting, and the like.

THE MECHANICAL THEORY, which recognised " *lentor and morbid viscidity of the blood,*" as the principal cause of all diseases, introduced attenuant and diluent medicines, or substances endued with some mechanical force; thus Fourcroy explained the operation of mercury by its specific gravity, and the advocates of this doctrine favoured the general introduction of the preparations of iron, especially in schirrus of the spleen, or liver, upon the same hypothetical principle; for, say they, whatever is most forcible in removing the obstruction, must be the most proper instrument of cure; such is *Steel*, which, besides the attenuating power, with which it is furnished, has still a greater force, in this case, from the *gravity* of its particles, which, being seven times specifically heavier than any vegetable, acts in proportion, with a stronger impulse, and therefore is a more powerful deobstruent. This may be taken as a specimen of the style in which these mechanical physicians reasoned and practised.

THE CHEMISTS, as they acknowledged no source of disease, but the presence of some hostile acid, or alkali, or some deranged condition in the chemical composition of the fluid, or solid parts, so they conceived all remedies must act by producing chemical

changes in the body; we find Tournefort busily engaged in testing every vegetable juice, in order to
discover in it some traces of an acid or alkaline ingredient, which might confer upon it medicinal activity.
Unlike the mechanical physicians, they explain the
beneficial operation of iron by supposing that it encreases the proportion of red globules in the blood,
on the erroneous* hypothesis that iron constitutes the
principal element of these bodies. Thus has iron,
from its acknowledged powers, been enlisted into the
service of every prevailing hypothesis; and it is not a
little singular, as a late writer has justly observed,
that theories however different, and even adverse, do
nevertheless, often coincide, in matters of practice, as
well with each other, as with long established empirical usages, each bending, as it were, and conforming,
in order to do homage to truth and experience. And
yet iron, whose medicinal virtues have been so generally allowed, has not escaped those vicissitudes in
reputation which almost every valuable remedy has
been doomed to suffer; at one period the ancients
imagined that wounds, inflicted by iron instruments,
were never disposed to heal, for which reason, Por-
senna, after the expulsion of the Tarquins, actually
stipulated with the Romans that they should not use
iron, except in agriculture; and Avicenna was so
alarmed at the idea of its internal use as a remedy,
when given in substance, that he seriously advised the
exhibition of a magnet after it, to prevent any direful

---

* The animal nature of the colouring matter of the blood was first
pointed out by Dr. Wells, but Fourcroy and Vauquelin considered it to
be owing to *subphosphate of iron*. Mr. Brande, in 1812, demonstrated
he fallacy of this opinion, and proved, by satisfactory experiments, its
itle to be considered as a peculiar animal principle; the subsequent
experiments of M. Vauquelin have confirmed Mr. Brande's results.

consequences. The fame even of Peruvian bark has
been occasionally obscured by the clouds of false
theory; some condemned its use altogether, "because
it did not evacuate the morbific matter," others, "because it bred obstructions in the viscera," others again,
"because it only bound up the spirits, and stopped the
paroxysms for a time, and favoured the translation of
the peccant matter into the more noble parts." It was
sold first by the Jesuits for its weight in silver; and
Condamine relates that in 1690, about thirty years
afterwards, several thousand pounds of it lay at Piura
and Payta for want of a purchaser.

But the most absurd and preposterous hypothesis
that has disgraced the annals of medicine, and bestowed
medicinal reputation upon substances of no intrinsic
worth, is that of the DOCTRINE OF SIGNATURES, as
it has been called, which is no less than a belief that
*every natural substance which possesses any medicinal
virtue, indicates, by an obvious and well marked external
character, the disease for which it is a remedy, or the
object for which it should be employed!* This extraordinary monster of the fancy has been principally
adopted and cherished, by Paracelsus, Porta, and
Crollius, although traces of its existence may be certainly discovered in more ancient authors; the supposed virtues of the *Lapis Ætites*, or *Eagle stone*,* described by Dioscorides, Ætius and Pliny, who assert,
that if tied to the arm, it will prevent abortion, and
if fixed to the thigh, forward delivery, were, as we
learn, from ancient authority, solely suggested by the
manner in which the nodule, contained within the
stone, moves and rattles, whenever it is shaken.

---

* This mineral derives its name from the ancient belief that it was
found in the nests of the eagle. It is a variety of iron ore, which is
commonly met with in the argillaceous iron mines of this country.

" *Ætites lapis agitatus*, *sonitum edit*, *velut ex altero lapide prægnans*." The conceit however did not assume the importance of a theory, until the end of the fourteenth century, at which period we find several authors engaged in the support of its truth, and it will not be unamusing to offer a specimen of their sophistry; they affirm that since man is the lord of the creation, all other creatures are designed for his use, and *therefore*, that their beneficial qualities and excellencies must be expressed by such characters as can be seen and understood by every one; and as man discovers his reason by speech, and brutes their sensations by various sounds, motions, and gestures, so the vast variety and diversity of figures, colours, and consistencies, observable in inanimate creatures, is certainly designed for some wise purpose. It *must be*, in order to manifest these peculiar qualities and excellencies, which could not be so effectually done in any other way, not even by speech, since no language is universal. Thus, the lungs of a fox must be a specific for asthma, *because* that animal is remarkable for its strong powers of respiration. *Turmeric* has a brilliant yellow colour, which indicates that it has the power of curing the jaundice; for the same reason, *Poppies* must relieve diseases of the head; *Agarius* those of the bladder; *Cassia fistula* the affections of the intestines, and *Aristolochia* the disorders of the uterus.

The blood-stone, the *heliotropium* of the ancients, from the occasional small specks, or points of a blood red colour, exhibited on its green surface, is even at this day employed in many parts of England and Scotland, to stop a bleeding from the nose. It is also asserted that some substances bear the SIGNATURES of the humours, as the petals of the red rose that of the blood, and the roots of rhubarb, and the flowers of saffron, of the bile.*

I apprehend that John of Gaddesden, in the four-teenth century, celebrated by Chaucer, must have been directed by some remote analogy of this kind, when he ordered the son of Edward the First, who was dangerously ill with the small-pox, to be wrapped in scarlet cloth, as well as all those who attended upon him, or came into his presence, and even the bed and room in which he was laid were covered with the same substance, and so completely did it answer, say the credulous historians of that day, that the Prince was cured without having so much as a single mark left upon him.

DEVOTION TO AUTHORITY, AND ESTA-BLISHED ROUTINE.

This has always been the means of opposing the progress of reason—the advancement of natural truths—and the prosecution of new discoveries; whilst, with effects no less baneful, has it perpetuated many of the stupendous errors, which have been al-ready enumerated, as well as others, no less weighty, and which are reserved for future discussion.

To give general currency to an hypothetical opi-nion, or medicinal reputation to an inert substance, requires only the talismanic aid of a few great names; when once established upon such a basis, ingenuity, argument, and even experiment, may open their in-

---

* For a farther account of this conceit, see Crollius, in a work ap-pended to his " Basilica Chymica," entitled, " *De Signaturis internis rerum, seu de vera et viva Anatomia majoris et minoris mundi.*"

effectual batteries. It is an instinct in our nature,
to follow the track pointed out by a few leaders; we
are gregarious animals, in a moral as well as a physical sense, and we are addicted to routine, because
it is always easier to follow the opinions of others
than to reason and judge for ourselves. " The mass
of mankind," as Dr. Payley observes, " act more
from habit than reflection." What, but such a temper
could have upheld the preposterous system of Galen
for more than thirteen centuries ? and have enabled
it to give universal laws in medicine to Europe—
Africa—and part of Asia ?   What, but authority,
could have inspired a general belief, that the sooty
washings of rosin* would act as a universal remedy ?
What, but a blind devotion to authority, or an insuperable attachment to established custom, and
routine, could have so long preserved from oblivion
the absurd medicines which abound in our earlier
dispensatories ? for example, the " *Decoctum ad
Ictericos,*" of the Edinburgh College, which never
had any other foundation than the doctrine of signatures, in favour of the *Curcuma* and *Chelidonium
Majus* ; and it is only within a few years, that the
Theriaca Andromachi, in its ancient absurd form, has
been dismissed from the British Pharmacopæiæ.
The CODEX-MEDICAMENTARIUS of Paris, recently

* This practice of Bishop Berkley has been ridiculed with great point
and effect, in a pamphlet, entitled " *A Cure for the Epidemical madness of
drinking Tar Water,*" by Mr. Reeve ; in which, addressing the Bishop,
he says, " thus in your younger days, my Lord, you made the surprising discovery of the unreality of matter, and now in your riper age,
you have undertaken to prove the reality of a universal remedy; an
attempt to talk men out of their reason, did of right, belong to that
author, who had first tried to persuade them out of their senses."

edited, still cherishes this many-headed* monster of pharmacy, in all its pristine deformity, under the appropriate title of " *Electuarium Opiatum Polupharmacum.*"

It is, however, evidently indebted for this unexpected rescue from oblivion, to a cause very remote from that which may be at first imagined ; not from any belief in its powers, or reliance upon its efficacy, but from a disinclination to oppose the torrent of popular prejudice, and to reject what has been established by authority, and sanctioned by time ; for the same reason, and in violation of their better judgment, the editors have retained the absurd formula of Diest, for the preparation of an extract of opium, which, after directing various successive operations, concludes by ordering the decoction to be boiled incessantly for six months, supplying the waste of water at intervals ! Many of the compound formulæ in this new CODEX, it is frankly allowed, possess an unnecessary, and unmeaning, if not an injurious complexity, and yet, such force has habit, and so paramount are the *verba magistri,* that the editors rest satisfied by distinguishing the more important ingredients by printing them in *Italics,* leaving the rest to be supplied at the whim and caprice of the

---

* This preparation contains 72 ingredients, which are arranged under 13 heads—viz. ACRIA, of which there are 5 species. AMARA, of which there are 8. STYPTICA vulgo ASTRINGENTIA, 5 in number. AROMATICA EXOTICA, 14. AROMATICA INDIGENA, 10. AROMATICA EX UMBELLIFERIS, 7. RESINOSA ET BALSAMA, 8. GRAVE-OLENTIA, 6. VIROSA, *seu quæ Narcosin inducunt,* there is under this head but one species, which is opium. TERREA INSIPIDA ET INERTIA. This comprises only the *Lemnian Earth* GUMMOSA, AMYLACEA, &c. 4 species. DULCIA, *liquorice and honey.* VINUM, *Spanish.*

Upon no principle of combination can this heterogeneous ferrage be vindicated.

dispenser, and thus is the grand object, and use of
a national Pharmacopœia defeated, which should above
all things, ensure uniformity in the strength, and
composition of officinal preparations.

The same devotion to authority, which induces us
to retain an accustomed remedy with pertinacity, will
always oppose the introduction of a novel practice
with asperity, unless indeed it be supported by
authority of still greater weight and consideration.
The history of various articles of diet and medicine
will prove, in a striking manner, how greatly their
reputation and fate have depended upon authority;—
it was not until many years after *Ipecacuan* had been
imported into Europe, that Helvetius, under the
patronage of Louis XIV, succeeded in introducing it
into practice.

That most extraordinary plant, *Tobacco*, notwithstanding its powers of fascination, has suffered romantic vicissitudes in its fame and character; it has
been successively opposed, and commended by physicians—condemned, and eulogised by priests—and
proscribed, and protected by governments; whilst at
length, this once insignificant production of a little
island, or an obscure district, has succeeded in diffusing itself through every climate, and in subjecting
the inhabitants of every country to its dominion; the
Arab cultivates it in the burning desart—the Lap-
landers and Esquimaux risk their lives to procure a
refreshment so delicious in their wintry solitude—the
Seaman, grant him but this luxury, and he will
endure with cheerfulness, every other privation, and
defy the fury of the raging elements; and, in the
higher walks of civilized society, at the shrine of
fashion, in the palace, and in the cottage, the fasci-
nating influence of this singular plant commands an

equal tribute of devotion and attachment. The history of the Potatoe is perhaps not less extraordinary,
and is strikingly illustrative of the omnipotent influence of authority; the introduction of this valuable
plant received, for more than two centuries, an un-
exampled opposition from vulgar prejudice, which
all the philosophy of the age was unable to dissipate,
until Louis the XVth wore a bunch of the flowers of
the potatoe, in the midst of his court, on a day of
festivity; the people then, for the first time, ob-
sequiously acknowledged its utility, and began to
express their astonishment at the apathy which had
so long prevailed with regard to its general cultivation; that which authority thus established, time and
experience have fully ratified, and scientific research
has extended the numerous resources, which this plant
is so wonderfully calculated to furnish; thus, its stalk,
considered as a textile plant, produces, in Austria, a
cottony flax—in Sweden, sugar is extracted from its
root—by combustion, its different parts yield a very
considerable quantity of potass,—its apples, when
ripe, ferment and yield vinegar by exposure, or
spirit by distillation—its tubercles made into a pulp,
are a substitute for soap in bleaching,—cooked by
steam, the potatoe is the most wholesome, and nutritious, and at the same time, the most economical of
all vegetable aliments,—by different manipulations, it
furnishes two kinds of flour, a gruel, and a paren-
chyma, which, in times of scarcity, may be made into
bread, or applied to encrease the bulk of bread made
from grain,—to the invalid, it furnishes both aliment
and medicine. Its starch is not in the least inferior
to the Indian arrow root, and our worthy President
has lately shewn, that an extract may be prepared

from its leaves and flowers, which possesses valuable properties as an anodyne remedy.

There is moreover a certain fashion in medicine, as in the other affairs of life, regulated by the caprice, and supported by the authority, of a few leading practitioners, which has been frequently the occasion of dismissing from practice valuable medicines, and of substituting others less certain in their effects, and more questionable in their nature. As years and fashions revolve, so have these neglected remedies, each in its turn, risen again into favour and notice, whilst old receipts, like old almanacks, are abandoned, until the period may arrive, that will once more adapt them to the spirit and fashion of the times; thus it happens that most of our *New Discoveries* in the Materia Medica have turned out to be no more than the revival and adaptation of ancient practices. In the last century, the root of the *Asphidium Filix,* the Male Fern, was retailed as a secret nostrum by a French empiric, for the cure of tape worm; the secret was purchased, for a considerable sum of money, by the French King, and the physicians then discovered that the same remedy had been administered in that complaint by Galen.

The history of popular medicines, for the cure of gout, will also furnish us with ample matter for the illustration of this subject. The celebrated Duke of Portland's Powder was no other than the *Diacentaureon* of Cælius Aurelianus, or, the *Antidotos ex duobus Centaureæ generibus* of Ætius;* the receipt

---

* DUKE OF PORTLAND'S POWDER FOR THE GOUT.—Equal quantities of the roots of *Gentian*, and Birthwort (*Aristolochia rotunda*) the tops and leaves of Germander ((*chemadrys*) Ground Pine (*chamæpitys*) and lesser centaury, (*Chironea Centaurium*) powdered, and mixed together.

for which a friend of his Grace brought from Switzerland; into which country it had been probably introduced by the early medical writers, who had transcribed it from the Greek volumes, soon after their arrival into the western parts of Europe. The active ingredient of a no less celebrated remedy for the same disease, the *Eau Medicinale*, has been discovered to be the *Colchicum Autumnale*, or Meadow Saffron; upon investigating the properties of this medicine, it was observed, that similar effects in the cure of the gout were ascribed to a certain plant, called *Hermodactylls*, by Oribasius and Ætius, but more particularly by Alexander Trallian, a physician of Asia Minor, in the fourth century; an enquiry was accordingly instituted after this unknown plant, and upon procuring a specimen of it from Constantinople, it was actually found to be a species of *Colchicum*.

The use of Prussic acid, in the cure of Pthisis, which has been lately proposed by Dr. Majendie, and introduced into the *Codex Medicamentarius* of Paris, is little else than the revival of the Dutch practice in this complaint; for Linnæus informs us, in the fourth volume of his " *Amœnitates Academicæ*," that distilled Laurel water was frequently used in Holland, for the cure of pulmonary consumption.

The celebrated fever powder of Dr. James, was evidently not his original composition, but an Italian nostrum, invented by a Mr. Lister, a receipt for the preparation of which is to be found, at length, in *Colborne's Complete English Dispensatory, for the year* 1756.

c

THE ASSIGNING TO ART THAT WHICH
WAS THE EFFECT OF UNASSISTED NA-
TURE.

Our inability, upon all occasions, to appreciate the
efforts of nature, in the cure of disease, must always
render our notions, with respect to the powers of art,
liable to numerous errors, and multiplied deceptions.
Nothing is more natural, and at the same time more
erroneous, than to attribute the cure of a disease to
the last medicine that had been employed ; the advocates of amulets and charms have even been thus
enabled to appeal to the testimony of what they call
experience, in justification of their superstitions ; and
cases, which in truth and justice, ought to be considered most lucky escapes, have been triumphantly
pronounced as skilful cures ; and thus have medicines,
and practitioners alike, acquired unmerited praise, or
unjust censure. Upon Mrs. Stephens offering her
remedy for the stone, to Parliament, a committee of
professional men was nominated to astertain its efficacy ; a patient with stone was selected, and he took
the remedy ; his sufferings were soon relieved, and
upon examining the bladder in the usual way, no stone
could be felt, it was therefore agreed that the patient
had been cured, and that the stone had been dissolved ;
sometime afterwards, this patient died, and on being
opened, a large stone was found in a little pouch,
formed by a part of the bladder, and which communicated with it.

AMBIGUITY OF NOMENCLATURE.

It has been already stated that we are, to a great degree, ignorant of the Simples used by the ancient Physicians; we are often quite unable to determine what the plants are, of which Dioscorides treats, and yet no labour has been spared to clear the subject of its difficulties; Cullen even laments that so much pains should have been bestowed upon so barren an occasion. The early history of botany presents us with such a chaos of nomenclature that it must have been impossible for the herbarist and physician to have communicated their mutual lights, every one was occupied with disputes upon words and names, and every useful enquiry was suspended, from an inability to decide what plant each author intended; thus, it seems very doubtful whether the plant which we denominate *Hemlock* was the poison usually administered at the Athenian executions, and which deprived Socrates and Phocion of life; Pliny informs us that the word *Cicuta*, amongst the ancients, was not indicative of any particular species of plant, but of vegetable poisons, in general; this is a circumstance to which I am anxious to fix your attention; it is by no means uncommon, to find a word which is used to express general characters, subsequently become the name of a specific substance, in which such characters are predominant; and we shall find, that some anomalies in nomenclature may be thus explained. The term ' Αρσενικον,' from which the word *Arsenic* is derived, was an ancient epithet, applied to those natural substances, which possessed strong and acrimonious properties, and as the poisonous quality of arsenic was found to be remarkably powerful, the term was

especially applied to Orpiment, the form in which
this mineral more usually occurred. So the term
Elaterium was used by Hippocrates, to signify various
internal applications, especially purgatives, of a violent and drastic nature, (from the word, ' Ελαυνω,'
agito, moveo, stimulo), but by succeeding authors, it
was, exclusively, applied to denote the active matter,
which subsides from the juice of the *wild cucumber*.
The word *Fecula*, again, originally meant to imply
any substance, which was derived by spontaneous
subsidence, from a liquid, (from *fœx*, the grounds or
settlement of any liquor) ; afterwards it was applied
to *Starch*, which is deposited in this manner, by agitating the flour of wheat in water ; and lastly, it has
been applied to a peculiar vegetable principle,
which, like *starch*, is insoluble in cold, but completely
soluble in boiling water, with which it forms a gelatinous solution ; this indefinite meaning of the word
fecula has created numerous mistakes in pharmaceutic
chemistry ; Elaterium, for instance, is said to be a
fecula, and in the original sense of the word it is
properly so called, inasmuch as it is procured from a
vegetable juice by spontaneous subsidence, but in the
limited and modern acceptation of the term, it con-
veys an erroneous idea, for instead of the active
principle of the juice residing in *fecula*, it is a peculiar
proximate principle, *sui generis*, to which I have
ventured to bestow the name of *Elatin*. For the same
reason, much doubt and obscurity involve the meaning of the word *Extract*, because it is applied *generally*
to any substance obtained by the evaporation of a
vegetable solution, and, *specifically*, to a peculiar
proximate principle, possessed of certain characters,
by which it is distinguished from every other elementary body. See *Extracta*.

The progress of BOTANICAL SCIENCE, by furnishing a strictly philosophical language, which is independent of all theory, because it is founded upon
natural structure, which is beyond the control of
opinion, will prevent the recurrence of those doubts
and difficulties, which have formerly embarrassed the
history of vegetable remedies: and the advancement
of chemical knowledge, by enabling us better to distinguish and identify the different substances we employ, will also materially assist in preventing the
confusion which has formerly oppressed us. At the
same time, I am unwilling to join in the commendations
which have been so liberally bestowed upon our chemical
nomenclature, nay, I am disposed to consider it as a
matter of regret, that the names of our medicinal
compounds should have any relation to their chemical
composition, for in the present unsettled state of this
science, such a language must necessarily convey
theory instead of truth, and opinions rather than facts;
in short, it places us at the mercy and disposal of
every new hypothesis, which may lay our boasted
fabric in ruins, and, in its place, raise another super-
structure, equally frail in its materials, and ephemeral
in its duration: thus CORROSIVE SUBLIMATE was a
muriate of Mercury, or an *oxy-muriate*, until Sir H.
Davy established his new theory of chlorine, and then
it became a *bi-chloride;* at some future period, Chlorine
will be found to be a compound, and then it must
have another name; for the same reason the term
CALOMEL,* is surely to be preferred to *submuriate*, or

* Calomel.—There is some doubt respecting the original meaning of
this word, literally it signifies, *fair, black,* καλος, μελας. Sir Theodore
Mayerne is said to have given the name to it, in consequence of his
having had a favorite black servant who prepared it, but is it not more
probable that its name was derived from the change of colour which it
undergoes, from *black* to *white*, during its preparation?

Chloride. TARTARIZED ANTIMONY, again, has been called by our nomenclatural reformers the *Tartrate of Antimony and Potass;* but is it a triple compound? Gay Lussac thinks not, and considers it as a combination, in which *cream of tartar* acts the part of a simple acid. The French in their new *codex,* are still more extravagant in their application of chemical nomenclature; thus, the sub-carbonate of potass is called by them *sub-deuto-carbonas potassii.* The first part of this quadruple name indicates the comparative quantity of acid in the salt, the second that of oxygen contained in the base, the third announces the acid, and the fourth the basis of the base.

THE PROGRESS OF BOTANICAL SCIENCE.

It has been just stated that we have derived from botanical science, a philosophical language which enables us to describe the structure and habits of any plant with a luminous brevity and an unerring perspicuity; but we are moreover indebted to botany for another service, no less important to the successful investigation of the materia medica, that of throwing into well defined groups, those plants which possess obvious natural affinities, and which will be found, at the same time, to present certain medicinal analogies; indeed, as a general rule, we may admit the axiom, " *Quæ genere conveniunt, virtute conveniunt.*"

The *Umbelliferæ* which grow on dry ground are aromatic, whilst the aquatic species are among the most deadly of poisons. The *Cruciform* plants are aromatic and acrid in their nature, containing essential oils,* which are obtainable by distillation; and Linnæus

* Hence the peculiar smell of cabbage water, &c.

asserts that "among all the *Leguminous* or *Papiliona-ceous* tribe there is no deleterious plant to be found:" this however is not exactly true. Some of the indivi-duals in these natural orders, although very nearly related, do nevertheless possess various, and even opposite qualities; in the leguminous tribe above mentioned, which is as consistent as any one we possess, we have the *Cytisus Laburnum*, the seeds of which are violently emetic, and those of *Lathyrus Sativus*, which have been supposed at Florence to soften the bones and cause death.

In the subdivision even of a genus there is often a remarkable difference in the properties of the species; there are for instance, *Solanums*, *Lettuces*, *Cucumbers*, and *Mushrooms*, both esculent and poisonous; the plants of the natural family of *Contortæ* abound with a highly acrid, milky juice, but Dr. Afzelius met with a shrub of this order at Sierra Leone, the milk of whose fruit was so sweet, as well as copious, as to be used instead of cream for tea; this is certainly what no one could have guessed from analogy. The same individual will vary from culture, or other circum-stances, as much as any two plants which have no botanic affinity; the Chamomile, *Anthemis Nobilis*, with which we are all acquainted, by cultivation, may have its whole disk changed to ligulate white florets, destitute of medicinal properties. But what is more embarrassing the different parts of the same plant have often very different powers; yet notwithstanding all these difficulties, botany is capable of furnishing us with analogies which will lead to just conclusions with respect to the medicinal properties of different vegetables.

The system of Linnæus, although in a great degree artificial, corresponds in a surprising manner with the natural properties of plants; thus a plant whose *calyx* is a double valved *glume*, with three *stamina*, two *pistills*, and one *naked seed*, bears seeds of a farinaceous and nutritious quality; a flower with twelve, or more *stamina*, all of which are inserted in the internal side of the *calyx*, will furnish a wholesome fruit; whereas a plant whose flower has five *stamina*, one *pistil*, one *petal*, and whose fruit is of the *berry* kind, may at once be pronounced as poisonous.

It is also in a great degree true that the sensible qualities of plants, such as *taste*, *colour* and *smell*, have an intimate relation to their properties, and may often lead, by analogy, to an indication of their powers; we have an example of this in the dark and gloomy aspect of the *Luridæ*, which is indicative of their narcotic and very dangerous qualities, as *Datura*, *Hyoscyamus*, *Atropa*, and *Nicotiana*. So again, a peculiar heavy odour, which is well known, but is with difficulty defined, is a sure indication of narcotic properties. Bitterness, when not extreme, denotes a tonic quality, which will stimulate the stomach and intestines, and promote the process of digestion.*

---

* *Bitter Extractive* seems to be as essential to the digestion of herbivorous, as salt is to that of carnivorous animals. It acts merely as a natural stimulant, for it has been shewn by a variety of experiments, that it passes through the body without suffering any diminution in its quantity, or change in its nature. No cattle will thrive upon grasses, which do not contain a portion of this vegetable principle; this has been most satisfactorily proved by the late researches of Mr. Sinclair, gardener to the Duke of Bedford, which are recorded in that magnificent work, the "HORTUS GRAMINEUS WOBURNENSIS." They shew, that if sheep are fed on *yellow turnips*, which contain little or no *bitter extractive*, that they instinctively seek for, and greedily eat any provender which may contain it, and that if they cannot obtain it, they become diseased, and die. We are ourselves conscious of the invigorating effect of slight bitters upon our stomach; and their presence in malt liquors not only tends materially to diminish the noxious effects of such potations, but to render them, when taken in moderation, promoters of digestion.

When the bitterness is more intense and pungent,* as in *Aloes*, *Colocynth*, &c. we may infer that such substances will produce a more active effect upon the *primæ viæ*, and that catharsis will ensue. Linnæus, however, in his PHILOSOPHIA BOTANICA, has carried these analogies much too far, when he asserts that " from the colour, taste and smell, the virtues of plants may be generally known ;" to which he adds, that " the sapid and sweet smelling are generally innocent, and that such as are nauseous, and of a rank and disagreeable smell, are hurtful." It is certainly reasonable to suppose, that those bodies which produce upon the organs of taste a sensible and pungent effect, may occasion an impression, corresponding in degree, upon the stomach, or intestines, which are but an extension of the same structure. But what numerous exceptions are there to such a law ? nay, some of the most poisonous substances affect in a very slight degree the organs of taste, especially those that belong to the mineral kingdom, as *Arsenious Acid, Oxyd of Antimony, Calomel, &c.*

THE APPLICATION AND MISAPPLICATION OF CHEMICAL SCIENCE.

Amongst the researches of different authors, who, animated with a sacred zeal for ancient learning, have endeavoured to establish the antiquity of chemical science, we find many conclusions deduced from an ingenious interpretation of the mythological fables,

---

* Lord Bacon attributes the operation of purgatives to three causes, viz. *extreme bitterness, loathsomeness and horrible taste*, as in Agaric and black Hellebore, and *a secret malignity*, as in antimony, &c.

which are supposed to have been transmitted by the
Egyptians, who, previous to the invention of letters,
adopted this method of perpetuating their discoveries
in natural philosophy. Thus, wherever Homer studi-
ously describes the stolen embraces of Mars and
Venus, they recognise some chemical secret, some
combination of iron with copper, shadowed in the
glowing ornaments of fiction. Lord Bacon* conceived
that the union of spirit and matter was allegorised in
the fable of Proserpine being seized by Pluto, as she
was gathering flowers; an allusion, says Dr. Darwin,
which is rendered more curiously exact by the late
discovery, that pure air, (oxygen) is given out by
vegetables; and that in this state it is greedily absorbed
by inflammable bodies. The same ingenious Poet
supposes that the fable of Jupiter and Juno, by whose
union the vernal showers were said to be produced,
was meant to pourtray the production of water, by
the combination of its two elements, an opinion, which,
says he, is strongly supported by the fact that, in the
ancient mythology, the purer air, or æther, was always
represented by Jupiter, and the inferior, by Juno. Were
the elegant author of the botanic garden now living,
he would no doubt, with a taste, and delicacy, peculiarly
his own, avail himself of the singular discovery of Mr.
Smithson, who has detected in the juice of the mulberry
two distinct species of colouring matter;—the mingled
blood of the unfortunate Pyramus and Thisbe :

" Signa tene cædis : pullosque et luctibus aptos
Semper habe fætus, *gemina* monumenta cruoris."
Ovid. Metamorph. Lib. iv. 160.

---

* Bacon's works, vol. v. p. 470. Editio, 4to. London, 1778.

But with whatever ingenuity and success the antiquity of chemical knowledge may be advocated, as it relates to the various arts of life, yet it must be allowed, that not the most remote trace of its application to physic can be discovered in the medical writers of Greece or Rome. The operation of distillation* is not even mentioned by Hippocrates, or Galen; and the waters of different plants, as described by some later authors, are to be understood, as we are informed by Gesner, merely as simple decoctions, and not as the products of any chemical process.

Upon the downfall of the Roman Empire, all the sciences, the arts, and literature, were overwhelmed in the general wreck, and the early Mahometans, in the first paroxysms of their fanaticism, endeavoured to destroy every record of the former progress of the human mind, consigning to destruction, by the conflagration of the Alexandrian library, no less than seven hundred thousand volumes, which comprised the most valuable works of science and literature. It is not a little extraordinary that this same people were destined at a more advanced period, to rekindle the light of letters, which they had taken such pains to extinguish, and to become the inventors and cultivators of a new science, boundless in its views and inexhaustible in its applications. The medical profession too was more particularly selected as an object of reward and encouragement; and we may say, with much truth, that our *Materia Medica* is more indebted to the zeal and industry of the Arabians, than to the learning of the Greeks, or to the refinement of

---

* Dioscorides and Pliny describe a process, which may be considered that of distillation in its infancy, it consists in obtaining oil from pitch, by spreading over it, while boiling, fleeces of wool, which receive the vapour, and afterwards yield it by expression.

the Romans. From this source we have acquired the milder purges of *Manna*, *Cassia*, *Senna* and *Rhubarb*, and many plants and oriental aromatics, amongst which we may notice *Musk*, *Nutmeg*, *Mace*, and *Cloves;* and although Archigenes and Aretæus had long before applied *Blisters*, yet it is to the Arabian physicians that we are indebted for a practical acquaintance with their value, for in general, the Greeks and Romans prescribed acrid *Sinapisms* for such a purpose. We are also indebted to the Arabians for our knowledge respecting Camphor, as its name imports, for the original word was *Cafur* or *Canfur.** They are also the first upon record, who speak of sugar, and sugar candy, extracted from the sugar cane, which they call *honey of cane;* and they ushered into practice *Syrups*, *Juleps*, and *Conserves*. At the same time it is but just to allow that from the disgusting ostentation of this people, and their strong attachment to the marvellous, many absurd medicines have been introduced. Gold, Silver, Bezoars, and precious stones were received into their materia medica, and surprising virtues were attributed to them. Amongst a people thus disposed to magnificence, and - from the very spirit of their religion, credulous and romantic, it is not a matter of surprise that their first researches into the nature of bodies, should have raised a hope, and excited a belief, that the baser metals might be converted into gold.*

* Garcias as well as Geoffroy and Hill say that Ætius mentions camphor, but it cannot be found, as Dr. Alston has observed, in that, or in any other Greek author. There is a *Camphoræ herba* in Myrepsus, but this is evidently a very different thing.

* Those who advocate the antiquity of chemistry, conceive that the alchemical secret is metaphorically concealed in the fable of the GOLDEN FLEECE of the Argonauts, rejecting the more probable solution of this story by Strabo, who says that the Iberians, near neighbours of the

They conceived that gold was the metallic element. in a state of perfect purity, and that all the other metals differed from it, in proportion only to the extent of their individual contamination, and hence the origin of the epithet *base*, as applied to such metals; this hypothesis explains the origin of alchemy: but, in every history, we are informed that the earlier alchemists expected, by the same means that they hoped to convert the *baser* metals into gold, to produce a universal remedy, calculated to prolong, indefinitely, the span of human existence.

It is difficult to imagine what connection could exist in their ideas between the " *Philosopher's stone,*" which was to transmute metals, and a remedy which could arrest the progress of bodily infirmity: upon searching into the writings of these times, it clearly appears that this conceit originated with the alchemists from the application of false analogies, and that the error was subsequently diffused, and exaggerated, by a misconstruction of alchemical metaphors.

An example of reasoning by false analogy, is presented to us by Paracelsus, in his work *de vita longa,* wherein, speaking of antimony, he exclaims, " *Sicut antimonium finit aurum, sic, eadem ratione et forma, corpus humanum purum reddit.*"

The processes of alchemy were always veiled in the most enigmatic and obscure language; the earliest alchemist whose name has reached posterity, is Geber, an Arabian prince of the seventh century, whose language was so proverbially obscure, that Dr. Johnson supposes that the word gibberish, or *geberish* was derived from this circumstance; sometimes the pro-

Colchians, used to receive the gold, brought down from the high lands by the torrents, into sieves and sheep skins, and that from thence arose the fable of the Golden Fleece.

cesses of alchemy were expressed by a figurative and
metaphorical style of description, thus Geber exclaims,
" *Bring me the six lepers that I may cleanse them;*"
by which he implied the conversion of the six metals,*
the only ones then known, into gold. From the
works of later alchemists it also appears that they
constantly represented *gold* as a sound, healthy, and
durable man, the imperfect metals as diseased men,
and the means or processes by which the latter were
to be transmuted into the former, they designated by
the name of *medicines*, and hence, those who were
anxious to dive into the secrets of these magicians
or 𝔄𝔡𝔢𝔭𝔱𝔰, as they termed themselves, without possessing a key to their language, supposed that these
descriptions were to be understood in a literal sense,
and that the imperfect metals might be changed into
gold, and the bodies of sick persons into healthy ones,
by one and the same chemical preparation.

This hieroglyphical style of writing adopted by
the earlier alchemists, was in a great degree supported
by the prevailing idea that the elements were under
the dominion of spiritual beings, who might be submitted to human power; and Sir Humphry Davy has
observed that the notions of fairies, and of genii,
which have been depicted with so much vividness of
fancy, and liveliness of description in THE THOUSAND
AND ONE NIGHTS, seem to have been connected with
the pursuit of the science of transmutation, and the
production of the elixir of life. That the Arabian
Nights' Entertainment admits of a mystic interpretation, is an opinion which I have long entertained.
How strikingly is the effect of fermented spirit, in
banishing the pressure of the melancholy which occurs

* Silver, Mercury, Copper, Iron, Tin, Lead.

in solitude, depicted in the story of Sinbad when he encountered the withered and decrepid hag, on the uninhabited island—but, to return from this digression to the subject of medical chemistry.

It was not in fact, until several years had elapsed in the delusive researches of alchemy, that the application of chemical knowledge became instrumental in the advancement of the chemical art. RHASES and AVICENNA, who were the celebrated physicians of the age, are the first who introduced pharmaceutical preparations into their works, or made any improvement in the mode of conducting pharmaceutical processes. Avicenna describes, particularly, the method of conducting *Distillation*; he mentions also, for the first time, the three *Mineral Acids*, and distinguishes between the *vegetable* and *mineral Alkalies*; he speaks likewise of the *Distilled Water of Roses*, of *Sublimed Arsenic*, and of *Corrosive Sublimate*.

In the year 1226, ROGER BACON, a monk of Westminster Abbey, laid the foundations of chemical science in Europe; his discoveries were so extraordinary that he was excommunicated by the Pope, and imprisoned ten years, for supposed dealings with the devil; it appears that he was a believer in a universal Elixir, for he proposed one to Pope Clement the Tenth, which he extolled highly, as the invention of Petro de Maharncourt.

This wonderful man was succeeded, at the end of the same century, by Arnoldus de Villa Nova, a Frenchman, or as others assert, a Spaniard, who deserves to be noticed on this occasion, as being the first to recommend the distilled spirit of wine, impregnated with certain herbs, as a valuable remedy; from which we may date the introduction of *Tinctures* into medical practice; for, although Thaddæus, a

Florentine, who died in 1270, at the age of eighty, bestows great commendation upon the virtues of *Spirit of Wine,* yet he never used it as a solvent for active vegetable matter.

It was not however until the end of the thirteenth century, that Chemistry can be said to have added any considerable power to the arm of Physic.

BASIL VALENTINE, a German Benedictine monk, led the way to the internal administration of metallic medicine, by a variety of experiments on the nature of *Antimony,* and in his " *Currus Triumphalis Antimonii,*" a work written in high Dutch, he has described a number of the combinations of that metal. If however we may credit a vague tradition, he was extremely unfortunate in his first experiments upon his brother monks, all of whom he injured if not killed ; those who have keen ears for etomological sounds will instantly recognise, in this circumstance, the origin of the word *Antimony,* 'αντι Μονοχυς.

It appears that the ancients were ignorant of the internal use and administration of the metals, with the exception of iron, although they frequently used them in external applications ; Oribasius and Ætius added " *Lithargyrium*" to several plaisters, and the composition of the " *Snow-like plaister,*" from *Minium,* was long preserved amongst their more valuable secrets. Whether antimony is the *Stimmi* or *Stibium* of the ancients has been a matter of conjecture, for Pliny, in speaking of its preparation observes, " Ante omnia urendi modus necessarius, ne *Plumbum* fiat." This plumbum however was evidently the revived metal of *Antimony,* with which the ancients were unacquainted, and therefore mistook it for *Lead;* besides, the word *Plumbum,* like many others which I have before mentioned, was used as a general term, thus, according to Pliny, Tin was called *Plumbum album*.

The question however is unimportant, for this *Stibium* was never used, but as an external Astringent, especially for the purpose of contracting the eye-lids, and thereby of making the eyes appear very large, which has been considered from the most remote antiquity, as a feature of great beauty; thus the epithet βοῶπις is constantly applied by Homer to Juno. This practice appears also to have been followed by the Jews, for Jezebel is said to have painted her eye-brows to make the eyes appear big;* the expression also shews that the drug employed was the *Stimmi*. ''Εσίιμμισαίο Ίυς οφθαλμυς 'αυίης.

To BASIL VALENTINE we are moreover indebted for the discovery of the *Volatile Alkali*, and of its preparation from *Sal Ammoniac*; he also first used mineral acids, as solvents, and noticed the production of *Ether* from Alcohol.

In the year 1493, was born near Zurich in Switzerland, PARACELSUS, or as he termed himself, Philippus, Theophrastus, Bombastus, Paracelsus de Hoheinheim, a man who was destined to produce a greater revolution in the Materia Medica, and a greater change in medical opinions and practice, than any person who had ppeared since the days of Galen. He travelled all over the Continent of Europe to obtain knowledge in chemistry and physic, and was a great admirer of Basil Valentine; declaring that Antimony was not to be equalled, for medicinal virtue, by any other substance in nature : this op nion however does not deserve our respect, for it was not founded upon observation and experiment, but on a fanciful analogy, derived from a property which this metal possesses,

* ii Kings, chap. ix. verse 30.

d

of refining gold, as I have before related. He also used *Mercury* without reserve, and appears to have been the first who ventured to administer it internally ; for, although Avicenna asserts that it was not so poisonous as the ancients had imagined, yet he attributes to it no virtues ; he merely says, " Argentum quidem vivum, plurimi qui bibunt, *non læduntur eo.*" Its effects, when applied externally, were well known to Theodoric the friar, in the twelfth century, who describes the salivation which mercurial frictions will produce.

Paracelsus, thus armed with opium, mercury, and antimony, remedies of no trifling importance, travelled in all directions, and performed many extraordinary cures, amongst whom was the famous printer, Frobenius of Basil, a circumstance which immediately brought him acquainted with Erasmus, and made him known to the magistracy of Basil, who elected him professor of chemistry in the year 1527, which was the first professorship that was established in Europe for the promotion and dissemination of chemical science.

While seated in his chair, he burnt with great solemnity the writings of Galen and Avicenna, and declared to his audience, that if God would not impart the secrets of physic, it was not only allowable but even justifiable, to consult the Devil. His cotemporary physicians he treated with the most sottish vanity, and illiberal insolence ; in the preface to his work entitled " Paragranum," he tells them, "that the very down of his bald pate had more knowledge than all their writers, the buckles of his shoes more learning than Galen and Avicenna, and his beard more experience than all their Universities." With such a temper it could not be supposed that he would long

retain his chair, in fact, he quitted it in consequence
of a quarrel with the magistrates, after which he
continued to ramble about the country, generally in-
toxicated, and seldom changing his clothes, or even
going to bed; and, although he boasted of possessing
a *Panacea*, which was capable of curing all diseases
in an instant, and even of prolonging life to an indefinite length, yet this drunkard and prince of empirics
died, after a few hours illness, in the forty-eighth year
of his age, at Saltzburgh in Bavaria, with a bottle of
his immortal *Catholicon* in his pocket.

In contemplating the career of this extraordinary
man, it is difficult to say whether disgust or astonishment is the most predominant feeling; his insolence, and unparalled conceit, his insincerity, and
brutal singularities, and his habits of immorality
and debauchery, are beyond all censure; whilst the
important services he has rendered mankind, by opposing the bigotry of the schools, and introducing
powerful remedies into practice, cannot be recorded
without feelings of gratitude and respect: but in
whatever estimation Paracelsus may be held, there
can be no doubt but that his fame produced a very
considerable influence on the character of the age, by
exciting the envy of some—the emulation of others—
and the industry of all.

A prejudice in favour of chemical remedies having
been thus introduced, the merited success which attended their operation, and the zeal and perseve-
rance which distinguished the votaries of that science,
soon kindled a more general enthusiasm in its favour.
It is impossible to reduce into miniature the historical features of these chemical times, so as to bring
them within the compass of a lecture; I must therefore rest satisfied with delineating a few of the more

prominent outlines. The Galenists, who were in
possession of the schools, and whose reasonings were
fettered by the strongest predilection for their own
doctrines, instantly took the alarm; and the celebrated contest ensued between the *Galenical* and *Chemical* sects, which has given such a controversial tone
to the writers of the fifteenth and sixteenth centuries.
As this revolt from orthodox authority was in a great
degree attributed to the mischievous introduction,
and unmerited success, of Antimonial remedies, so
were the preparations of this metal denounced
with all the virulence of party spirit; and upon this
occasion, in order to support their ground, and oppress and persecute their adversaries, the Galenists
actually solicited the assistance of secular power; the
Supreme Council of Paris accordingly proscribed its
use, by an edict in 1566; and Besnier was expelled
the faculty of medicine in 1609, for having administered it to a patient. In 1637, *Antimonial wine* was,
by public authority, received into the number of purgatives; and in 1650, a new *arret* rescinded that of
1566, and again restored Antimony to public favour,
and general reputation; before this period the invention of *Calomel* had taken place; this preparation
is first mentioned, although very obscurely, by Os-
wald Crollius, in his *Basilica Chemica*, in 1608, and
in the same year, Beguin described it most fully and
clearly, under the title of *Draco Mitigatus*, in his
Tirocinium Chemicum, which he published in Paris.

Chemistry, at this period,* began to take possession of the schools, and whilst it was gradually grafted
into the theory of medicine, it soon became the only

* In the year 1644 Schroeder published a *Chemico*-medical Pharmacopœia, which delineates with accuracy, the pharmacy of these times, and
enumerates almost all the chemical medicines that were known towards
the close of this period.

guide to its practice, the absurdity of which has been already dwelt upon.

In tracing the march of chemical improvement during the last century, we cannot but be struck with the new and powerful remedies which it has introduced, and the many unimportant and feeble articles which it has dismissed from medical practice.

In the present century, the rapid progress of Chemistry has outstripped the anticipations of its most sanguine votaries ; and even in the department of vegetable analysis, a correctness has been attained, the very attempt at which had been abandoned by the most illustrious chemists of the former age, as hopeless and chimerical : let us for instance only compare the results obtained by the Academicians of Paris, and published by Geoffroy, in their analyses of several hundred plants, by the operation of heat, with the elegant and satisfactory researches in this branch of science, lately conducted in the same country ; whilst the former failed in establishing any distinction between the most inert and the most poisonous plants, the latter have succeeded in detecting, separating, and concentrating several of their more subtile constituents. *Opium* has been at length compelled to confess its secret source of action, and *Ipecacuan* to yield its emetic element in a state of perfect purity.

Our Pharmacopœias and Dispensatories* have cautiously kept pace with the scientific progress of the age ; and in tracing them from their origin to the present time † it is gratifying to observe the gradual

* The Dispensatories of London, and Edinburgh, the former by Mr. A. T. Thomson, and the latter by Dr. Duncan, are works which reflect credit on the age and country in which they were written.

† In the year 1618 the London College published their first Pharmacopœia, and successive editions in the following years, viz. 1650, 1677, 1721, 1745, 1787, 1809.

influence of knowledge in reducing the number of
their articles—simplifying the composition of their
formulæ—and improving the processes for their preparation.* Chemistry has also been the means of
establishing the identity of many bodies, which were
long considered specifically different; thus an extensive
list of animal substances has been discarded, since it is
known that they owe their properties to one and the
same common principle, as to *gelatine, albumen, carbonate of lime,* &c. so again, the fixed alkaline salt, produced by the incineration of different vegetables, has
been found to be potass, from whatever plant it may
have been obtained, with the exception of sea plants,
and perhaps some of the Tetradynamia, the former of
which yield *Soda,* and the latter *Ammonia.* Previous
to the Pharmacopœia of 1745, every vegetable was
supposed to yield a salt essentially different, and
therefore a number of alkaline preparations were recommended, each bearing the name of the particular
plant from which it had been procured, as salt of
Wormwood—salt of *Broom,* &c.

But from the very nature and object of a Pharmacopœia, it cannot be supposed to proceed, *pari passu,*
with the march of chemical science, indeed it would
be dangerous that it should, for a chemical theory
must receive the seal and stamp of experience before
it can become current: a Pharmacopœia however, is

---

* What would be the surprise and gratification of the Pharmaceutist
who lived a hundred years ago, if he could now visit Apothecaries Hall?
the application of steam for the various purposes of pharmacy, and for
actuating machinery, for levigation, trituration, and other mechanical
purposes is no less useful, in ensuring uniform results, than it is in
abridging labour and economising time. The greatest credit is due to
those gentlemen, under whose guidance this national laboratory is conducted, and more especially to their worthy and public spirited Trea-
surer, William Simons, Esq. whose zeal and liberality suggested and
promoted the fitting up of the Steam Laboratory.

always an object of abuse, because it is a national
work of authority, which is quite a sufficient reason
why the ignorant and conceited should question its
title to respect, and its claims to utility. " *Plures
audivi,*" says Huxham, " *totas blaterantes Pharmacopœias, qui tamen ne intellexerint quidem quid vel ipse
pulsus significabat.*"

It is very evident, that the greater number of these
attacks has not been levelled with any view to elicit
truth, or to advance science, but to excite public attention, and to provoke unfair discussion for individual, and unworthy advantage ; their obscure and
presumptuous authors vainly hope, that they may
gain for their ephemeral writings some share of importance, and for themselves some degree of reputation, if they can only obtain notoriety, by provoking a
discussion with the College, or with some of its re-
sponsible members, though such a combat should be
sure to terminate in their defeat. Like the Scythian
Abaris, who upon being wounded by Apollo, plucked
the arrow from his side, and heedless of the pain and
disgrace of his wound, exclaimed in triumph, that the
weapon would in future enable him to deliver Oracles.

It is not to such persons that the observations which
are contained in this work are addressed, for with
them I am most anxious to avoid a contest, in which,
as a worthy Fellow of our College expresses it,
" *Victory itself must be disgraceful.*"

When, however, we are assailed, upon every occasion, by a gentleman, whose talents entitle him to respect, and whose public situation commands notice, I
apprehend that a humble individual like myself, may,
in the conscientious discharge of a public duty,
deliver his sentiments from the chair, to which he has
been called by his professional brethren, without any

risk of compromising the dignity of the College, or
of drawing upon himself the charge of an unnecessary
and injudicious interference.

The attack to which I chiefly allude, is contained
in an historical preface by Mr. Professor Brande, to
the *Supplement of the Fourth and Fifth Editions of
the Encyclopædia Britannica*; in which, speaking of
the writings of BOERHAAVE, he says, " The observations which he has made upon the usefulness of
Chemistry, and of its necessity to the medical practitioner, may be well enforced at the present day;
for, except in the schools of London and Edinburgh,
Chemistry, as a branch of education, is either entirely
neglected, or, what is perhaps worse, superficially,
and imperfectly taught ; this is especially the case in
the English Universities, and the London Pharmacopœia is a record of the want of chemical knowledge,
where it is most imperiously required."

The learned Professor of Oxford, Dr. Kidd, naturally anxious to repel a charge which he considered,
individually, unfair, and to vindicate his University
from an aspersion, which he felt to be, generally,
unjust, published an animated, but at the same time,
a cool and candid defence, to which I have much
pleasure in referring you. With respect to the Sister
University, my own *Alma Mater*, I feel that I should
be the most ungrateful of her sons, were I, upon this
occasion, to omit expressing similar sentiments with
respect to the course of chemistry, and that of its
collateral branches, which are annually delivered in
the crowded schools at Cambridge Is Mr. Brande
acquainted with the discipline of our University?—
Is he aware that the chemical chair has been successively filled by BISHOP WATSON—MILNER—WOL-
LASTON—and the late lamented Mr. TENNANT?

To say that such men have been the lecturers, is surely a sufficient testimony to shew that the science of chemistry heretofore *could not* " have been neglected, or what perhaps is still worse, imperfectly taught;" and the zeal and ability displayed by the present Professor, ought to have shielded him from any such attack. Is Mr. Brande aware that the eloquent appeal of BISHOP WATSON from the chair at Cambridge,* on the general importance and utility of chemistry, gave the first impulse to that public taste for this science, which so eminently distinguishes our Augustan age, and which has been the means of founding and supporting the Royal, and other Public Institutions in this Metropolis, as well as in the other towns of the British Empire ?

I need make no farther remark upon this part of Mr. Brande's assertion ; the sequel, judging from the construction of the sentence, is evidently intended to be understood as a consequence, viz. and *therefore* " the London Pharmacopœia is a record of the want of chemical knowledge, where it is most imperiously required," *because Oxford and Cambridge Physicians were its Editors.* Is not this the obvious construction ?

It appears from Mr. Brande's laconic answer to Dr. Young, published in " *The Journal of Science and*

---

* The Chemical Laboratory at Cambridge has produced some valuable discoveries. *Ex pede Herculem*, let me remind the chemist of the formation of Nitrous Acid, by passing a current of ammoniacal gas through the heated Oxyd of Manganese, for which we are indebted to Dr. Milner. I mention it merely as a whimsical circumstance, that the greatest degree of cold ever produced, was effected at Oxford, and the highest temperature, lately, at Cambridge. The researches of Dr. Clarke are highly interesting and important, a succinct account of them has been published by him in a small work, entitled " *The Gas Blow-pipe, or the Art of Fusion, by burning the Gaseous Constituents of Water.*"

the Arts," that his objections are those of Mr.
Phillips, contained in his experimental examination
of the Pharmacopœia, a work which, I confess, appears to me to furnish a testimony of the experimental tact, subtile ingenuity, and caustic style of
criticism, which its author so eminently possesses,
rather than a proof of any fatal or material inac-
curacy in the Pharmacopœia; and I may urge this
with greater force and propriety, when it is considered that at the time of its publication, I was not
a Fellow of the College, and therefore had no voice
upon the subject of its composition, and consequently
must be *personally* disinterested in its reputation.

I cannot conclude these observations upon Mr.
Brande's attack, without expressing a deep feeling of
regret, that a gentleman, whose deserved rank in
society, and whose talents and acquirements must
entitle him to our respect, should have condescended
to countenance and encourage that vile and wretched
taste of depreciating the value and importance of our
most venerable institutions, and of bringing into contempt those acknowledged authorities, which must
always meet with the approbation of the best, and
the sanction and support of the wisest portion of
mankind.

And I shall here protest against the prevailing
fashion of examining, and deciding upon, the pretensions of every medicinal compound to our confidence,
by a *mere chemical* investigation of its composition,
and of rejecting, as fallacious, every medical testimony which may appear contradictory to the results
of the Laboratory; there is no subject in science to
which the maxim of Cicero more strictly applies, than
to the present case; let the *Ultra* Chemist therefore

cherish it in his remembrance, and profit by its application—PRÆSTAT NATURÆ VOCE DOCERI, QUAM
INGENIO SUO SAPERE."
Has not experience fully established the value of
many medicinal combinations, which, at the time of
their adoption, could not receive the sanction of any
chemical law? We well remember the opposition,
which, on this ground, was for a long time offered to
the introduction of the *Anti-hectic Mixture* of Dr.
Griffith,—the *Mistura Ferri Composita* of the present
Pharmacopœia, and yet, subsequent enquiry has confirmed, upon scientific principles, the justness of our
former practical conclusion; for it has been shewn,
that the cnemical decompositions, which constituted
the objection to its use, are in fact the causes of its
utility; *(see Mist. Ferri,)* the explanation, moreover,
has thrown additional light upon the theory of other
preparations; so true is the observation of the celebrated Morveau, that " *We never profit more than by
those unexpected results of Experiments, which con-
tradict our Analogies and preconceived Theories.*"
Whenever a medicine is found by experience to be
effectual, the practitioner should listen, with great
circumspection, to any *chemical* advice for its correction or improvement.* From a mistaken notion of

* Great credit is due to Dr. Scudamore for the steadiness with
which he rejected the expostulations of the *Ultras*, on the unchemical
and contradictory nature of his formula for the administration of the
Colchicum. Experience led him to the conclusion, that the *Acetum
Colchici* generally proved more efficacious, when exhibited in combination with some medicine that will relax, without occasioning any
uneasiness in the bowels or stomach; and he accordingly found, that
the following formula is the best adapted for such a purpose. ℞
Magnesiæ, gr. xv. *Magnesiæ Sulphat:* ℥iss. *Aceti Colchici*, f℈j. *Aquæ
Cinnamomi*, f℥x. *Extract: Glychrrh.* gr. x. At this formula, it appears,
the *Ultra* Chemists were terribly disconcerted. What—combine an

this kind the *Extractum Colocynthidis compositum*,
with a view of making it chemically compatible with
Calomel, has been deprived of the *Soap* which formerly entered into its composition, in consequence of
which, its solubility in the stomach is considerably
modified, its activity is therefore impaired, and its
mildness diminished.

On the other hand, substances may be medically
inconsistent, which are chemically compatible, as I
shall have frequent opportunities of exemplifying.
The stomach has a chemical code of its own, by which
the usual affinities of bodies are frequently modified,
often suspended, and sometimes entirely subverted;
this truth is illustrated in a very striking manner by
the interesting experiments of M. Drouard, who found
that Copper, swallowed in its metallic state, was not
rendered poisonous by meeting with oils, or fatty
bodies; nor even with *Vinegar*, in the digestive
organs. Other bodies, on the contrary, seem to possess the same habitudes in the stomach as in the
Laboratory, and are alike influenced, in both situa-
tions, by the chemical action of various bodies, many
examples of which are to be found under the consideration of the influence which solubility exerts
upon the medicinal activity of substances; so again,
acidity in the stomach is neutralized by *Alkalies*, and
if a *Carbonate* be employed for that purpose, we have
a copious disengagement of *Carbonic acid gas*, which

alkaline earth with an acetic solution of an active vegetable? to which
Dr. Scudamore very justly replies, that the Colchicum, brought to the
state of a mere solution in water, by having its acid menstruum neutra-
lised, is in the most favourable state of preparation, in which is can be
possibly administered. This explanation agrees perfectly with the
views I have long entertained respecting the operation of Colchicum.
(See *Colchici Radix.*)

has been frequently very distressing; lastly, many bodies taken into the stomach undergo decompositions and changes *in transitu*,* independent of any play of chemical affinities, from the hidden powers of digestion, some of which we are enabled to appreciate. (*See Potassæ Acetas.*)

The powers of the stomach would seem to consist in decomposing the *Ingesta*, and reducing them into simpler forms, rather than, in complicating them, by favouring new combinations.

But every rational physician must feel in its full force, the absurdity of expecting to account for the phænomena of life, upon principles deduced from the analogies of inert matter, and we therefore find that the most intelligent physiologists of modern times, have been anxious to discourage the attempt, and to deprecate its folly. Sir Gilbert Blane, in his luminous work on MEDICAL LOGIC, when speaking of the different theories of digestion, tells us that Dr. William Hunter, whose peculiar sagacity and precision of mind detected at a glance the hollowness of such delusive hypotheses, and saw the danger which theorists run in trusting themselves on such slippery ground, expressed himself in his public lectures, with that solidity of judgment, combined with facetiousness of expression, which rendered him unparalleled as a public teacher. "Gentlemen," said he, "Physiologists will have it that the stomach is a mill—others, that it is a fermenting vat—others again, that it is a stew-pan,—but in my view of the matter, it is neither

---

* What can illustrate in a more familiar and striking manner, the singular powers of *Gastric Chemistry*, than the fact of the shortness of time in which the aliment becomes acid in depraved digestion? A series of changes is thus produced in a few hours, which would require in the laboratory as many weeks.

a mill, a fermenting vat, nor a stew-pan—but a
STOMACH, Gentlemen, a STOMACH."

From what has been said, it is very evident that
the mere chemist can have no pretensions to the art
of composing or discriminating remedies; whenever
he arraigns the scientific propriety of our Prescriptions,
in direct contradiction to the deductions of true medical experience,—whenever he forsakes his laboratory,
for the bed-side, he forfeits all his claims to our respect,
and his title to our confidence. It is amusing to see
the ridiculous errors into which the chemist falls, when
he turns physician; Seguin found that Peruvian bark
contained a peculiar principle that precipitated *Tannin*,
he immediately concluded that this *could not be any
other* than *Gelatine*, and upon the faith of this blunder,
the French and Italian physicians gave their patients
nothing but *Clarified Glue*, in intermittent fevers!
But I desist—not however without expressing a
hope, in which I am sure my medical brethren will
concur, that, should Mr. Brande again condescend
to favour us with a commentary upon Boerhaave, he
will select that passage in his work, where, alluding
to the application of Chemistry to Physic, he emphatically exclaims, " EGREGIA ILLIUS ANCILLA
EST, NON ALIA PEJOR DOMINA."

THE INFLUENCE OF CLIMATE AND
SEASON.

So few facts have hitherto been collected upon this
subject, that I introduce its consideration in this
place, rather with a wish to excite farther enquiry, than
with any hope of imparting additional information.

There can be little doubt but that Climate and
Season may modify the properties and operation of
a remedy, as well as the type and character of a disease; unless this be admitted, it will be difficult to
explain the diversity of testimony which the physicians of different climates have furnished with respect
to the efficacy of various remedies. It is probable
that in southern countries some vegetables enjoy more
energetic properties than in the north ; and vice versa,
whether this observation will apply to *Hemlock*, as
some have supposed, I have no means of deciding :
on the other hand, some remedies appear to succeed
in cold climates, which produce little or no benefit
in the same diseases, in warmer latitudes; this is a
fact with respect to chronic rheumatism ; soon after
the publication of the first edition of my Pharmacologia, I received a letter from Dr. Halliday of
Moscow, upon the subject of the *Eau-Medicinale*,
and as it offers a striking proof of the powers of
the *Rhododendron Crysanthum* in curing the rheumatism of the north, whilst in this country the plant
has been repeatedly tried without any signal proof
of success, I shall beg to subjoin an extract from the
letter of my correspondent. "In reading your account of the ' *Eau Medicinale*,' I perceive, that upon
the authority of Mr. James Moore, you state it to be
a preparation of the *white hellebore*; may I be allowed
to suggest the probability of its being made from the
leaves of the *Rhododendron Crysanthum*, for so far as
I can learn, the effects of the French medicine are
precisely those which are experienced from an infusion of the above plant, which the Siberians and
Russians regard as an infallible specific in the cure of
chronic rheumatism and gout, and from which I
myself, as well as other physicians in Russia, have

witnessed the most desirable and decided effects, whenever we had it in our power to administer the remedy with confidence and courage; we have seldom given it in any other form or dose than that adopted by the Siberians themselves, which is to infuse in a warm place, generally near a furnace, during the night, two drachms of the fresh leaves in about twelve ounces of boiling water, taking care that the liquid never boils. This dose is to be taken in the morning upon an empty stomach, and during its nauseating operation, which generally commences in about a quarter of an hour after it has been swallowed; neither solids nor liquids of any description are allowed; after an interval of three or four hours, I have seen the patient obtain a copious and black fœtid stool, and get up free from all pain. Should it happen that the patient does not recover from the first dose, another is administered on the succeeding day, and I have known it to be taken for three days in succession, when the severest fits of gout have been removed.* Is it not then probable that some cunning Frenchman has availed himself of this Siberian specific, and concentrated it in such a form, as to defy all the learned to find it out ?"

Dr. Halliday adds, " The Siberians denominate the leaves of this plant, when infused in water, *Intoxicating Tea ;* and a weaker infusion is in daily use, especially for treating their neighbours, just as the Europeans do with tea from China."

---

* This plant was first described by Gmelin in his *Flora Siberica.* iv. 121. It has obtained a place in the Edinburgh Pharmacopœia. Besides the effects stated by Dr. Halliday, it is said by different authors to excite a peculiar creeping sensation in the pained part.

THE IGNORANT PREPARATION AND FRAUDULENT ADULTERATION OF MEDICINES.

The circumstances comprehended under this head certainly deserve to be ranked amongst the more powerful causes, which have operated in affecting the reputation of many medicinal substances. The subject is copious, and full of importance, and I have taken considerable pains to collect very fully, the various modes in which our remedies are thus deprived of their most valuable properties, and to suggest the best tests by which such frauds may be discovered; very few practitioners have an idea of the alarming extent to which this nefarious practice is carried, or of the systematic manner in which it is conducted: there can be no doubt but that the sophistication of medicines has been practised in degree in all ages, but the refinements of chemistry have enabled the manufacturers of the present day not only to execute these frauds with greater address, but unfortunately, at the same time to vend them with less chance of detection. It will be scarcely credited, when I affirm, that many hundred persons are supported in this metropolis by the art of adulterating drugs, besides a number of women and children who find ample employment, and excellent profit, in *counterfeiting* Cochineal, with coloured dough, Isinglass with pieces of bladder, and the dried skin of soles, and by filling up with powdered Sassafras the holes which are bored in spice and nutmegs, for the purpose of plundering their essential oils.

THE UNSEASONABLE COLLECTION OF VEGETABLE REMEDIES.

Vegetable physiology has demonstrated, that during the progress of vegetation, most remarkable changes occur in succession, in the chemical composition, as well as in the sensible qualities of a plant; time will not allow me to be prodigal of examples, take therefore one which is familiar and striking,—the aromatic and spicy qualities of the unexpanded flowers of the Caryophyllus Aromaticus, *(Cloves)* are well known to every body, but if the flower-bud be fully developed it loses these properties altogether, and the fruit of the tree is not in the least degree aromatic. The *Colchicum autumnale* may be cited as another example in which the medicinal properties of the vegetable are entirely changed during the natural progress of its developement. See also *Inspissated Juices*, under the article *Extract*.

THE OBSCURITY WHICH HAS ATTENDED THE OPERATION OF COMPOUND MEDICINES.

It is evident that the fallacies to which our observations and experience are liable, with respect to the efficacy of certain bodies, as remedies, must be necessarily multiplied when such bodies are exhibited in a state of complicated combination, since it must be always difficult, and often impossible, to ascertain to which ingredient the effects produced ought to be attributed.

How many frivolous substances have from this cause alone gained a share of credit which belonged exclusively to the medicines, with which they happened to be accidentally administered? Besides, in the exuberance of mixture, certain reactions and important changes are mutually produced, by which the identity of the original ingredients is destroyed; this however will be more properly introduced for discussion in my next essay.

The practice of mixing together different medicinal substances, so as to form one remedy, may boast of very ancient origin, for most of the prescriptions which have descended from the Greek physicians are of this description; the uncertain and vague results of such a practice appear also to have been early felt and often condemned, and even Erasistratus declaimed with great warmth against the complicated medicines which were administered in his time; the greater number of these compositions present a mass of incongruous materials, put together without any apparent order or intention; indeed it would almost appear as if they regarded a medical formula as a problem in *Permutation*, the only object of which was to discover and assign the number of changes that can be made in any given number of things, all different from each other.

At the same time, it must in justice be allowed, that some of the earlier physicians entertained just notions with regard to the use and abuse of combination, although their knowledge of the subject was of course extremely limited and imperfect.

ORIBASIUS recommends in high terms certain combinations of *Evacuant* and *Roborant* medicines, and the remarks of ALEXANDER TRALLIAN, on a remedy which he exhibited in paralysis, serve to shew that he

was well acquainted with the fact, that certain substances lose their efficacy when they stimulate the
bowels to excess, for he cautions us against adding a
greater proportion of *Scammony* to it; many, he observes, think that by so doing, they increase the force
of the medicine, whereas in fact they make it *useless*,
by carrying it immediately through the bowels, instead
of suffering it to remain and be conveyed to the
remote parts.

The curious law, that a combination of similar
medicines is more powerful than an equivalent dose
of any single one, does not appear to have been known
to the ancient physicians. The earliest mention of it
that I can find, is by VALLISNIERI, the favourite
pupil of Malpighi, who was professor at Padua in
1711, nearly ninety years before Fordyce published
his memoir on the Combination of Medicines. He
states, as the result of experiment, that twelve drachms
of *Cassia Pulp* are about equivalent in purgative
strength to four ounces of *Manna;* and yet, says he,
if we give eight drachms of *Cassia Pulp*, in combination with four drachms of *Manna*, we obtain double
the effect! How, adds the professor, can this possibly
happen? Surely the very contrary *ought* to obtain,
for four drachms of Cassia are much more than equivalent to an equal weight of manna, the strength of
the former being to that of the latter as 8 to 3.

To Fordyce however we are first indebted for the
generalization of this fact, and for the successful
application of it to practice, as will appear more fully
in the succeeding essay.

In modern Europe, the same attachment to lux-
uriancy of composition has been transmitted to our
own times: there are several prescriptions of Huxham
extant, which contain more than *four hundred* ingre-

dients. I have already observed, that all extravagant
systems tend, in the course of time, to introduce practices of an opposite kind; this truth finds another
powerful illustration in the history of medicinal combination, and it becomes a serious question, which it
will be my duty to discuss, whether the disgust so
justly excited by the *poly-pharmacy* of our predecessors, may not have induced the physician of the
present day, to carry his ideas of simplicity *too far*,
so as to neglect and lose the advantages, which, in
many cases, beyond all doubt, may be obtained by
scientific combinations.

In the year 1799 Dr. Fordyce, in a valuable
paper, published in the second volume of the Transactions of the Medical Society, has investigated this
subject with much perspicuity and success: unfortunately, however, this memoir terminates with the
investigation of *similar* remedies, that is to say, of
those which produce upon the body similar effects,
and he is entirely silent upon the advantages which
may be obtained by the combination of those medicines, which possess *different*, or even *opposite* qualities; it must be also remembered, that at the time
this memoir was composed by its eminent author,
Chemistry had scarcely extended its illuminating rays
into the recesses of physic. Under such circumstances, I am induced to undertake the arduous task
of enquiring into the several relations, in which each
article of a compound formula may be advantageously
situated with respect to the others; and I am farther
encouraged in this investigation, by a conviction of
its great practical importance, as well as by feeling
that it has hitherto never received the share of attention which it merits. " I think," says Dr. Powell,
" it may be asserted, without fear of contradiction,

that no medicine compounded of five or six simple
articles, has hitherto had its powers examined in a
rational manner." If this attempt should be the
means of directing the attention of future practitioners
to the subject, and thereby, of rendering the Art of
Composition more efficient, by placing it upon the
permanent basis of science, I shall feel that I have
profitably devoted my time and attention to the most
useful of all medical subjects. " *Res est maximi
momenti in arte medendi, cum, Formula, in se con-
siderata, possit esse profecto mortis vel vitæ sententia.*"

INTRODUCTORY ESSAY.

AN ANALYSIS,

&c.

INTRODUCTORY ESSAY.

AN ANALYSIS

OF

THE OBJECTS TO BE ATTAINED BY MIXING AND COMBINING MEDICINAL SUBSTANCES.

THE objects to be attained, and the resources which are furnished by MEDICINAL COMBINATION, together with the different modes of its operation, and the laws by which it is governed, may with much practical advantage be arranged in the following order.

I.

TO PROMOTE THE ACTION OF THE BASIS, OR PRINCIPAL MEDICINE.

A.—*By combining it with Substances which are of the* SAME NATURE, *that is, which are* INDI-VIDUALLY *capable of producing the same effects, but with less energy than when in combination with each other.*

Dr. Fordyce first demonstrated the existence of the singular and important law, that *a combination of similar remedies will produce a more certain, speedy, and considerable effect, than an equivalent dose of any single one ;* thus

A

EMETICS are more efficient when composed of
Ipecacuan united with *Tartarized Antimony*, or *Sulphate
of Zinc*, than when they simply consist of any
one of such substances in an equivalent dose. See
Formulæ, 1, 3.

CATHARTICS not only acquire a very great increase
of power by combination with each other, but they
are at the same time rendered less irritating in their
operation, the *Extractum Colocynthidis Compositum*
affords a very good example of a compound purgative
mass, which is much more active and manageable, and
less liable to irritate than any one of its components
separately taken. Additional examples are furnished
by *Formulæ* 14, 15, 16, 17, 18, 22.

DIURETICS. Under this class of medicinal-agents
it may be noticed that *whenever a medicine is liable to
produce effects different from those we desire, its combination
with similar remedies is particularly eligible*,
by which the action of the basis may be directed and
fixed : thus the individuals which compose the class of
Diuretics, are uncertain in their operation, and disposed,
when exhibited singly, to produce diaphoretic,
and other contrary effects : it is therefore in such cases,
highly judicious to unite several of them in one Formula,
by which we encrease their powers, and are
more likely to ensure their operation. Formulæ
29. 31 36, 37, 38, 39, are constructed upon this principle.

EXPECTORANTS. More is to be gained by the co-
operation of these remedies than can be obtained by
the exhibition of any of them separately, as in Formulæ
48, 49.

DIAPHORETICS are under the influence of the same
law. Formulæ 58, 59, 60.

EMMENAGOGUES. Formulæ 70, 71, 72.

3

STIMULANTS. There is no class of remedies which receives greater benefit by combination, acquiring encreased efficacy, and at the same time losing much of their acrimony : if, for instance, any one spice, as the dried capsule of the *Capsicum*, be taken into the stomach, it will excite a sense of heat and pain ; in like manner will a quantity of pepper ; but if an equivalent quantity of these two Stimulants be given in combination, no such sense of pain is produced, but on the contrary, a pleasant warmth is experienced, and a genial glow felt over the whole body ; and if a greater number of spices be joined together, the chance of pain and inflammation being produced is still farther diminished; the truth of this law is also strikingly illustrated, as Dr. Fordyce has observed, by that universal maxim in cookery, *never to employ one spice if more can be procured;* the object being to make the stomach bear a large quantity of food without nausea. This principle also finds an illustration of its importance, as it regards the class of Stimulants, in the following preparations of our Pharmacopœia : *Pulvis Cinnamomi compositus. Infusum Armoraciæ compositum. Infusum Aurantii compositum. Spiritus Lavendulæ compositus. Tinctura Cinchonæ composita. Tinctura Cardamomi composita*, and the *Confectio Opii*, the elegant and scientific substitute for the celebrated *Mithridate* and *Theriaca*. The practitioner is also referred to Formulæ 103. 106.

LOCAL STIMULANTS are under the dominion of the same law, and perhaps the origin of the custom, so long observed, of mixing the varieties of snuff, may thus receive a plausible explanation ; certain it is that by such combination the harsh pungency of each ingredient will be diminished, whilst its stimulating properties will in the same ratio be encreased, but

A 2

4

rendered more grateful; the same principle will direct
the formation of safe and efficient plaisters and lotions,
the *Emplastrum Cumini* of the London, and the *Emplastrum Aromaticum* of the Dublin Pharmacopœia,
offer examples of its judicious application.
BITTER TONICS are also thus exalted. Formulæ
94, 96.

NARCOTICS. The intention of allaying irritation
and pain, will be better fulfilled by a combination of
these substances in different proportions, than by any
single one, notwithstanding its dose be considerably
encreased. See Formulæ 117, 118.

ALTERATIVES. Our maxim " VIS UNITA FORTIOR " certainly applies with equal truth and force to
this obscure class of medicinal agents.

DEMULCENTS do not appear to obtain any other
benefit from combination, than occasionally a convenience and efficacy of application, by deriving a proper degree of consistence and solubility. See Article
Trochismi, in the Pharmacologia.

It may be observed that it is frequently judicious
to combine, in one Formula, several of the different
preparations of the same substance, by which we shall
more completely ensure the full and general effect of
all its principles; thus, where the bark is required in
the cure of an Intermittent, and the stomach will not
allow the exhibition of the powder, it will be eligible
to conjoin the Tincture, Decoction, and Extract.
(Formulæ, 37, 62, 63.) As a general rule it may be
stated that such a combination is advantageous, *whenever the chemical nature of the medicinal substance
will not admit of the full solution of all its active principles in any one Solvent, and at the same time its exhibition in substance is ineligible.*

The operation of the law which has thus formed the first object of this enquiry, will be found, like every other, to have a natural and well defined limit; it is easy to perceive that by multiplying the number of ingredients too far, we shall either so encrease the quantity and bulk of the medicine, as to render it nauseous and cumbersome, or so reduce the dose of each constituent as to fritter away the force and energy of the combination. There is also another important precaution respecting the application of this principle which demands our most serious attention; that in combining substances in the manner, and for the object just related, the practitioner should be well satisfied that their medicinal virtues are in reality perfectly SIMILAR, or he will fall into an error of the most fatal tendency. He must remember that medicines are not necessarily similar because they have been arranged in the same artificial class of remedies; but that, in order to establish a perfect similarity, their operation must be found by experience to continue similar under every condition of the human body; and that, moreover, they must owe such similarity to modes of operation which are compatible with each other, and consonant with the general plan of cure; thus *Squill, Calomel,* and *Digitalis,* are each powerful Diuretics, but nevertheless they cannot be considered similar remedies, since *Digitalis* will entirely fail in its effects in the very cases that *Calomel* and *Squill* succeed; and *Squill* will prove inert, when *Digitalis* is capable of producing the most powerful influence; this arises from their modes of operation being dissimilar, and consequently requiring for their success, different states of the living system.

Dr. Blackall, in his " Observations upon the Cure of Dropsies," has offered some remarks so valuable in themselves, and so illustrative of this important subject, that I beg leave to quote the passage. " Many Physicians, he observes, are fond of combining *Squill, Calomel,* and *Digitalis,* as a Diuretic in Dropsy ; a practice often unsafe, and not very decidedly possessing the merit even of being consistent. Digitalis greatly depresses the action of the heart and arteries, and controls the circulation, and it seems most unreasonable to believe that its curative powers can be independent of such an effect ; on the other hand, Mercury, if it does not pass off quickly, is always exciting fever, and raising and hardening the pulse ; speaking from experience, where the urine is coaguable, and *Digitalis* agrees, both the others are, often at least, positively injurious. On the contrary, where the urine is foul, and not coaguable, and *Squills* with *Calomel* render service, I have on that very account made less trial of Digitalis, and cannot therefore speak of it from much experience."

The same observations will apply, in some respects at least, to the operation of Cathartic remedies ; a long list of substances might be produced, all of which have the general property of acting upon the alimentary canal, but it does not follow that they are on that account similar remedies, since they act with different degrees of force, and upon different portions of the *primæ viæ* ; and whilst some produce watery evacuations, others are distinguished by the feculent discharges which they excite.

B.—*By combining the Basis with Substances of a* DIFFERENT NATURE, *and which do not exert any Chemical influence upon it, but are found by experience to be capable of rendering the Stomach, or System, or any particular organ, more susceptible of its action.*

Thus it is that the system is rendered more susceptible of the influence of Mercury, by combining it with Antimony and Opium. Where the stomach is insensible to impressions, the exhibition of Opium previous to, or in combination with, any active medicine, often assists its operation ; this is frequently seen in Mania, when emetics will fail, unless the stomach be previously influenced and prepared by a Narcotic ; so again, the system, when it is in that particular condition which is indicated by a hot and dry skin, is unsusceptible of the expectorant powers of Squill, unless it be in union with antimony or some powerful diaphoretic, (48). Squill is by no means disposed to act upon the urinary organs, when exhibited singly, but calomel, and some other mercurial preparations, when in conjunction with it, appear to direct its influence to the kidneys, and to render these organs more susceptible of its operation, (31. 34). Upon the same principle, *Antimonial Wine* quickens the operation of saline cathartics (8.) ; *Opium* encreases the sudorific powers of *Antimony* (60) ; and the purgative operation of *Jalap* is promoted by *Ipecacuan*, (21).

The solutions of saline cathartics appear likewise to receive an accession of power, and a celerity of operation by impregnation with *Carbonic acid gas*, depending

probably upon the Intestines thus receiving a degree
of distention favourable to the action of the salt,
(19. 23).

In enumerating the methods to be adopted for encreasing the energies of a remedy, by rendering the
system more susceptible of its action, it is right to
observe that under certain circumstances, Venesection
deserves a distinguished rank amongst the A D J U V A N -
T I A. This fact is strikingly discovered in the exhibition of *Mercurial* **Preparations**, and some other Alterative Medicines. Whether the " *Vis Conservatrix*,"
which Nature when in a state of health and vigour
opposes to the admission of poisonous substances into
the circulation, be overcome by blood-letting, is a
question which I shall leave others to decide, but
thus much reiterated practice has taught me, that the
system in a strong and healthy condition frequently
offers a resistance to the operation of mercury, which
is overcome the moment the stomach becomes deranged, the circulation languid, or the general tone
of the system impaired. I have frequently seen this
during my Hospital practice : if a patient, who has
been using mercurial friction, or taking the preparations of that metal without effect, be transferred into
a close and unhealthy ward, his appetite soon fails,
the tongue becomes furred, and the system instantly
yields to the influence of the remedy. Nauseating
doses of *antimony* frequently repeated, or the accidental supervention of any disease of debility, will be
attended with the same phenomena. My practice has
also afforded me an opportunity of appreciating the
debilitating effects of despondency in a case of this
description ; a patient had been taking mercurial medicines, and using frictions for a considerable period,
without any apparent effect; under these circumstances

he was abruptly told that he would fall a victim to his disease; the unhappy man experienced an unusual shock at this opinion, and in a few hours became violently salivated. The effects of CATHARTIC MEDICINES are likewise encreased by previous venesection. I have often noticed this fact in contending with a plethoric diathesis; whenever the bleeding preceded the purgative, the effects of the latter have been uniformly more speedy and considerable; in obstinate constipation the same fact has been observed, and mild remedies have been known to act more powerfully, when preceded by blood-letting, than potent ones have when exhibited antecedent to it. The effects of *Bark*, *Steel*, and other tonics, are certainly influenced in the same manner; whether in any case it may be prudent or judicious, to have recourse to such a practice, is a question not connected with the present inquiry.

PURGATIVES also seem capable of exalting the efficacy, and indeed of accelerating the benefit to be derived from many Alteratives, when administered previous to the exhibition of these latter substances; the advantages of a course of Steel medicines are undoubtedly encreased by such means. The febrifugous and antiseptic properties of diluted muriatic acid (see Form. 85.) are inconsiderable, unless its exhibition be accompanied with cathartics, I beg to refer the practioner to some cases published by me in *the Medical and Physical Journal for December*, 1809, in further illustration of these views. Experience enables me also to state that *Diuretics* are considerably assisted by similar means, having many instances in my case book of the failure of these agents before, and their successful operation after, the exhibition of a cathartic. Dr. Darwin observes that " *Absorptions are always encreased by Inanition,* and in support of this position refers to the frequent advantage derived from evacuations in the cure of ulcers. I have certainly seen obstinate sores in the leg cured by small and repeated bleedings.

CHANGE OF DIET AND OF HABITS may be also classed amongst the *Adjuvantia,* but the young practitioner must be warned that he is not to exercise his *Caduceus* as Sancho's Doctor did his wand. I have seen a young disciple of Esculapius so vex his patient, that his food became more nauseous to him than his medicine, and I verily believe his Physician was more irksome than his disease.

II.

TO CORRECT THE OPERATION OF THE BASIS, BY OBVIATING ANY UNPLEASANT EFFECTS IT MIGHT BE LIKELY TO OCCASION, AND WHICH WOULD PERVERT ITS INTENDED ACTION, AND DEFEAT THE OBJECTS OF ITS EXHIBITION.

The virtues of the most important remedies are frequently lost, or much invalidated for want of proper attention to the circumstances comprehended in this section. It may be almost admitted as an axiom, that, *whenever an Alterative medicine acts with violence upon the primæ viæ, its energies are uselessly expended; and the objects of its exhibition defeated.* So again, *Diaphoretics, Diuretics,* and many other remedies suffer a diminution in their effects, whenever they stimulate the stomach or bowels to excess. *Guaiacum* loses its anti-arthritic, *Squill* its diuretic, and *Antimony* and *Ipecacuan* their diaphoretic virtues under such circumstances. The action of these substances therefore requires correction, and a medicine must be selected capable of fulfilling that intention. *Opium* has very extensive powers as a corrigent. Formulæ 28. 34, 38, 89.

The griping and nauseating tendency of some remedies receives correction by the addition of *aromatics* or essential oils, (10, 15, 16, 21,) or by small portions of a corresponding tincture, (9, 14.) The drastic operation of *Colocynth* may be mitigated by trituration with *Camphor:* the griping from *Senna* and resinous purgatives is prevented by the addition of *soluble Tartar,* or alkaline salts, by which their solubilities are increased, (15.) There are many other substances which receive a much pleasanter mode of operation by having their solubilities encreased or diminished, but the farther consideration of this question will be resumed under the fourth section of the Analysis. It has been already shewn in the first section that the operation of a purgative substance is frequently rendered milder by combining it with several others of the same nature.

There are several substances which are deprived of their acrimonious qualities by trituration with mucilage, milk, barley-water, &c. The tendency which mercurial preparations possess of affecting the bowels is, with the exception of *corrosive sublimate*, corrected by *Opium*, but the acrid operation of this latter salt is more securely guarded against by the decoction of *Guaiacum* or *Mezereon*, or by the plentiful exhibition of mucilaginous drinks and broths; the enfeebling influence of *Digitalis*, *Tobacco*, and of other narcotics, is successfully opposed by aromatics and stimulants.

Sometimes the unpleasant or perverse operation of a medicine may be obviated by changing the form of its exhibition, the period at which it is taken, or the extent of its dose; thus the inconvenience arising from the too easy solubility of *Gamboge*, and its consequent action upon the stomach, Dr. Cullen found might be obviated by repeating small doses at short intervals, (26).

The scientific physician, from his knowledge of the chemical composition of a medicine, and of the principles upon which its different qualities depend, is enabled to remove, or render inert the element which imparts to it a deleterious operation ; thus it has been found that the peculiar principle in the *Spanish Fly*, which so frequently irritates the urinary organs, is soluble in boiling water ; ebullition in water therefore offers the means of depriving them of the power of thus acting upon the kidneys, whilst it does not effect any alteration in their vesicatory properties. It is upon the same principle that many vegetable substances of a very acrid nature, become harmless by boiling, and some of them might even in times of scarcity and want, be introduced as wholesome and nutritious articles of diet.

Under this head it ought also to be noticed, that there is frequently a *chemical* condition of the stomach, which may interfere with the mild operation of a medicine, and may therefore require consideration ; this is particularly exemplified in the action of those antimonial preparations which are liable to become emetic and drastic by the presence of an acid ; it is, for this reason, very eligible to guard such substances with antacid adjuncts. See *Antimonii Sulphuretum*, and Formulæ 61, 64.

The vinous infusion of *Colchicum* appears to act more violently when acid is present in the stomach; small doses of magnesia ought therefore to precede and accompany its exhibition.

III.

TO OBTAIN THE JOINT OPERATION OF TWO OR MORE MEDICINES WHICH HAVE DIFFERENT POWERS, AND WHICH ARE REQUIRED TO OB-VIATE DIFFERENT SYMPTOMS, OR TO AN-SWER DIFFERENT INDICATIONS.

Arrangements constructed upon this principle con-stitute some of the most valuable remedies with which we are acquainted; they are in general *extempo-raneous*, because their very value depends upon their being varied and modified according to the symptoms and circumstances of each particular case. Dr. Fordyce observes, that combinations of this kind are often in-dicated in cases of Diarrhœa, where it is necessary to astringe the vessels of the intestines, and at the same time to relax those of the skin: such an indication, he says, may be fulfilled by exhibiting *Tormentil root*, or any other vegetable astringent, with *Ipecacuan*.

The practice suggested by Drs. Stoll and Warren in the treatment of *Cholica Pictonum*, affords a striking example of the expediency of combinations of this nature. It is found in that disease, as well as in others attended with spasmodic constriction of the intestinal canal, that purgatives produce no effect unless the

spasm be allayed by combining them with *Opium,*
(Form. 13, 14.) In the treatment of Dropsies we have
often two indications to fulfil—to evacuate the water,
and to support the strength of the patient ; hence the
necessity of combining brisk and stimulating purges,
such as *Scammony, Jalap,* &c. with active tonics,
(10, 20,) : hence also the value of combinations composed of diuretics with the preparations of Steel. (10.)
In Chlorosis again, cardialgia is not unfrequently a
vexatious attendant, and solicits the union of *Emmenagogues* with *Antacids,* or *Absorbents,* (72). In the
cure of Dyspepsia, it is frequently desirable to
strengthen at the same time the tone of the system in
general, and that of the stomach and organs of digestion in particular, an indication which demands the
use of *Steel, Bark* or *Bitter tonics,* conjoined with active
stimulants, as *Ammonia, Æther,* &c. In my own
practice I have repeatedly found combinations of Steel,
and fixed alkalies, highly beneficial in certain chronic
affections of the liver.

In the exhibition of Tonic medicines it is frequently
essential to accompany their operation with purgation ; in Intermittent fevers, for instance, when attended with a redundant secretion of bile, or any obstruction of the viscera, the *Bark* must be given in
combination with some laxative, for which purpose
Boerhave has recommended *Muriate of Ammonia* ;
Mead, *Rhubarb* ; whilst, in many cases, experience
suggests the propriety of selecting some of the warmer
cathartics, especially the aloetic. Arrangements of
this nature are also continually necessary during the
progress of an alterative plan, in order to remedy any
incidental symptom which may occur : thus the addition of *Magnesia* may be required to obviate constipation, or cretaceous powder to check a too great

relaxation of the intestines. In the exhibition of *Cathartics* how frequently it happens that the patient's strength will hardly allow the evacuation? In such a case, the addition of steel as a roborant, or of æther or ammonia as a diffusible stimulant, is loudly called for; the Cheltenham waters offer a natural combination of this character. In the cure of *cynanche Maligna*, the use of bark is indicated; but if the skin be hot and dry, it should be accompanied with a diaphoretic, (62.) In the treatment of the chronic and humid coughs of old men, I have generally witnessed the beneficial union of the warm and stimulating influence of myrrh, with the astringent tonic of *sulphate of Zinc*. Formula 105 presents the combination which I have usually adopted.

In the construction of these complex arrangements, the practitioner must of course take care that he does not fall into the error of CONTRA-INDICATION, combining substances, possessing properties essentially different, and which are at variance with, or opposed to each other; it is an error of the most serious description, and unfortunately, is one of too common occurrence in the lower walks of medical practice, " *crimine ab uno disce omnes.*" I lately met with a practitioner in the country, who upon being asked by a lady, whom he attended, the intention of three different draughts which he had sent her, replied, that one would warm, the second cool her, and that the third was calculated to moderate the too violent effects of either; thus it is that discredit and contempt fall upon the use of medicines, which ought only to attach to the ignorant pretenders, or designing knaves, who administer them.

IV.

TO OBTAIN A NEW AND ACTIVE REMEDY NOT
AFFORDED BY ANY SINGLE SUBSTANCE.

A. *By combining Medicines which excite different actions in the Stomach and System,
in consequence of which NEW, or modified
Results are produced.*

This constitutes by far the most obscure part of the
subject of medicinal combination, and must ever continue so until we become better acquainted with the
laws which govern the action of medicinal substances
upon the living system. That the most valuable
effects, however, are really produced by such arrangements, we have he testimony of long experience, and
examples are furnished in the valuable and well
known operation of many officinal preparations; thus
the "*Pulvis Ipecacuanhæ compositus*" contains as its
active elements, *Opium* and *Ipecacuanha ;* and yet, in
well regulated doses, it neither possesses the narcotic
operation of the former, nor the nauseating effects of
the latter; they appear to be mutually lost, and converted into a powerful diaphoretic : so again, the
emetic operation of *Sulphuret of Antimony*, and the
specific influence of *Calomel*, are changed by combination with each other, giving rise to a remedy, eminently distinguished for its powers as an Alterative.

B. *By combining Substances which have the property of acting chemically upon each other the result of which is the formation of* NEW COMPOUNDS, *or the decomposition of the original Constituents, and the developement of their more* ACTIVE ELEMENTS.

It may be safely asserted that the arm of Physic has derived more power, and greater energy, from a few chemical combinations, than from all the numerous simple bodies presented to us by Nature; or from the various compounds which Art has formed by their intermixture. And it is to the crucible and alembic that we must look for the future improvement, and extension of our remedies. That medicinal substances are actually capable of thus combining together, and of producing new compounds, or of effecting decompositions, and thereby of developing active elements, may be illustrated by many well known examples.

a. *Formation of New Compounds.*

Under this head, the class of Metals will immediately present itself to our consideration; all the individuals of which, with the exception perhaps of iron, are perfectly inert and harmless; even arsenic, lead, copper, and mercury, which in certain states of combination are the most virulent substances known, exert no action upon the living system, until they be in union with some other body; but when so united, how valuable do they become; what various medicinal effects may they not be made to produce? The preparation of one metal alone may be said, with much truth, to have preserved the human race from extinction.

B

The *Acetic acid* and *Volatile alkali* become neutralized by combination, affording a compound of new virtues.—*Sulphate of Zinc*, and *Super-acetate of Lead* when mixed together in solution, decompose each other, and the *Acetate of Zinc* which is formed, affords a more valuable remedy than either of the former salts for ophthalmia. The "*Mistura Ferri composita*" offers another example. I also beg to refer the reader to Formula 19, which presents an instance of an elegant purgative draught being created by chemical combination, in which the original properties of every element are entirely changed. See also *Formula 24*, the chemical actions of which are more complicated than the preceding one; thus, the free *Sulphuric acid*, together with that which exists in the *Sulphate of Iron*, is sufficient to saturate the *Carbonates of Soda*, and *Magnesia*, forming two *Sulphates*, and thereby disengaging a volume of *Carbonic acid gas*, which not only encreases the purgative operation of the new salts, as already explained, but by its excess, it holds in *solution* the *Carbonate of Iron*, which is formed by the decomposition of the Sulphate, and which in that state, is a very active tonic, might therefore afford an example of the species of chemical action which is considered in the following division, viz.

b.   *Developement of Active Elements.*

A more striking and instructive instance of the effect of chemical action in developing an active principle cannot be selected than that of the well known *Stimulant Plaister*, composed of *Muriate of Ammonia, Soap and Lead Plaister*, in which the alkali of the soap enters into combination with the *Muriatic Acid*, when the *Ammonia*, upon which the virtues of the plaister solely depend, is slowly disengaged in the form of gas, producing a powerful rubefacient and stimulant effect. The " *Cataplasma Fermenti*" or " *Yeast Poultice,* is indebted for its antiseptic properties to a similar agency, for they do not depend upon any virtue in the ingredients themselves, but upon their decomposition, and the consequent developement of an active element, which is *Carbonic Acid.* The practitioner unacquainted with the *modus operandi* of these combinations would inevitably fall into an error, by which their efficacy must be lost, he would hardly apply them as soon as they were formed, nor would he be aware of the necessity of repeating them at short intervals.

The decomposition of *Calomel* by lime water, forming the well known " *black wash,*" and that of *corrosive sublimate* in the same fluid, constituting the " *aqua phagadenica,*" furnishes remedies which derive all their peculiar efficacy from the developement of the mercury in different states of oxidation.

Many interesting and important illustrations of this principle may possibly be hereafter derived from an extended knowledge of vegetable chemistry ; the late researches of Serturner render it probable that we may be able to develope a new principle of extraordinary powers from opium, in which it appears to exist in a state of neutralization ; the same observations may be applied to the discoveries relative to the emetic principle of Ipecacuan.

C. *By Combining Substances between which no other Chemical change is induced than a diminution or encrease in the* Solubilities *of the Principles, which are the Repositories of their Medicinal virtues.*

The degree of solubility possessed by a medicinal substance may perhaps be regarded by some practitioners as a circumstance of but little, or no importance, it will however appear in many cases that *it not only influences the activity of a remedy, but like its dose goes far to determine its specific operation.* It is probably owing to the diversity which exists in the solubility of the active elements of purgatives, that so great a diversity occurs in their operation : it is for instance easy to conceive that a medicine may act more immediately and specially on the stomach, small, or large intestines, according to the relative facility with which its principles of activity enter into solution; that those which are dissolved before they pass the Pylorus are quick and violent in their effects, and liable to affect the stomach, as is exemplified by the action of *Gamboge, &c.* whilst some resinous purgatives, on the other hand, as they contain principles less soluble, seldom act until they have passed out of the stomach, and often not until they have reached the colon. *Colocynth* has a wider range of operation, since its principles of activity reside both in soluble and insoluble elements. *Aloes* again, being still further insoluble, pass through the whole alimentary canal before they are sufficiently dissolved, and act therefore more particularly upon the rectum, by which they are liable to produce piles, tenesmus, and the various effects which so usually attend their operation. The characteristic effects of *Rhubarb, Senna, Saline Carthartics,* and indeed of all the individual substances which compose the class of purgative medicines, will also admit of a satisfactory explanation from the application of these views. It ought moreover to enable the practitioner, by changing the solubilities of these substances, to change their medicinal effects. Experience shews that this is the fact, and that by combining *Aloes* with *Soap,* or an *Alkaline Salt,* we quicken their operation, and remove their tendency to irritate the rectum ; the *Compound Decoction of Aloes* affords a combination of this kind. *Gamboge*, whose too ready solubility it is an object to obviate, should be intimately incorporated with some insoluble purgative, as for instance *Aloes ;* a formula of this nature was introduced by Dr. George Fordyce, and it has been since simplified, and admitted into our Pharmacopœia, under the title of *Pilulæ Cambogiæ Compositæ.*" *Tartrate of Potash*, which on account of its comparative solubility has gained the name of *Soluble Tartar*, acts with corresponding briskness upon the small intestines, but if we encrease its proportion of *Tartaric Acid*, we convert it into a *super-tartrate* or " *Cream of Tartar*," which is a substance characterized by a comparative degree of insolubility, a correspondent change is produced in the medicinal activity of the salt, its purgative effects are considerably diminished, whilst its diuretic powers are rendered more considerable ; we may even extend this experiment by adding to the *Cream of Tartar*, *Boric Acid*, a substance capable of increasing to a certain extent its solubility, when we shall again find that its purgative properties are strengthened in an equal proportion.

It has been observed that a mixture of different saline cathartics is more efficient than an equivalent dose of any single one, a fact which is strikingly exemplified in the prompt and active operation of factitious Cheltenham Salts in comparatively small doses, as well as in that of sea water—I submit whether this may not in some degree depend upon encreased solubility ; for it is a law well known to the chemist that *when water has ceased to act upon a salt, in consequence of its having obtained the term of saturation, the solution may still take up another salt of a different kind.* I apprehend thàt an advantageous application of this law might be frequently made in practice, and the energies of a remedy thereby considerably extended.

Where the active principle of a cathartic is not sufficiently soluble, it is apt to vex and irritate the bowels, producing tormina instead of exciting a free and copious excretion, hence the reason why the operation of resinous purgatives are so commonly attended with griping, and why relief or prevention may be obtained by combining them with *neutral salts*; thus also *Senna*, whose virtues reside in extractive matter, is apt by decoction, or long exposure to the air, to act with griping, in consequence of the extractive matter becoming by oxidation, resinous and comparatively insoluble : this effect is best counteracted by the addition of *soluble Tartar*.

It appears then to be established as a pharmaceutical axiom, that *the intensity and even specific action of a purgative medicine may be modified or changed, by changing the degree of solubility possessed by the principles in which its activity resides.*

The application of this principle is highly important in practice, directing us in the choice of the different purgatives, according to the objects which we may wish to fulfil by them, and pointing out safe and easy methods by which we may encrease, diminish, retard, or accelerate their operation : it thus enables us to construct new and powerful combinations, by imparting to established remedies fresh activity, or by mitigating the acrimony and violence of arrangements, in other respects efficacious and eligible.

In the exhibition of solid substances, their mechanical state of division may be capable of modifying their operation, from the influence which this condition must necessarily exert upon their solubilities, although I am by no means disposed to assign to it the importance which Gaubius has ventured to express, " *Sunt quæ ruditer pulverata alvum, subtilius vero urinas, aut alios humores movent.*" I have endeavoured under the article *Pulveres* to establish some useful precepts upon this subject.

Of remedies composed of vegetable tonics and astringents, the useful application of this principle is farther apparent. Thus the addition of *alkalies*, or *lime water* to the infusions of *Gentian*, &c. or to the decoctions of *Bark*, by rendering their extractive and resinous principles more soluble, encrease their elegance, and exalt their virtues. (Formulæ, 94, 96.) A knowledge of this principle likewise offers many useful hints connected with the successful exhibition of active remedies; it points out the medicines which require dilution in order to promote their operation, and those whose too speedy and violent effects may be retarded and checked by an abstinence from all potation. Thus in the exhibition of *Diuretics* likely to become cathartic or diaphoretic, no liquid should be given for at least an hour after their administration; the same caution applies with respect to the *Compound Powder of Ipecacuan*, which has a strong tendency to excite vomiting. When the remedy has passed out of the stomach, then the ingestion of fluids may, and ought to be encouraged.

To Sir Francis Milman the Profession is highly indebted for hints concerning the importance of accompanying the exhibition of *Diuretics* with plentiful dilution, the arguments which he adduces elucidate in a very satisfactory manner the view which has been just taken of the *INFLUENCE OF SOLUBILITY*.

Whenever a poisonous substance has been received into the stomach we should religiously avoid administering any thing which may be likely to favour its solubility. In the selection of *Emetics* this admonition must not be forgotten, *Vomiting ought never to be provoked by preparations containing water, nor by liquids, which are capable of acting as solvents ;* hence we perceive the propriety of that practice, to which so much importance has been attached, of producing vomiting by the mechanical irritation of the fauces.

Late experiments* have shewn that *Magnesia,* as well as the *fixed Alkalies,* encrease the virulence of arsenic, by forming with it a soluble salt; whereas *Lime* or its *Carbonate,* has an opposite tendency, in consequence of the insolubility of *Arsenite of Lime.* I confess that these results agree with the views I have long entertained upon this subject : *destroy the solubility of a poisonous substance, and you will probably disarm it of its virulence.* *Nitrate of Silver,* by coming in contact with a *Muriatic Salt,* is rendered quite inert, and may be discovered unaltered in the fæces of persons to whom it has been administered. See *Argenti Nitras.* Orfila has accordingly found that a solution of common salt is a complete counter-poison to *lunar caustic,* and he has also shewn that the pernicious qualities of the *Muriate of Barytes* are counteracted by any soluble *Sulphate.*

Under the article *Plumbi Superacetas* the practitioner will find that the conjunction of this substance with any sulphuric salt, at once deprives it of its valuable properties as a remedy in *Hæmopthysis.* At the same time it is right to acknowledge that in the medical treatment of a case of poison, there are circumstances which might render it even judicious to administer a solvent, in order to remove the particles of the substance which sometimes adhere with such obstinacy to the coats of the stomach, as to defy the ex-

* London Medical Repository, August, 1817.

ertions of an emetic, especially if the poison be *Arse-nic;* but this practice should not be allowed until all that can be fairly ejected by vomiting or purging has been pr..viously removed, then the ingestion of *Magnesia,* or an *Alkaline Salt,* as proposed by Mr. Marshall* might be admissible, but it should be quickly followed up by fresh emetics, or purgatives. The propriety of administering *vinegar, lemonade,* and different acid potations, in order to counteract the baneful effects of *Opium* and other narcotics, which has been so often questioned, receives ample explanation from the same views : they shew that if any quantity of the substance of opium remain in the primæ viæ, that acid, or muci-laginous drinks, by favouring its solution and absorption, must accelerate its fatal effects,+ but should it have been previously removed from the stomach, that then the antinarcotic influence of a vegetable acid may remove the consequent stupor and delirium, and thus realize the expectations which Virgil has so poetically raised.

——————— quo non præsentius ullum
(Pocula si quando sævæ infecere novercæ
miscueruntque herbas, et non innoxia verba)
Auxilium venit, ac membris agit atra venena.

" When the drug'd bowl mid witching curses brew'd
Wastes the pale youth by step-dame hate pursu'd,
It's powerful aid unbinds the mutter'd spell
And frees the victim from the draught of hell."‡

* Remarks on Arsenic, to which are added Cases of Recovery from its Poisonous Effects, by John Marshall, Surgeon, &c. Lond. 8vo. 1817·
+ The Reader is referred to a work lately published by M. Orfila, entitled " Toxocologie générale considérée, sous les Rapports de la Physiologie, de la Pathologie, et de la Medicine légale." Paris, 1815.
‡ Mr. Parkes, author of the Chemical Catechism and other works, suggested the probability of this passage being an allusion to the anti-narcotic powers of a vegetable acid.

V

TO AFFORD A CONVENIENT, AGREEABLE, AND EFFICACIOUS FORM.

After the views which have been submitted, it is evident that the form in which a remedy is exhibited may exert some influence upon its medicinal effects; in general it must be adapted to the extent of the dose—the nature of the remedy—its degree of solubility—the objects it is to fulfil—and, as far as can be attained with propriety, to the caprice of the patient. For more particular directions, see *Decocta, Infusa, Tincturæ, Misturæ, Pilulæ, Pulveres,* &c.

When a substance, or a combination of substances, requires the addition of some other one for the purpose of imparting a convenient, agreeable, or efficacious form, *a vehicle should always be selected, whose effects will be likely to correspond with the intention of the other ingredients.* This precept may be exemplified by a reference to *Formulæ* 1, 17, 33, and others, the key letters of which will shew the *modus operandi* of their respective *vehicles.*

Some medicines are more grateful to the stomach, as well as more efficacious in their operation, when exhibited in a state of effervescence, we must however be careful that their properties are not injured by such a combination; see Formulæ 19, 23, 24.

Such are the objects which are to be obtained by combining several substances in one *Formula,* and such are the laws by which these compositions are to be regulated; but unless a physician can satisfactorily trace the operation of each element in his prescription to the accomplishment of one or more of the objects which I have enumerated, SIMPLICITY should be regarded by him as the greatest desideratum. I was once told by a practitioner in the country that the quantity, or rather complexity of the medicines which he gave his patients, for there never was any deficiency in the former, was always increased in a ratio with the obscurity of their cases; " if," said he, " I fire a great profusion of shot, it is very extraordinary if some do not hit the mark." A patient in the hands of such a practitioner has not a much better chance than the Chinese Mandarin, who upon being attacked with any disorder, calls in twelve or more physicians, and swallows in one mixture all the potions which each separately prescribes!

Let not the young practitioner however be so deceived; he should remember that unless he be well acquainted with the mutual actions which bodies exert upon each other, and upon the living system, it may be laid down as an axiom, that *in proportion as he complicates a medicine, he does but multiply the chances of its failure.* SUPERFLUA NUNQUAM NON NOCENT: let him cherish this maxim in his remembrance, and in forming compounds, always discard from them every element which has not its mode of action clearly defined, and as thoroughly understood.

The perfection of a Medicinal Prescription may be defined by three words; it should be PRECISE (in its *directions,*) CONCISE (in its *construction,*) DECISIVE (in its *operation.*) It should carry upon its very face an air of energy and decision, and speak intelligibly the indications which it is to fulfil. It nay be laid down as a position which is not in much danger of being controverted, that *where the intention of a medicinal compound is obscure, its operation will be imbecile.*

A Medicinal Formula has been divided into four
constituent parts, a division which will be found to
admit of a useful application to practice, in as much as
it was evidently suggested with a view of accomplish-
ing the more prominent objects which have been related in the preceding pages; or in the language of
Asclepiades of enabling the BASIS to operate "CITO,"
" TUTO," et "JUCUNDE." Quickly, Safely, and Plea-
santly.—thus

I. THE BASIS, or Principal Medicine.

II. THE ADJUVANS; that which assists and promotes its operation.
  (" Cito.")

III. THE CORRIGENS; that which corrects its operation.
  (" Tuto.")

IV. THE CONSTITUENS; that which imparts an
  agreeable form.
  (" Jucunde.")

These elements however are not all necessarily
present in every scientific formula, for many medicines do not require any addition to promote their
operation, and the mild and tractable nature of others
renders the addition of any corrective unnecessary;
whilst many again are in themselves sufficiently manageable, and do not therefore require the *intermede*
of any *vehicle* or *constituent*. It also frequently occurs that one element is capable of fulfilling two or
more of the objects required; the ADJUVANS for instance, may at the same time act as the CORRIGENS,

or CONSTITUENS; thus the addition of *Soap* to *Aloes* or *Extract of Jalap* mitigates their acrimony, and at the same time quickens their operation (17.) So again *Neutral Salts* both quicken and correct the griping which attends the operation of resinous purgatives. The disposition of the key letters placed opposite to the elements of the following *Formulæ*, will furnish the practitioner with a farther elucidation of these principles, viz. 1, 9, 10, 14, 15, 29, 30, 33, 49, &c. This coincidence, if possible, should be always attained, for it simplifies the formula, and by decreasing the bulk of the remedy, renders it less nauseous and more elegant.*

This division also affords the best general rule for placing the ingredients of a formula in proper order; for the order should correspond with that of the arrangement; and those elements intended to act in unity should be marshalled together. The chemical and mechanical nature however of a medicinal substance will occasionally offer exceptions to any general rule; thus the volatile ingredients should be those last added, and the constituent or *vehicle* should be placed next the particular element to which it is intended to impart convenience or efficacy of form, or a capability of mixing with the other ingredients, as may be seen in Formulæ 8, 10, 50, 63, &c. If any substance require decoction or infusion, a question then arises,

---

* It appears from what has been stated under Section I. A. with respect to DIURETICS, that some medicines not only *assist*, but actually DIRECT the operation of the substances with which they may be associated, and that many remedies act in unison with those they are joined with; thus *Nitre* in conjunction with *Squill* is diuretic; in conjunction with *Guaiacum*, diaphoretic; for these reasons I hesitated, whether I ought not to have added a fifth *constituent*, and restored the " *Dirigens*" of Ancient authors.

determinable only by a knowledge of its chemical composition, whether the remaining ingredients should be added previous to, during, or subsequent to that operation; *Formula* 95, which is recommended by Pringle as a remedy in Typhus fever, may serve to exemplify this principle. The preparation of the ingredients is resolved into three distinct stages, and it is easy to discover that by any other arrangement their several virtues could not be fully obtained, and secured from change. The *Cinchona*, for instance, yields its full powers only by decoction, a process which would necessarily impair those of *Serpentaria*, which are connected with an essential oil; whilst the addition of the acid at any other stage of the process than that directed, would produce decompositions in the vegetable substances; and it is evident, that were the *Spirit of Cinnamon* added previously, it would be entirely lost by vaporization.

COMPOUND MEDICINES have been divided into two Classes, *viz.*

I. OFFICINAL PREPARATIONS,
which are those ordered in the Pharmacopœias, and kept ready prepared in the shops. No uniform class of medicines however can answer the indications of every case, and hence the necessity of

II. MAGISTRAL OR EXTEMPORANEOUS FORMULÆ.
These are constructed by the practitioner at the moment, and may be either arrangements altogether new, or officinal preparations with additions, or modifications. *Extemporaneous* are also preferable to *Officinal Formulæ*, whenever the powers of the compound are liable to deterioration from being kept;

for examples, see *Mistura Ferri composita ; Infusum Sennæ ; Liquor Hydrargyri Oxy-muriatis,* &c.

THE CHEMICAL AND PHARMACEUTICAL ERRORS, WHICH MAY BE COMMITTED IN THE COMPOSITION OF EXTEMPORANEOUS FORMULÆ, ARE REFE- RABLE TO THE FOLLOWING SOURCES.

1.—*Substances are added together which are in- capable of mixing, or, of forming Com- pounds of uniform and suitable consistence.*

This may be termed an error in the *Mechanism* of the Prescription, and has been generally regarded as being more inconvenient than dangerous, more fatal to the credit of the Prescriber, than to the case of the Patient; the observations however which are offered in this work, especially under the article *Pilulæ*, must satisfy the practitioner, that this error is more mis- chievous in its effects than has been usually supposed; it is so palpable, and self-evident in its nature, that it will be unnecessary to illustrate it by more than one or two examples. *Calomel,* for instance, has been ordered in an aqueous vehicle ; and certain *resinous tinctures* have been directed in draughts, without the necessary intervention of mucilage ; so again, an intermixture of substances has been formally ordered in powder that possess the perverse property of becoming liquid by triture (see *Pulveres.* p. 349.) and bodies have been prescribed in the form of pills, whose consistence renders it impossible that they should preserve the globular form.

II.—*Substances are added together which mutually
decompose each other, whence their original
virtues are changed, or destroyed.*

This is a more serious, but not a less frequent
source of error; it has been already shewn in this
Analysis (IV. B) that the judicious and scientific application of chemical science has furnished new and
endless resources to the physician, by exalting the
efficacy, and correcting the acrimony of established
remedies, or by combining inert substances, so as to
create new and powerful medicines. With equal
truth and confidence it may be asserted, that the
abuse of these means not only destroys the virtues of
the most valuable articles in the *Materia Medica,*·but
that the mildest remedy may be thus converted into
an instrument of torture, and even of death. In a
lecture delivered at Apothecaries' Hall, Mr. Brande
stated, that he had seen a prescription in which the
blue, or mercurial pill, was ordered in conjunction
with nitric acid, and that the patient was brought to
" death's door," from the formation of *nitrate of mercury* in his stomach! I have myself lately seen a
Recipe, professing to afford a preparation similar to
the " *Black Drop,*" and which directed a mixture of
a *Tincture of Opium,* made with rectified spirit, with
Nitric Acid; in this case, it may be very safely inferred, that the author was not only ignorant of the
chemical habitudes of these bodies, but that he never
performed the experiment in question, or he would
have learnt from dire experience, that in consequence
of the rapid evolution of *nitric ether,* the contents of
the phial will explode with violence, to the imminent
hazard of the operator's eye-sight. During the course
of my professional practice, 1 have witnessed more

than an ordinary share of consumptive cases, and I
can confidently state, that in the treatment of Hæmopthysis, the styptic properties of *super-acetate of
lead* are entirely invalidated by combination with
alum, or, by its exhibition being accompanied with
that of the acidulated *infusion of roses,* or, with small
doses of *sulphate of magnesia,* and yet, I would ask,
whether this practice is not usual, and general ? The
practitioner however cannot be too often reminded,
that he is not to reject a remedy whose value has
been ascertained by experience, merely because it
appears to be unchemical : the popular and certainly
useful pill, consisting of calomel, rhubarb, and soap,
may be adduced as an example of this kind. Of the
Mistura Ferri Composita, I will only say, that it is a
most valuable combination ; and whether it be the
product of accident, or the result of philosophical induction, it equally deserves a distinguished place in
our list of tonic remedies : but, it cannot be denied
that many of our esteemed arrangements, which are
in apparent contradiction to all the laws of composition, owe their efficacy to the operation of affinities
altogether blind, and fortuitous.

It is impossible to furnish any general rule that
may enable the practitioner to avoid mixing together
substances which are incompatible with each other;
a knowledge of their chemical habitudes, must in
every case direct him, and these are enumerated in
the present work, under the history of each medicinal
substance. The Physician however will find it useful
to retain in his remembrance the simple and beautiful law, which has been so ably developed by the
eminent author of the " STATIQUE CHIMIQUE," that,
*whenever two salts in a state of solution are brought
together, which contain, within themselves, elements ca-*

pable of producing a soluble, and insoluble salt, a de-composition must necessarily arise; he illustrates this law by the example of *Nitrate of Silver,* and *Muriate of Potass,* whose elements are capable of forming, within themselves a soluble salt, *Nitrate of Potass,* and an insoluble salt, *Muriate of Silver.*

III.—*The Methods directed for the preparation of the Ingredients are either inadequate to the accomplishment of the object, or they change and destroy the efficacy of the Substances.*

The observations already offered upon *Formula* 95, will sufficiently explain the nature of the various errors comprehended under this head: so, again, if the virtues of a plant reside in *essential oils,* which are easily volatilized, or in *extractive matter,* which readily becomes oxidized, DECOCTION must necessarily destroy its efficacy ; a striking example of this fact is presented us in the history of the *Laurel* and *Bitter Almond,* the poisonous influence of the essential oil and distilled water of these vegetable substances, is well known, but their watery extracts are perfectly innocuous. On the other hand, an er-ror equally injurious would be committed, by direct-ing a simple infusion of a vegetable, whose medicinal properties depended upon resino-mucilaginous princi-ples. See *Decocta, Infusa, Extracta.*

An instance of the baneful effects which may arise from an erroneous method of preparation, happened some time ago to fall under my immediate notice and care ; it was in preparing an infusion of the root of the *Veratrum* with *Opium,* as directed by Mr. James Moore, when the dispenser ignorantly substituted a spirituous for a vinous menstruum.

A very common error may be here noticed, which is that of prescribing a substance in such a form, as not to be acted upon with any effect by the solvent; as an example it may be stated, that in preparing an Infusion of *Juniper Berries*, unless pains be taken, by strong contusion, to break the seeds, it will contain but little powers as a medicine. It is unnecessary to multiply examples in proof of the numerous errors into which a physician must unavoidably fall, who presumes to compose prescriptions without a knowledge of the chemical habitudes of the different substances which he combines. The file of every apothecary would furnish a volume of instances, where the ingredients of the prescription are fighting together in the dark, or at least, so adverse to each other, as to constitute a most incongruous and chaotic mass.

" Obstabat aliis aliud : quia corpore in uno
Frigida pugnabant calidis, humentia siccis,
Mollia cum duris, sine pondere habentia pondus."

THE DOSES OF MEDICINAL SUBSTANCES are specific with respect to each, and can therefore be only learnt from experience; the young and eager practitioner however is too often betrayed into the error of supposing, that the powers of a remedy always encrease in an equal ratio with its dose, whereas THE DOSE ALONE VERY OFTEN DETERMINES ITS SPECIFIC ACTION. " *Medicines* " says Linnæus, " *differ from poisons, not in their nature, but their dose,* " which is but a paraphrase of the well known aphorism of Pliny, " *Ubi virus, ibi virtus.*"—Five grains of *Camphor* act as a mild sedative, and slight diaphoretic, but twenty grains induce nausea, and act as a stimulant; so again, *Opium,* in too large doses, instead of promoting, prevents sleep, and rather stimulates the bowels, than acts as a narcotic. Two ounces of any neutral salt are apt to be emetic, one ounce even of *Alum,* to be cathartic, and two drachms to be refrigerant; in like manner the preparations of *Antimony* either vomit, purge, or sweat, according to the quantity exhibited.

Would it not appear that *powerful doses rather produce a local than general effect?* Experience seems to prove in this respect, that the effect of an internal application is similar to that of an external impression; if violent, it affects the part only, as pinching does that of the skin, whereas titillation, which may be said to differ only from the former in degree, acts upon the whole system, and occasions itching, and laughter, and if long continued, weakness, sickness, vomiting, and convulsions; in like manner *Digitalis,* if given in large doses, acts immediately upon the stomach or bowels, becoming emetic, and cathartic, but in smaller proportions, it produces a GENERAL effect, encreasing all the excretions, especially that of urine. I am well satisfied that the regulation of the dose of a medicine is even more important than it is usually supposed to be. *Substances perfectly inert and useless in one dose, may prove in another, active and valuable.* Hence may be explained the great efficacy of many mineral waters, whilst the ingredients which impart activity to them are found comparatively inert, when they become the elements of an artificial combination; and hence probably the failure of many *alterative* medicines, when no other rational cause can be assigned for it. We need not seek far for an example of the very different and opposite effects which the same substance can produce in different doses; the operation of *Common Salt* is familiar to us all; Sir John Pringle has shewn that in quantities such as we usually take with our food, its action is highly septic, softening and resolving all meat to which it is applied, whereas in larger quantities it actually preserves such substances from putrefaction, and therefore, when so taken, instead of promoting, destroys digestion.

It is moreover probable that medicinal, like nutritive substances, are more readily absorbed into the circulating system when presented in small quantities, than when applied in more considerable proportions. It is upon this principle that a large quantity of food taken seldom, does not fatten so much as smaller quantities, at shorter intervals, as is exemplified in the universal good condition of cooks and their attendants. It is not pressing the principle of analogy too far to suppose that the action of *alteratives*, which require to be absorbed, may be more effectually answered by similar management, that is, *by exhibiting small doses at short intervals.*

The operation of medicines is influenced by certain general circumstances, which should be also kept in mind when we apportion their dose; e. g. AGE—SEX —TEMPERAMENT—STRENGTH OF THE PATIENT— HABIT — DIET — CLIMATE— DURATION OF THE DISEASE—STATE OF THE STOMACH — IDIOSYN- CRASY — and THE VARIABLE ACTIVITY OF THE MEDICINAL SUBSTANCE.

Women in general require smaller doses than men. Habit, or the protracted use of a medicine, generally diminishes its power, although saline cathartics appear to offer an exception, for when long continued, their activity is proportionally encreased, as is well known to every person who is familiar with the operation of the Cheltenham waters.

In apportioning the dose of a very active medicine, it is of the greatest moment to determine the relative degrees of power between the system and the remedy, and to know to what extent the latter is likely to be carried, compatible with the powers of life to resist it; thus after a patient has been exhausted by protracted and severe suffering, and watching, a different dose is necessary than at the commencement of the disease. The importance of this precept is impressed upon my mind from having witnessed, in the course of my practice, several instances of the mischief which has arisen from a want of attention to it; but this is a question connected rather with THERAPEUTICS than PHARMACOLOGY.

THE VARIABLE ACTIVITY OF A MEDICINE should also be attended to, and perhaps the practitioner would act cautiously if he were to reduce the dose, should it be a very considerable one, whenever a fresh parcel of the medicine is commenced, especially of the powders of active vegetables, liable to deterioration from being kept, as *Digitalis, &c.*

THE TIME OF THE DAY at which remedies should be administered, deserves likewise some attention. *Evacuating Medicines* ought to be exhibited late at night, or early in the morning. It would seem that during sleep the bowels are not so irritable, and consequently, not so easily acted upon, which allows time for the full solution of the substance; the same observation applies to *Alterative*, and other medicines which are liable to suffer from a vexatious irritability of the bowels; it is on this account eligible to exhibit *Guaiacum, Pilula Hydrargyri,* &c. when they are not intended to purge, at bed time. On the other hand, where the effects of a remedy are likely to be lost by perspiration, as is the case with *Diuretics*, many of which, are by external heat, changed into *Diaphoretics*, it may become a question with the judicious practitioner whether he cannot select some more favourable period for their exhibition.

In fevers it is of importance to consult in all respects the quiet and comfort of the patient ; Dr. Hamilton therefore, in his valuable work on Purgatives, very judiciously observes, that on this account, the exhibition of purgative medicines should be so timed, that their effects may be expected during the day.

The Intervals between each Dose must be regulated by the nature of the remedy, and of the objects which it is intended to fulfil, and whether it be desirable or not that the latter dose should support the effects of the preceding one, or whether there be any fear of a reaction, or collapse taking place after the effect of one dose has subsided, unless immediately repeated. There is a caution also which it is very necessary to impress upon the practitioner, respecting the power which some medicines possess of accumulating in the system ; this is notorious with regard to Lead and Mercury, and probably with the preparations of Arsenic, and some other metallic compounds. Dr. Withering has observed that the repetition of small doses of *Digitalis*, at short intervals, till it produces a sensible effect, is an unsafe practice, since a dangerous accumulation will frequently take place, before any signals of forbearance present themselves.

Constitutional Peculiarities, or Idyosyncrasies, will sometimes render the operation of the mildest medicine poisonous, " *Virum novi*," says Gaubius, " *qui cum fatuum lapidum cancrorum pul-*

visculum ingessit, vix mitius afficitur quam alii ab Arsenico." I have seen a general Erysipelas follow the application of a blister, and tormina of the bowels, no less severe than those produced by the ingestion of *Arsenic*, attend the operation of purgatives composed of *Senna!* It is unnecessary to dwell upon this subject, since a knowledge of such peculiarities can alone enable the practitioner to avoid the particular medicines which are so unaccountaby liable to disturb the constitution.

The popular scheme of Gaubius, for adapting the doses of medicines to different ages, which was published in the former editions of this work, is now omitted, as being less easy of application, than the following simple formula by Dr. Young.

RULE.

For Children under twelve years, the doses of most Medicines must be diminished in the proportion of the Age to the Age increased by 12.

thus at two years to $\frac{1}{7}$—viz.

$$\frac{2}{2+12} = \frac{1}{7}$$

At 21 the full dose may be given.

Every general rule however respecting the doses of medicines will have exceptions. Thus Children will bear larger doses of *Calomel* than even Adults, and many medicines which do not affect Adults, although exhibited in considerable quantities, prove injurious, even in small doses, to Children.

41

A

SYNOPSIS

OF THE PRINCIPLES INVESTIGATED

IN THE INTRODUCTORY ESSAY,

FOR THE SAKE OF ABRIDGING THE LABOUR ATTENDING THE
FREQUENT REFERENCES REQUIRED FOR THE
EXPLANATION OF THE

MEDICINAL FORMULÆ.

OBJECT I.

TO PROMOTE THE ACTION OF THE BASIS.

Key
Letters

A.—*By combining it with Substances which are
of the* SAME NATURE, *i. e. which are indi-*

a   *vidually capable of producing the same effects,
but with less energy than when in combination
with each other.*

NOTE. *It is often eligible to combine the*

a*   *different Preparations of the* SAME SUB-
STANCE, *in order to ensure the full effects
of its Principles.*

B.—*By combining the Basis with Substances of
a* DIFFERENT NATURE, *and which do not
exert any Chemical Influence upon it, but are*

b   *found by experience, or inferred by analogy,
to be capable of rendering the Stomach, or
System, more susceptible of its action.*

Key
Letters

OBJECT II.

c

TO CORRECT THE OPERATION OF THE BA-
SIS, BY OBVIATING ANY UNPLEASANT
EFFECTS IT MIGHT BE LIKELY TO OC-
CASION, AND WHICH WOULD PERVERT
ITS INTENDED ACTION, AND DEFEAT THE
OBJECTS OF ITS EXHIBITION.

OBJECT III.

d

TO OBTAIN THE JOINT OPERATION OF
TWO, OR MORE MEDICINES, WHICH HAVE
DIFFERENT POWERS, AND WHICH ARE
REQUIRED TO OBVIATE DIFFERENT
SYMPTOMS, OR TO ANSWER DIFFERENT
INDICATIONS.

OBJECT IV.

TO OBTAIN A NEW AND ACTIVE REMEDY
NOT AFFORDED BY ANY SIMPLE SUB-
STANCE.

e

A.—*By combining Medicines which excite different actions in the Stomach and System, in
consequence of which,* NEW, *or* MODIFIED
RESULTS, *are produced.*

B.—*By combining Substances which have the
property of acting* CHEMICALLY *upon each
other,* the Results of which are,

43

f   **a.** *The formation of New Compounds.*

g   **b.** *The Decomposition of the Original Constituents, and the developement of their more active elements.*

h   **C.**—*By combining Substances, between which no other chemical change is induced than a diminution, or encrease in the* SOLUBILITIES *of the principles in which their Medicinal virtues reside.*

OBJECT V.

i TO AFFORD SUCH A FORM AS MAY BE EFFICACIOUS,

k AGREEABLE OR CONVENIENT.

A COLLECTION OF FORMULÆ.

INTENDED TO ILLUSTRATE THE FOREGOING PRECEPTS,

And to furnish the inexperienced Prescriber

WITH A SERIES OF

USEFUL AND INSTRUCTIVE LESSONS.

EXPLANATION OF THE KEY LETTERS.

The *Modus Operandi* of the different elements of
each formula is designated by a KEY LETTER, which
is placed in the margin opposite to them. This letter
refers to a corresponding one in the Synopsis, and
thereby shews the division containing an exposition
of the principle upon which the operation of the
ingredient is supposed to depend.

Two or more KEY LETTERS denote that the element against which they are so placed has several
modes of operation, whilst the order in which the
letters succeed each other, serves to shew the relative
importance of them.

Where any one of the letters is smaller and placed
above another, thus, b^a, it denotes that the operation
which it is intended to express is only *incidental* to,
or very subordinate in, the general scheme of the
combination.

When any number of elements are included within
a *vinculum* or bracket, it is intended to shew that they
operate but as one substance, or, that the virtues of
each are not independent of the other; in this case
the KEY LETTER within the bracket expresses upon
what principle this unity depends, whilst that on the

exterior shews the action of such a combination upon the base, or the part which it performs in the general scheme of the Formula.

Let us exemplify it by a reference to *Formula 16*, which presents us with a Purgative, in conjunction with a Stimulant. The base is *Aloes*, which is succeeded by *Scammony, and Extract of Rhubarb*; these substances appear by the bracket, to act in unity, a concurrence which the interior letter (a) shews to depend upon their being SIMILAR REMEDIES; the letter also on the exterior shews that its operation upon the base depends upon the same principle. We next come to powdered *Capsicum, and Oil of Cloves*; these ingredients are also shewn by a bracket to act in unity, and the letter *a*, in the interior, denotes that it is in consequence of their possessing a similar mode of action, whilst the letter *d*, on the exterior, announces that they act in the general scheme for the purpose of fulfilling a second indication; at the same time, the position of the smaller letter, ^c informs us that the combination acts, at the same time, as a *corrector* to the base.

EMETICS.

1. ℞. Vini Ipecacuanhæ f3j.
   Antimonii Tartarizati gr.j   a.
   Infus. Anthemid. Flor. tepid. fℨjss. a.k
   Fiat Haustus.

2. ℞. Antimonii Tartarizati gr. ij.
   Aquæ distillatæ fℨiv.   h.
   Solve. Hujus danda sunt cochlearia duo medioc: singulis horæ quadrantibus donec vomitus excitatus sit.

EMETICS.

3. ℞. Pulveris Ipecacuanhæ ʒss
Antimonii Tartarizati gr. j
Tinct: Scillæ f ℥ j   a. ⟩ a.
Aquæ distillatæ f ℥ viiss h.k.

Fiat Mistura, cujus sumat quamprimum cochlearia majora quatuor, et cochl : duo, sexta quaque, parte horæ, donec supervenerit vomitus.

4. ℞. Zinci Sulphatis   ℈ j
Confect : Rosæ canin : q, s   i.

ut fiat Bolus ex pauxillo Infusi Anthemidis hauri-endus. Post quamlibet vomitionem superbibantur cyathi aliquot Infusi ejusdem tepidi.

5. ℞. Tabaci Foliorum ℥ j
Aquæ fontis   q. s,   i.

simul contunde in cataplasm : et regioni epigastricæ admoveatur.

6. ℞. Cupri sulphatis gr. x
Aquæ distillatæ f ℥ ij   i.
Fiat pro haustu emetico.

℞. This sign, which is prefixed to Medicinal Formulæ, and now generally understood to mean *Recipe*, is in truth, a relict of the astrological symbol of Jupiter, viz. ♃, which probably derived its origin in the days when the physician was tinctured with the tenets of astrology, and therefore considered some such invocation essential to the salutary operation of the medicine.

47

CATHARTICS.

7. ℞, Extracti Colocynthidis comp : ʒj
   Opii puri   gr. iij   d.
   Olei Nucis Moschat : m iv   c.
Fiat Massa in Pilulas duodecem dividenda, quarum
capiat duas omni hora donec bis dejecerit Alvus.
Bilious Cholic.

8. ℞. Magnesiæ Sulphatis
      et Sodæ Sulphatis āā ʒvj   a. } a.h.
      Infus : Ros : fℨv   k.h.
      Liquoris Antimonii Tart : fʒj   b.
Fiat Mistura de qua sumantur cochlearia duo ampla ter quotidie.

9. ℞. Infusi Sennæ fℨj
      Træ Sennæ
      Træ Jalap : āā fʒi   a. } a.c.
      Potassæ Tart : ʒj   a.c.
      Syrup : Sennæ fʒj   k.ᵃ
Fiat Haustus primo mane sumendus.

10. ℞. Magnesiæ Sulphatis
       et Sodæ Sulphat : āā ℨss   a li.
       Misturæ Camphoratæ fℨviij   d.k.ᶜ
       Ferri Sulphatis gr. v   d.
Fiat Mistura de qua sumantur cochlearia duo amplæ
bis indies.

11. ℞. Jalapæ Rad. Contrit : gr. xv
       Hydrargyri Sub-muriatis gr. v   a.
       Confect : Ros : gall : q. s   k.
ut fiat bolus.

48

CATHARTICS.

12. ℞. Confect: Sennæ ℥iss
 Sulphuris præcipitat: ℥ss   d.
 Syrup : Ros: q. s   i.
Ut fiat Electuarium, de quo ter vel quater de die ad
nucis moschatæ magnitudinem capiatur, donec alvus
commode purgetur.   *In Hæmorrhoids.*

13. ℞. Olei Ricini f℥ss
 Vitelli Ovi q, s.   k.
 tere simul et adde
 Syrupi Papaveris f℥ij   a. ⎬ d.
 Træ Opii *m* v
fiat Haustus, tertiis vel quartis horis sumendus.
In Cholic from the ingestion of Lead.

14. ℞. Magnesiæ Sulphatis ℥vj
 Infus : Sennæ f℥iss   h. a.
 Træ Jalap : f℥j   aᶜ.
 Træ Opii *m*x
 Træ Castorei f℥j   a. ⎬ a.
Fiat Haustus, ut supra, dandus.

15. ℞. Infus : Sennæ f℥ij
 Sodæ Tart: ℥vi   a.c.
 Aquæ Cinnamomi f℥vj   k.ᶜ
Fiat Solntio duabus vicibus sumenda.

CATHARTICS.

16. ℞. Aloës Spicata : ℈j
 Scammoneæ gr. xij   a.⎱ a.
 Extract : Rhei ℈ij   ⎰
 Baccarnm Capsici pulv : gr. vj   a.⎱ dᶜ.
 Olei Caryophyll : m v   ⎰
fiant Pilulæ xij, e quibus sumantur binæ, hora decubitus, pro re nata.

17. ℞. Pulv : Aloes comp : ℥j
 Pulveris Antimon : gr. v   b.
 Saponis duri gr. x   i. h.
 Decoct : Aloes comp : q. s,   iª.
fiat massa in Pilulas xx dividendà, e quibus capiantur binæ, ad alvum, officii immemorem, excitandum.

18. ℞. Extracti Colocynth : comp : gr. xxiv.
 Pil : Aloes cum Myrrha ℥j   a.
 Hydrargyri Sub-muriatis gr. xv a.
Fiat Massa in Pilulá xij dividenda, e quibus sumantur una vel binæ, p. r. n.

19. ℞. Sodæ Sub-carbonat : crystall : ℥iss ⎱
 Crystallorum Tartari ℥iij   t.g.⎰
 Aquæ puræ ℥viij   ⎰
Stent in lagena bene obturata per triduum, et deinde sit in promptu, pro potu cathartico.
Young's Medical Literature; p. 445.

20. ℞. Scammonæ gr. x
 Pulv : Rhei gr. xv   a.
 Ammoniæ Sub-carbonat : gr. v   a.
fiat pulvis, ex vehiculo aliquo idoneo sumendus.

D

CATHARTICS.

21. ℞. Pulveris Jalap : gr. xv
       Pulv : Ipecacuan : gr. v   b
       Olei Cinnamomi *m* ij   c.k
fiat pulvis ut supra dandus.

22. ℞. Pulveris Rhei gr. xv
       Potassæ Super-sulphat : ʒi   a.c.
       Aquæ Cinnamomi fʒi   h.i.
fiat Haustus.

23. ℞. Sodæ Tartarizat; ʒij
       Sodæ Carbonatis ʒi
       Aquæ puræ fʒiss   f g
       fiat haustus cum Cochl : j amplo
         Succi Limonum
In impetu ipso effervescentiæ sumendus.   Quotidie
mane.
A grateful aperient.

24. ℞. Sodæ Carbonatis ʒij
       Ferri Sulphatis gr. iij
       Magnesiæ Sub-carb ; ʒi   f.g
       Aquæ puræ oss
       Acidi Sulphurici diluti fʒx
Infundatur primum lagenæ aqua, dein immittantur
salina, et denique Acidum Sulphuricum ; illico obtu-
retur lagena, et in loco frigido servetur.

NOTE.—*The decompositions which take place in this formula, are described in the Analysis, page* 18.—*There is a
precaution respecting the proportion of the Sulphuric Acid
which it is essential to remember, viz. that it should never be
added in excess; for in that case the Sulphate of Iron will
not undergo decomposition.—A farther account may be found
in one of the early numbers of Nicholson's Journal.*

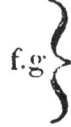

CATHARTICS.

25. ℞. Hydrargyri Sub-muriat: gr. x
 Pil: Cambogiæ co
 et Extract: Colocynth co āā gr. xv
 Syrupi Zingiberis q. s

a. ? a.
k.ᶜ·

ut ft. Pilulæ xij, e quibus
sumantur binæ, hora decubitus, vel summo mane, ad
alvum officii immemorem excitandam.

26. ℞. Cambogiæ in pulverem tritæ gr. iij
 Sacchari purificati Ʒi   i.
tere optime simul, et fiat pulvis tertia quaque hora
sumendus, donec alvus commode purgetur.

27. ℞. Foliorum Sennæ ʒiij
 Sodæ Sulphatis ʒi   a.
 Aquæ ferventis oj   h i.
Infunde, et Cola, ut fiat Enema.

DIURETICS.

28. ℞. Scillæ Radicis exsiccat: gr. iij
 Pulveris Opii gr. ss   c.b.
 Cinnamomi Corticis gr. x   k.c.
fiat Pulvis bis quotidie sumendus.

29. ℞. Potassæ Sub-carbonatis gr. x
 Infus: Gentian: comp: ʒss   d.h.
 Spir: Etheris comp; ʒss   a.
 Træ Cinnamomi fʒi   k.
fiat Haustus.
Diuretic and Stimulant.

D 2

DIURETICS.

30. ℞. Scillæ Radicis exsiccat. gr. xij
Potassæ Nitratis ʒi   a.c.
Sacchari purificat :   i.
et Cinnamomi cort: contrit :   k.
āā ʒi. fiat pulvis in sex partes æquales dividend : sumatur una bis indies.

31. ℞. Scillæ Rad : exsiccat : gr. iv
Digitalis Foliorum gr. x   a.
Hydrargyri Sub-muriat : gr. vj   b.
Myrrhæ Pulv : ℈i
simul tere et adde   a } d.
Assafœtidæ ʒss
Extract : Gentian q, s   k.
fiat massa in Pilulas xij, e quibus sumatur una, nocte maneque.

32. ℞. Massæ Pill. Scillæ ʒi
Hydrarg : Sub-muriat : gr. v   b.
fiat massa in Pilulas xv dividenda, quarum sumantur duæ singulis noctibus.

33. ℞. Sodæ Carbonat : exsiccat : ʒi
Saponis duri ℈iv   k.ᵃ·
Olei Juniperi   k.ᵃ·
Syrupi Zingiberis q. s   k.ᶜ·
fiat massa in Pilulas xxx dividenda, e quibus capiat tres, indies, contra calculos renum.

34. ℞. Scillæ Radicis exsiccat : gr. ij
Pilulæ Hydrargyri gr. v   d.ᵇ·
O ii gr. ss.   c.ᵇ·
Fiat Pilula hora decubitus per tres vel quatuor noctes consequentes capienda.

53

DIURETICS.

35. ℞. Potassæ Sub-carbonat : ℈i
    Succi Limonum : f℥ss, vel q, s   f.⎰
    Aquæ Cinnamomi f℥i
    Aceti Scillæ f℥iss   a.
    Tinct : Opii *m* v   b.
    Syrupi Aurantii f℥ss   k.
Fiat Haustus bis indies sumendus.

36. ℞. Potassæ Acetatis ℥i
    Oxymel : Colchici f℥ij   a.
    tere simul c̄ aquæ puræ f℥i   i.
    Spir : Juniperi comp : f℥ss   a.
Fiat Haustus, ut supra dandus.

37. ℞. Baccarum Juniperi contus : ℥ij
    Semin : Anisi contus : ℥ij
    Aquæ ferventis oj
macera per tres horas, dein cola.

    ℞. Colaturæ f℥xij
        Spir : Junip : comp : f℥ij   a*⎰
        Træ Scillæ f℥i   a.
        Potassæ Nitratis ℈ij   a.
Fiat Mistura, de qua sumatur cyathus subinde.

38 ℞. Infus : Digitalis f℥vij
      Træ Digitalis f℥i   a*⎰
      Potassæ Acetat : ℥i   a.
      Tinct : Opii *m* iv   c.b.
Fiat Mistura, de qua sumantur coch : ij ampla bis terve indies.

54

DIURETICS.

39. ℞. Liquoris Ammoniæ Acetat: f℥i
Potassæ Acetatis ʒi
fiat Haustus ter quotidie sumendus.

40. ℞. Potassæ Supertartratis ʒi
Pulveris Scillæ exsiccat: ℈iij   a.
Pulveris Zingiberis gr. v   c.
ft. pulvis, sexta quaque hora capiendus.

41. ℞. Spartii cacum: concis: ℥i
Aquæ puræ oj
Decoque ad octarium dimidium, et cola.

℞. Colaturæ f℥j
Spir: Etheris Nitrici m x,   a.c.
sumatur alternis horis.

42. ℞. Tinct: Ferri Muriat: m xv
Infus: Quassiæ f℥i   i d.
Fiat Haustus tertia quaque hora sumendus.

43. ℞. Potassæ Nitratis ʒi
Misturæ Ammoniaci f℥vj   i.a.
Spir: Juniperi comp: ℥iss   a. } a.
Aceti Scillæ f ʒvj
Fiat Mistura de qua capiat cochl: j amplum quartis
horis.

44. ℞. Tincturæ Lyttæ m x
Spiritus Ætheris Nitrici f ʒi   a.
Misturæ Camphoræ f ʒxij   i.a.
Syrup: Zingiberis f ʒi   ʀ.a.
Fiat Haustus ter in die sumendus.
A highly stimulating Diuretic.

EXPECTORANTS.

45. ℞. Assafœtidæ ℈ij
trituratione solve in
Aquæ Menthæ vir: f℥iij i.
addeque Syrupis Tolu: f℥j k.d.
Fiat Mistura, de qua sumatur cochl: unum amplum tertia quaque hora.

46. ℞. Myrrhæ gum-resin: ʒss
Sacchari purificati ℥ss
tere optime simul ut fiat Pulvis, partitis dosibus, quotidie sumendus, in vehiculo aliquo idoneo.

47. ℞. Extract: Myrrhæ ʒiss
Scillæ exsiccat: ʒss
Extract: Hyoscyami ℈ij a
Aquæ q, s ut fiant Pil xxx. d.
e quibus sumantur binæ, nocte maneque.

48. ℞. Scillæ exsiccatæ gr. viij
Pulveris Ipecacuanhæ gr. v a.
Camphoræ ℈j
Pulv: Antimon: gr. vj } a. b.
Sacch: purificat: ʒj k.
Tere in pulverem, in quatuor partes æquales dividendum; pars una sumatur bis quotidie, ex haustu decocti hordei.

49. ℞. Oxymel Scillæ
Syrupi Altheæ
Mucilag: Acaciæ } a. a.k.
āā f℥ss, misce, et fiat linctus, de quo lambat sæpe.

EXPECTORANTS.

50. ℞. Misturæ Ammoniac :
    et Aquæ Cinnamomi āā f℥ij   i.
    Syrupi Totut : f℥ss   k.ᵃ
    Træ Castorei f℈ij
    Træ Opii *mv.*   a. } d.

Fiat Mistura, cujus sumatur Cochl : unum amplum subinde, ac repetatur dosis p, r, n.
Expectorant and Antispasmodic. Houghing Cough.

51. ℞. Mist : Amygdal : f℥j
    Vini Ipecacuanhæ *mx*
    Potassæ Carbonatis gr. x.
Sumatur c̄ Succi Limon : f℈iij   g. }
in impetu ipso effervescentiæ.

52. ℞. Pulveris Myrrhæ gr. xij
    Pulv : Ipecacuanhæ gr. vj   a.
    Pulv : Potassæ Nitrat : ℨss   ā.c.
Misce et divide in doses æquales quatuor, quarum sumat unam quartis horis.

———

DIAPHORETICS.

53. ℞. Misturæ Camphoræ f℥iss
    Liquor : Ammon : Acet : f℥ss   a.
    Liquor : Antimonii Tart : *m* xx.
    Træ Opii *m* x.   b. } a.

DIAPHORETICS.

54. ℞. Potassæ Sulphureti **gr. xv.**
Saponis duri ʒj.   **i.c.**
Balsam : Peru : q. s.
ut ft : Pilulæ **xxx**; sumat tres quarta quaque hora
ex cyatho Infusi calidi Juniperi baccarum.
In Cutaneous Affections.

55. ℞. Pulveris Antimon : ʒss ⎫
Opii Pulv : Ɵss   **e** ⎬
Hyrdrargyri Sub-muriat : gr. v. ⎭
Confect : Opii q, s.   **i.a.**
ur fiant Pilulæ decem, quarum capiat unam hora de-
cubitus, et repetatur p. r. n

56. ℞. Pulveris Ipecacuanhæ comp : gr. **xv.**
Pulv : Trag : comp : Ɵij   **i.**
divide in partes quatuor æquales, quarum sumaʈ unam
quavis hora.

57. ℞. Pulv. Ipecacuanhæ comp : gr. **xv**
Pulv : Antimon : ij   **a.**
ft : pulvis hora decubitus sumend : superbibendo Haus-
tulum tepidum.

58. ℞. Guaiaci gum-resinæ Ɵss
Pulv : Ipecacuanhæ comp : gr. v **a.**
Confect : Rosæ q. s   **k.**
ut fiat Bolus, h. s. sumendus.

59. ℞. Potassæ Carbonatis gr. **x** ⎫
Mist : Camphoræ : fℨj **f.g.** ⎬
ft : Haust : cum Succi Limonum   ⎭
Cochleari uno amplo, in impetu ipso effervescentiæ
sumendus.

58

DIAPHORETICS.

60. ℞. Guaiaci Resinæ Ʒj
    Antimonii Tart :
        et   e. } a.
    Opii puri āā gr. j
    Syrupi q. s   k.
    fiat Bolus bis quotidie sumendus.

61. ℞. Camphoræ
    et Pulveris Antimon : āā gr. iij   e. } a.
    Opii puri gr. j
    Confect : Aromat q. s.   k.ᶜ·
    fiat Bolus, h, s, sumendus.

62. ℞. Liquor : Ammoniæ Acetat : f ʒ i j
    Decoct. Cinchonæ f ʒx   a* } d.
    Tinct : Cinchonæ f ʒij
    Confect : Aromat : ʒss   a.k.
    Fiat Haustus, tertia vel quarta quaque hora sumendus.

63. ℞. Guaiaci ʒij
    Acaciæ gummi ʒij   k.
    Simul bene tritis adde
    Træ Opii f ʒss   h
    Pulv : Cinchonæ ʒj
    Træ Cinchonæ f ʒij   a.* } d.
    Decoct : Cinchonæ f ʒviij
    fiat Mistura cujus sumatur cyathus bis quotidie.
    Rheumatism.

64. ℞. Extracti Aconiti
    Antimonii Sulphureti
    Præcipitati āā gr. j   c. } a.
    Magnesiæ Carbonatis Ʒss
    tere simul ut fiat pulvis.

59

DIAPHORETICS.

65. R. Oxydi Antimonii
  Potassæ Sub-carbonatis āā Əss   c.
  Anthemid. Flor. exsiccat : Əj   k.
  M. Fiat Pulvis sexta quaque hora, per
  biduum vel triduum sumendus.

66. R. Pulveris Ipecacuanhæ gr. ij   e. ⎬
  Pulveris Opii
  Potassæ Nitratis gr. xvj   a.i.
Fiat Pulvis hora somni sumendus.

EMMENAGOGUES.

67. R. Sabinæ Foliorum exsiccat :
  Zingib : rad : contus : āā Əss   c.
  Potassæ Sulphatis ʒss   d.ᵇ
  M. Fiat Pulvis bis die sumendus.

68. R. Myrrhæ pulv : Əj
  Ferri Ammoniati gr. vj   d.
  tere simul et adde
  Syrup : Zingib : q s ut fiat Electuarium,
de quo sumatur ad myristicæ nuclei magnitudinem bis
quotidie.

69. R. Mist : Ferri comp : fʒss
  Aquæ Cinnamomi fʒij   k.
  ft. Haustus bis de die sumendus.

60

EMMENAGOGUES.

70. ℞. Tinct : Ferri Muriatis
    Tinct : Aloes comp : āā f℥ss   a
    Tinct : Castorei f℈ij   d.

M. de qua sumatur cochl : unum minimum ex cyatho Infus : Anthemid : Flor : ter quotidie.

Emmenagogue and *Antispasmodic.*

71. ℞. Pil : Aloes cum Myrrha
         et
    Pil : Galbani comp : āā ℈ij   a.

Divide in Pil : xxiv, e quibus sumantur binæ bis quotidie.

72. ℞. Pil : Aloes cum Myrrha
         et
    Pil : Ferri comp : āā ℈ij   a.
    Sodæ Sub-Carbonatis ℈j   d.

Divide Massam in Pilulas xxx e quibus sumantur binæ bis quotidie.

DEMULCENTS.

73. ℞. Olei Amygdal : f℥j
    Acaciæ gummi ℈iij   j
    tere simul, et dein gradatim adde
    Aquæ distillatæ f℥vij   j
    Syrup : Rhæados f℥ss   k.a.

Fiat Mistura, de qua sumantur Cochlearia duo ampla ter, quaterve indies.

61

DEMULCENTS.

74. ℞. Olei Amygdal : f ʒvj   f.}
      Liquoris Potassæ m L   h.
      Aquæ Rosæ f ʒviiss
Fiat Mistura, ut supra capienda.

75. ℞. Mistura Amygdal : f ʒj
      Potassæ Carbonatis gr. x
      Syrupi Rhæados f ʒj   f. }d
Ft : haust : cum cochl : Succ : Limon :
in impetu effervescentiæ sumend :
Demulcent & Febrifuge.

76 ℞. Pulv : Cetacei
      Pulv : Trag : co āā ʒss   a.i.
      Syrupi Papaveris q. s   d.k.
misceantur, et fiat Linctus. Dosis cochl : minimum
subinde.

77. ℞. Cetacei ʒij
      Pulv : Trag : comp : ʒj   a i.
      Potassæ Nitratis ʒss   d.
      Syrup : Papaveris   d.k.
      Syrupi Tolu : āā f ʒij   k.
      Confect : Ros : ʒvj   i.
Fiat Electuarium, de quo capiat · ad nucis moschatæ
magnitudenem.

78. ℞. Cetacei ʒij
      Vitelli ovi dimidium   i.k.
      Syrupi f ʒss   k a.
      Aquæ Cinnamomi f ʒij   k ᶜ
      Aquæ distillatæ f ʒiv   i.
Ì iat Mistura, de qua capiat æger cochleare amplum
frequenter.

DEMULCENTS.

79. ℞.   Amyli ʒiij
     Aquæ ferventis fʒiv   i
     Solve pro enemate, et adde,
     si opus fuerit,
     Tinct : Opii fʒss   d.

80. ℞.   Decoct : Lichenis oss
     Sumatur quotidie, cochleatim,
     ad instar potus communis.

ANTACIDS AND ABSORBENTS.

81. ℞.   Liquoris Potassæ fʒij
     Liquoris Calcis fʒvj   i.a.
M.   Cujus capiat æger, acido infestante, cochleare
amplum unum, vel alterum, ex poculo jusculi bovini.

82. ℞.   Magnesiæ ʒss
     Aquæ Menthæ Pip : fʒiiss
     Spir : Lav : comp : fʒss
     Spir : Carui fʒiv   a. d.
     Syrup : Zingib : fʒij
Sumatur cochleare unum mediocre, p, r, n.
Antacid & Carminative.

83. ℞.   Pulv : Cretæ co cum Opio Əj
     Pulv : Catechu Extract gr. xv   d.
Sit pulvis, post singulas sedes liquidas sumendus.
In Diarrhœa depending upon Acidity.

REFRIGERATNS.

84. ℞. Potassæ Nitratis gr. xv
Ft: Pulv: ex cyatho Aquæ perfrigidæ, illico post
solutionem sumend :

85. ℞. Acidi Muriatici f3j
Decoct: Hordei oj   i.
Syrupi f3ij vel q. s
ad acorem compescendum, et gustum conciliandum.
Sumatur quotidie, ad instar potus, et bibat quantum
sitis exigat.
In Typhus and other Fevers.
See Introductory Essay, p. 9.

86. ℞. Ammoniæ Muriat : 3ij
Acidi Acetici f3ij   h.
Spir : Camphor : f3ss   d.
misce ut fiat Lotio.

87. ℞. Liquor: Plumbi Acetat : f3ij
Acidi Acetici f3iv   h.a.
Spir : tenuior : f3j   d.
Aquæ distillatæ oj   i.
fiat lotio.

ASTRINGENTS.

88. ℞. Cort : Quercus contus : 3ss
Aquæ ferventis f3viij
macera per horam, et cola.
℞. Hujus Colaturæ f3iss
Pulv : Gallarum gr. x   a. } a.
Tinct : Catechu f3ss
Tinct. Cardamom : co f3ss   c.
Syrup : Cort : Aurant: f3ss   i.
Fiat Haustus —

ASTRINGENTS.

89. ℞. Plumbi Superacetatis gr. iij
Opii puri gr. j **e.**
fiat massa in Pilulas tres dividenda, quarum sumatur una bis quotidie, superbibendo Haustum ex acido acetico compositum.

90. ℞. Infus : Cuspariæ f℥j
Tinct : Catechu f℥j **a.**
Pulv : Ipecac : gr. iij b } d.
Opii Pulv : gr. ss
Fiat Haustus.

TONICS.

91. ℞. Ferri Ammoniati ℈j
Extract : Gentian : **a.**
Extract : Aloes āā ℈ss **d.**
contunde simul, et divide massam in Pilulas xxx quarum sumat binas ter quotidie.
Tonic and Purgative, in Dyspepsia, Hysteria, Mesenteric Obstructions, &c.

92. ℞. Cinchonæ pulv : subt : ℥ss
Magnesiæ Sulphat : ℨvj **d.**
terē simul, et divide in quatuor partes, ex quibus sumatur una, alternis horis.
Intermittents.

93. ℞. Ferri Carbonatis gr. v
Pulv : Valerian : ℈ss **d.**
Syrupi Zingib : q. s **c.k.**
fiat bolus.

TONICS.

94. ℞. Infus : Gentian : comp : f℥j
  Liquor : Potassæ sub-carb. f℈ss   h.
  Tinct : Cascarillæ f℈j   c.a.
  Fiat Haustus

95. ℞. Cinchonæ cort : contus : ℥iij
  Coque ex aquæ puræ f℥xvj
  ad consumpt : dimid : adjectis sub finem coctionis,
  Serpentariæ radicis contus : ℥ij   a.
  Stent per horam, et colaturæ admisce
  Spir : Cinnamomi f℥iss   k.
  Acidi Sulphuric : diluti. f℈iss
  Sumantur f℥ij sexta quaque hora.
  Pringle.

96. ℞. Decoct : Cinehonæ f℥ij
  Infus : Gent : co f℥j   a.
  Tinct : Cascarill : f℈ij   a.c.
  Liquor : Potassæ Sub-Carb : f℈j   h.d.
  Fiat Mistura —

97. ℞. Decoct : Cinchonæ f℥vj
  Træ Cinchonæ f℈ij   a.*
  Confect : Aromat : gr, x
  Spir : Ammoniæ Aromat : *m*x   a.⎰ d.
  Fiat Mistura, de qua sumr. cochl : ij ampla indies.
  Tonic & Stimulant.

98. ℞, Ferri Ammoniat : gr. v
  Rhei rad : contrit : gr. iij   d.
  Fiat pulvis, e quolibet vehiculo idoneo quotidie su-
  mendus.

E

TONICS.

99. ℞. Infusi Cascarillæ f℥iss
   Tinct: Cascarillæ   a.*
   Tinct: Zingiberis āā f℥j   d.c.
Fiat Haustus, ter in die sumendus.

In Dyspepsia from Intemperance.

100. ℞. Ferri Tartarizati gr. x
    Pulveris Calumbæ gr. xv   d.
Fiat pulv : quarta quaque hora sumendus.

———————

STIMULANTS.

101. ℞. Lyttæ in pulv : trit : gr. i
    Ammoniæ carbonat :   a.⎱ a.
    Confect : Aromat : āā ℈j   ⎰
    Syrupi q. s   k.
ut fiat bolus, quartis vel sextis horis sumendus, cum
haustu Infusi Armoraceæ.

102. ℞. Ammoniæ Carbonat : ℈ss
       Aquæ Menth : Piperithid : f℥rij   i.a.
       Syrupi Aurantii f℥ss   k.
Sumatur octava pars in languoribus.

103. ℞. Mist : Camphoræ f℥j
       Spir : Etheris Sulphurici · f℥ij ⎤
       Tinct : Cardamom : comp : f℥iv |
       Spir : Anisi f℥vj   a. ⎬a.
       Olei Carui m xij |
       Syrupi Zingib : f℥ij |
       Aquæ Menthæ Pip : f℥vss   ⎦
Fiat Mistura, cujus sumatur cochlearia duo ampla ur-
gente flatu.

Flatulent Cholic.

67

STIMULANTS.

104. ℞. Ammoniæ Gum Resinæ
in pulv : trit : ℥ij
Aceti Scillæ q. s   h.i.
simul bene contritis, sit Emplastrum, scuto pectori.

105. ℞. Myrrhæ, in pulv : trit : ℈iss
Zinci Sulphat : gr. x   d₀
Confect : Rosæ q. s   i.
ut fiant Pil : xvij, e quibus sumantur binæ bis quotidie.

106. ℞. Sinapeos semin : contus :
Armoraceæ Radicis āā ℈vj   a
Aquæ ferventis oj,   i
macera per horam, et cola.
℞. Colaturæ f℥vij
Spir : Ammoniæ Aromat : f℈ss   a. ⎱ a,
Spir : Pimentæ f℥ss   ⎰
Fiat Mistura de qua sumantur cochl : duo ampla ter
die.
In Paralysis.

107. ℞. Olei Terebinth : f℈ij
Mellis despumati ℥j   k.
M. ut fiat linctus, de quo sumatur cochleare parvum,
nocte, maneque, cum haustu cujusvis potus tenuioris
tepefacti

E 2

ANTISPASMODICS.

108. R. Tinct: Castorei f3j
ÆEtheris Sulphurici *m* x   a.
Tinct: Opii *m* vij   a.
Aquæ Cinnamomi f℥iss   k.
Fiat Haustus ter quotidie sumend :

109. R. Moschi gr. xv
Camphoræ (Alcoholis pauxillo solutæ)   a.
gr. v.
Confect : Ros : canin : q. s. ut fiat bolus.

110. R. Moschi Ɖj
Acaciæ gummi 3ss   i.
tere optime simul, et adde gradatim.
Aquæ Ros : f℥j   k.
ÆEtheris Sulphurici f3j.   a.h.
Fiat Haustus p. r. n sumendus.

111. R. Assafœtidæ 3j
solve terendo cum
Aquæ Menth : Pip : f℥vj   k.
addeque
Tinct : Valerian : Ammoniat : f3ij ⎫
Tinct : Castorei f3iij   a. ⎬ a.
ÆEtheris Sulphuric f3j ⎭
Fiat Haustus, secundis horis sumendus.
Signetur.—*Antihysteric Draught.*

112. R. Pulv : Valerianæ Ɖj
Tinct : Valerian : Ammoniat :   a.*
Tinct : Castorei, āā f3j   a.
Misturæ Camphoræ : f3xij   a.i.
Fiat Haustus ter quotidie sumend :

69

ANTISPASMODICS.

113. ℞. Tabaci Folior: Ðij
  Aquæ ferventis f℥xij   i.
macera, et denique cola, fiat pro enemate

114. ℞. Opii puri gr. j
fiat Pilula —

NARCOTICS.

115. ℞. Camphoræ gr. xjj
  Extract: Hyoscyami gr. xviij a.
fiant pilulæ xij quarum sumantur tres, omni nocte.

116. ℞. Extracti Conii ʒj
  Folior Conii exsiccat :   a.⁎
et in pulverem tritorum, q, s
ut fiant pilulæ, singulæ grana duo pendentes.
Initio sumat æger pilulam unam pro dosi, mane ac
nocte, postea sumat binas, dein tres, et denique au-
geatur dosis quantum fieri potest.
In Scrophula, Schirrhus, and Cancer.

117. ℞. Tinct: Opii *m* xv
  Syrup: Papaveris f ʒij a.
  Spir: Cinnamomi f ʒj c.k.
  Aquæ puræ f ℥j   i.
Fiat Haustus, invadente paroxysmo caloris in febribus
intermittentibus sumendus.

70

NARCOTICS.

118. ℞. Opii gr. iv
Extract: Hyoscyami
Extract: Conii āā gr. xv   a.⎰ a.
Fiat massa in Pilulas sex dividenda, quarum sumat unam omni nocte.

119. ℞. Mist: Camphor: f℥j
Spir: Etheris comp: f3ss   a.
Tinct: Opii m x
Syrupi Papav: f3j   a.⎱ a.
Fiat Haustus hora decubitus sumendus.

120. ℞. Infusi Lini f℥vj
Tinct: Opii f3j
Fiat Enema —

ANTHELMINTICS.

121. ℞. Cambogiæ gr. viij
Hydrarg: Sub-muriat: gr. v   d.
Mucilag. Acaciæ q. s. ut fiat Bolus mane sumendus.
Contra Tœniam.

122. ℞. Pulv: Stanni ℥iij
Confect: Rosæ Gall: ℥iij   i.
Syrupi q. s. ut fiat Elect:
Capiat coch: amplum, quotidie mane, et repetatur dosis ad tres vices, et deinde capiat æger Haustum aliquem purgantem.

ANTHELMINTICS.

123. ℞ Sodæ Muriatis ʒij
        Coccinell : Ɂij   k
Fiat Pulvis, et detur drachma dimidia pro dosi, tempore matutino.

124. ℞ Ferri Carbonatis Ɂj
Sumatur ex vehiculo aliquo crasso, singulis auroris.

125. ℞ Camphoræ (Alcohole solutæ) ʒj
        Ol : Olivæ f ʒij   i
Misce, Fiat Enema.
Injiciatur h, s, tertia quaque nocte, ad tres vices; dein repetatur alternis noctibus, ad quartam usque vicem, si opus sit.
Contra Ascarides.

PHARMACOLOGIA

ABI.

ABIETIS RESINA. L. E. D. (Pinus Abies, *Resina concreta*). *Resin of the Spruce Fir.*

Olim, *Thus.—Frankincence. Burgundy Pitch.*

QUALITIES. *Form*, tears, or small brittle masses: *Odour*, very fragrant when burning. It has all the chemical properties of a *Resin* and is used only for external purposes. OFFICINAL PREPARATIONS. *Empl: Aromatic:* D. *Empl: Galban: comp:* L. *Empl: Opii* L. *Empl: Thuris.* D.

When distilled, it yields an oil, which is substituted for Oil of Turpentine, but is very inferior to it.

ABSINTHIUM. (Artemisia Absinthium) *Common Wormwood.*

QUALITIES. *Odour*, strong and peculiar. *Taste*, intensely bitter, slightly pungent and nauseous. CHEMICAL COMPOSITION. Extractive, a small portion of resin, and an essential oil, in the last of which its narcotic principle resides, which is therefore dissipated by decoction; its tonic and anthelmintic properties do not however appear to be impaired by the process. The essential oil of this plant is not in the least bitter. The whole plant is powerfully antiseptic. Infused in ale it forms the beverage known by the name of *Purl.* INCOMPATIBLE SUBSTANCES. Precipitates are produced in the decoction or infusion by *Sulphate of Iron*, *Superacetate of Lead*, and some other metallic salts; it is however rarely used. OFF: PREP: *Extract: Absinth: D.*

ACACIÆ GUMMI. L. (Acacia vera.) Mimosa Nilotica. E.D. *Gum Arabic.*

QUALITIES. It is dry, brittle and insipid; by exposure to the air, it undergoes no other change than loss of colour. SOLUBILITY. It is soluble in water in every proportion, forming a viscid solution, *mucilage.* One part dissolved in six of water affords a fluid of the consistence of syrup, and in two parts, a medium well calculated for the union of dry powders. Gum is also soluble in pure alkalies and lime water, as well as in vegetable acids, especially vinegar, with which it forms a mucilage that may be used as a cement, like the watery solution, and with the additional advantage of not being susceptible of mouldiness. It is insoluble in alkohol, as well as in æther and oils; for a farther history of its habitudes see *Mucilago Acaciæ.* OFFICINAL PREPARATIONS. *Mucilago Acaciæ. L.E.D. Emulsio mimosæ niloticæ. E. Emulsio Arabica. D. Mist. Corn. ust. L. D. Mist. Cretæ. L.D. Mist. Moschi. L. Confect. Amygdal. L. Pulv. Cret. co. L. Pulv. Tragacanth. co. L. Trochisci Carbonat. calcis E. Troch. Glycyrrh. Glab. E. Troch. Glycrrh. cum Opio. E. Troch. Gummos E.* ADULTERATIONS. Gum Sengal is not unfrequently substituted for it, but this may be distinguished by its clammy and tenacious nature, like the gum produced in this country from plumb or cherry trees, whereas genuine *gum arabic* is dry and brittle; the fraud is of no consequence in a medical point of view.

ACETICA. L.E.D. *Preparations of Vinegar.*

These preparations consist of vegetable principles dissolved in vinegar. OFFICINAL PREPARATIONS. *Acetum Aromaticum.* E. *Acidum Acetosum camphoratum.* E. Medicated vinegars were formerly much extolled; the first London Dispensatory contained no fewer than ten, at present the number is reduced to two, viz. *Acetum Colchici.* L. *Acetum Scillæ.* L.E.D.

ACETIS HYDRARGYRI. E. Acetas Hydrargyri. D. *Acetite of Mercury.*

QUALITIES. *Form,* small flaky crystals; *Colour,* silvery white; *Taste* acrid. CHEMICAL COMPOSITION. Acetic Acid, and Oxyd of Mercury. SOLUBILITY. It is soluble in hot, but very sparingly in cold water, and quite insoluble in Alcohol. FORMS OF EXHIBITION. It should be always given in pills,* it is however seldom used. DOSE, gr. j. As an external application, a solution of it, in the proportion of grs. ij. in f℥ij of rose water has been commended as a cosmetic.

ACETOSÆ FOLIA. L.E. Rumex Acetosa.
Common Sorrel Leaves.

QUALITIES. *Taste,* grateful, austere, and acidulous. CHEMICAL COMPOSITION. All its qualities depend upon the presence of *Super-oxalate of Potass.* In France the plant is commonly cultivated for the use of the table.

---

* KEYSER's ANTIVENEREAL PILLS, consist of this mercurial salt, triturated with Manna.

F 2

ACETOSELLA. L. Oxalis Acetosella.
Wood Sorrel.
The Qualities of this plant, like those of the preceding, depend upon *Super-oxalate of Potass.*

ACETUM. ⎛Acidum Aceticum⎞ *Vinegar,* L.
         ⎝   Impurum.   ⎠
Acidum Acetosum, E. Acetum Vini. D.

QUALITIES. Too well known to require description.
CHEMICAL COMPOSITION. Acetic Acid, largely diluted with water, vegetable gluten, mucilage, sugar, extractive matter, and frequently Malic and Tartaric Acids, together with small proportions of Sulphate of Lime, Sulphate of Potass, and Alcohol. Its composition however varies according to the fermented liquor from which it is obtained: e. g. wine yields a paler, purer, and stronger acid than fermented malt liquors, or solutions of sugar, hence the superiority of that prepared in France and Italy. Vinegar is liable to spontaneous decomposition, or to become mouldy, hence for the purposes of pharmacy it should be distilled; as however the change depends upon the presence of gluten, it may, if boiled, be kept for a much longer time, and if powdered charcoal be previously added, it will become quite colourless like distilled vinegar, and that without being impaired in strength, whereas it always becomes much weaker by distillation. It is a curious circumstance that this is the only vegetable acid, except the *Prussic,* that rises in distillation in combination with water.

ADULTERATIONS. Sulphuric acid, as it does not produce any turbid appearance in vinegar, is generally the acid selected for sharpening it; but here it is necessary to caution the chemist against inferring its presence from the mere occurrence of a precipitate by an *acetate of barytes*, as stated under *Acetic Acid*, since the sulphate of lime, or the sulphate of potass, so often present in common vinegar, would, as well as free sulphuric acid, produce with this test precipitates insoluble in nitric acid. To avoid therefore this fallacy, let the vinegar be assayed for sulphuric acid in the following manner; saturate a given quantity with chalk, add distilled water, and throw the whole upon a filtre; by these means if any sulphuric acid be present, an insoluble sulphate of lime will be formed, which may be recognised by the usual tests. For the purpose of making the vinegar appear stronger, acrid vegetables, as *grains of Paradise*, berries of *Spurge Flax*, *Capsicum*, *Pellitory of Spain*, &c. are sometimes infused in it, but by tasting it with attention, the pungency may be easily detected. For the other adulterations, see *Acidum Aceticum*.

A Vinegar has lately appeared in the market, produced from the distillation of wood, (*Pyro-ligneous acid*) but, notwithstanding its purification, which is effected by forming it into a salt, and then decomposing it by double affinity, it retains an empyreumatic taste, by which it may be recognised. The purest vinegar which I have ever examined is that manufactured from malt, by Mr. Macintosh of Glasgow.

ACETUM COLCHICI. L. *Vinegar of Meadow Saffron.*

Vinegar appears to be the best solvent of the acrid and medicinal principle which resides in the bulb of this plant. Dose ʒss to fʒij in any bland fluid. See *Colchici Radix*.

ACETUM SCILLÆ. L.E D. *Vinegar of Squill.*

This preparation is an acetic solution of the acrid matter of the Squill, upon which its medicinal efficacy depends   Dose f℥ss to f℥ij.   in cinnamon or mint water. See *Scillæ Radix.*   Form. 35. 43. 104.   This Preparation, as well as the *Oxymel,* deposits, when long kept, a precipitate consisting of *citrate of lime* and *tannin,* but its medicinal efficacy is not on that account impaired.

ACIDUM ACETICUM. L.   Acidum Acestosum Distillatum. E.   Acetum Distillatum. D.
Acetic Acid.

Qualities. *Odour,* fainter and less agreeable than common vinegar (*Acetum*) : *Taste,* less acrid ; *Colour,* none. Specific Gravity, varies from 1·006 to 1·0095. Chemical Composition. Acetic acid more largely diluted than that in vinegar, with very minute portions of uncombined mucilage and extrac tive. Solvent Powers. It is capable of dissolving all those vegetable principles which are soluble in water, and in some cases, as in *Squill, Colchicum,* and in several *Aromatics* and *Narcotics,* its acid appears to extend its solvent powers ; at the same time it often modifies or diminishes the medicinal virtues of the substances, as, for instance, those of *Narcotics ;* this circumstance very considerably limits its pharmaceutical application ; when however it is employed a portion of spirit should be always added, in order to counteract the spontaneous decomposition to which it is liable, and the acetic compound should be preserved in stopped bottles. Acetic acid does not dissolve true resins, but it has some action on gum resins. Dr. Powell states (*Translation of the Pharmacop: of London*, 1815) that one fluid ounce ought to dissolve, at least, thirteen grains of *white marble*. ADULTERA-TIONS. *Sulphuric Acid* may be detected by a precipitate being produced on the addition of acetate of barytes : this test however will not answer for its detection in common vinegar, for the reason stated under that article. See *Acetum*. The presence of *Nitric Acid* may be discovered by saturating the suspected sample with pure potass, evaporating to dryness, and then treating the product with a highly concentrated alcohol, the acetate of potass will be thus dissolved, but as it exerts no action on the *Nitrate* it will be found in the residuum, and may be recognized by its deflagration, when thrown upon burning charcoal. *Copper* may be detected by the acid assuming a blue colour, when supersaturated with ammonia ; and *Lead*, by a solution of sulphuretted hydrogen, producing a dark coloured precipitate.

CONCENTRATED ACETIC ACID. Acidum Acetosum Forte, E. Acidum Aceticum. D.

Radical Vinegar, has not retained its place in the London Pharmacopœia, as distilled vinegar, from which it differs only in the degree of concentration, is deemed sufficiently strong for all the purposes of medicine. Since however it possesses peculiar chemical habitudes, it claims some notice in this work. The concentrated acid may be obtained from the decomposition of acetic salts, by the action of sulphuric acid. It is pungent, acrid, and volatile, and when heated with free access of air, it takes fire very readily. Its solvent powers are much greater than those of distilled vinegar, it is capable of dissolving camphor

and essential oils copiously,* but they are precipitated
by dilution. Glass and gold can alone retain this acid
without being corroded.

ACIDUM BENZOICUM. L.E.D. *Benzoic Acid.*

QUALITIES. *See Powell's Translation of the Pharmacopœia.* OFFICINAL PREPARATIONS. *Tinctura
Camphoræ composita.* L.D. *Tinct: Opii Ammoniat :*
E. IMPURITIES. The crystals ought to possess a
brilliant white colour; they should be entirely soluble in alcohol, and when subjected to heat they should
be volatilized without leaving any residuum.

ACIDUM CITRICUM. L. *Citric Acid.*
Concrete Acid of Lemons.

QUALITIES. *Form,* crystals which are rhomboidal
prisms, white, semi-transparent, and persistent. *Taste,*
extremely acrid, almost caustic. SOLUBILITY. f℥j of
cold water dissolves ʒx, but if boiling, ℥ij. ℥j of the
crystals dissolved in a pint of water, is about equivalent to one pint of lemon juice, the solution however
if kept is liable to spontaneous decomposition. The
following table of equivalents may be found of prac-

────────────

* HENRY's AROMATIC VINEGAR is merely an acetic solution of camphor and some essential oil. A preparation of this kind may be extemporaneously made by putting ʒj of *Acetate of Potass* into a phial with a few
drops of some fragrant oil, and *m* xx of Concentrated Sulphuric Acid.

THIEVES VINEGAR, or MARSEILLES VINEGAR, is a pleasant solution of essential oils in vinegar; the Edinburgh Pharmacopœia has
given a formula for its preparation under the title of *Acetum Aromaticum.*
The repute of this preparation as a prophylactic in contagious fevers is
said to have arisen from the confession of four thieves, who, during the
plague of Marseilles, plundered the dead bodies with perfect security,
and who, upon being arrested, stated, on condition of their being
spared, that the use of *Aromatic Vinegar* had preserved them from the
influence of the contagion. It is on this account sometimes called
" *Le Vinaigre de quatre voleurs.*"

tical use; the author is aware that they do not exactly agree with the proportions of Dr. Haygarth, but they are the results of careful and repeated experiments, and as such they are submitted with confidence.

EQUIVALENT PROPORTIONS OF CONCRETE CITRIC ACID AND LEMON JUICE, NECESSARY FOR THE NEUTRALIZATION OF ALKALINE SALTS.

Citric Acid.	Lemon Juice.	A Scruple of Alkalies.
grs. x.	fʒiij.	Carbonate of Potass
grs. xv.	fʒiiij	Sub-Carbonate of Potass
grs. xxv.	fʒvij	SubCarbonate of Ammonia

These alkaline Citrates are decomposed by the *oxalic, tartaric,* and the stronger *mineral acids,* and by the solutions of *Lime* and *barytes.* FORMULÆ 35. 51. 59. 75.

Citric Acid decomposes the following salts, *viz. The Alkaline and Earthy Carbonates; the Alkaline and metallic Acetates; the Sulphurets of Earths and Alkalies, and Alkaline Soaps.* It curdles the milk of most animals, but it does not produce that effect on human milk, whether applied hot or cold. ADULTERATIONS. *Tartaric Acid,* with which it is sometimes mixed, may be detected by adding to the solution *Tartrate of Potass,* which will instantly form with it an insoluble super-tartrate, and precipitate in granular crystals. *Sulphuric Acid* is known by the superacetate of lead producing a precipitate, insoluble in Nitric acid. *Muriatic Acid* may be discovered in the same manner, substituting only an acidulous solution of nitrate of silver for the superacetate of lead. The presence of *Oxalic Acid* may be inferred, if the solution, when added to that of sulphate of lime, produce a precipitate. Malic acid has the power of precipitating silver, mercury, and lead, from their solutions in nitric acid, but no doubt or difficulty can arise from this circumstance, for the fact of its forming a soluble salt with lime will prevent every chance of accidental intrusion, and its price at once secures us against its fraudulent introduction; it might moreover be easily detected by throwing the suspected precipitate upon burning coals, when it would be decomposed. The juices of many other fruits besides the lemon and lime, will furnish the citric acid in abundance, and may be obtained from them by a similar process; e. g. VACCINIUM OXYCOCUS, the *Cranberry;* PRUNUS PADUS, the *Bird's Cherry*; DULCAMARA SOLANUM, the berry of the *Nightshade;* CYNOSBATUS, vel ROSA CANINA, the hep or fruit of the *Wild Briar.* There are many plants whose juices contain combinations of the CITRIC and MALIC acids, in considerable abundance, such as FRAGARIA VESCA, the *Wood Strawberry*, and the common *Raspberry;* RIBES RUBRUM, the *Red Gooseberry;* VACCINIUM MYRTILLUS, the *Bilberry;* CRATÆGUS ARIA, the *Hawthorn;* PRUNUS CERASUS, the *Black Cherry*, &c. This fact it interesting, since the juices of such fruits have been long known to possess the property of dissolving the *tartareous* incrustations on the teeth; whether they have any effect on ossification, or the formation of calculous concre tions, is a question which has hitherto not been investigated.

ACIDUM MURIATICUM. L. E. D. *Muriatic Acid.*

QUALITIES. *Form,* a liquid of the specific gravity 1·16, a fluidounce of which weighs about 527 grains, and according to Dr. Powell ought, when diluted, to dissolve 220 grains of limestone. *Odour,* strong and pungent; if exposed to the air it emits white fumes. *Taste,* intensely sour and caustic; it is however the weakest of the mineral acids; and no remarkable elevation of temperature is produced by dilution. CHEMICAL COMPOSITION. The liquid acid is a solution of muriatic acid gas in water, and ought therefore in conformity to our principles of nomenclature, to be be termed *Hydro*-muriatic acid; when of the sp. gr: 1.16, according to Davy, it contains 32.32 per cent. of the gas, which recent experiments have shewn to be a compound of *Chlorine* (*Oxy-muriatic acid*) and hydrogen in equal volumes; we accordingly find that the former element is disengaged from muriatic acid by adding any substance capable of uniting with its hydrogen. For an œconomical method of obtaining *Chlorine, see Powell's Pharmacopœia.* Accounts have been received from Spain, that in the midst of the dreadful contagion which reigned in that country, the inhabitants always escaped in those houses where fumigations of chlorine had been used. Muriatic acid gas has also been strongly recommended for the same purpose; it may be easily evolved by pouring sulphuric acid on common salt. If nitric and muriatic acids be mixed, a mutual decomposition takes place, of which water, chlorine, and nitrous acid are the results; this constitutes " nitro-muriatic acid," the *Aqua regia* of the older chemists. A bath acidulated with an acid of this kind has been recommended by Dr. Scott, as a powerful remedy for diseases of the liver in particular, and as a substitute for mercury in general. On the possible influence of this bath, I would beg to make one observation—that the extensive application of a dilute acid to the surface of the body, is capable of affecting the bowels. I have witnessed such an effect from sponging with vinegar and water. In this way the acidulated bath may occasionally produce benefit, but it is extremely difficult to conceive how it can be indebted for its utility to any other mode of operation. (See *Journal of Science and the Arts*, No. 2.) FORMS OF EXHIBITION. Muriatic acid should be administered in some bland fluid, as barley water, gruel, &c. *(Formula 85)*. I have uniformly exhibited it with success in the most malignant cases of typhus and scarlatina, during several years extensive practice in the Westminster Hospital, *see Introductory Essay, p.* 9. We should be careful not to apportion its dose in a leaden or pewter spoon. The antiseptic properties of this acid have been long known; Sir Wm. Fordyce relates that a dry salter acquired a large fortune from possessing a secret that had enabled him to send out provisions to India in a better state of preservation than any others of the trade; his secret consisted in adding a small quantity of muriatic acid to the contents of each cask. After a copious evacuation of the bowels, it is, in my experience, the best remedy for preventing the generation of worms; for which purpose the infusion of quassia, stronger than that of the Pharmacopœia, is the best vehicle. DOSE *m* x to xl. frequently repeated. It may be here

observed that where the permanent influence of an
acid is required, a mineral one should be always preferred, as such bodies appear to be beyond the control of the digestive process, and are incapable of
being decomposed by it; whereas on the contrary it
seems probable that the organs of assimilation have
command over those of a vegetable nature, and generally decompose them. Dr. Marcet has very judiciously noticed this fact, in his luminous work on the
treatment of calculi, and I have ventured to offer
some farther observations upon this subject, which
may be of practical value, under the article *Potassæ Acetas.* ADULTERATIONS. *Sulphuric acid* is
detected by diluting the acid with six parts of distilled
water, and adding a few drops of the muriate of
barytes, which occasions a white precipitate. *Iron*, by
saturating a diluted portion with pure carbonate of
soda, and adding prussiate of potass, which will indicate its presence by a blue precipitate. *Copper*, by
the production of a blue colour when supersaturated
with ammonia. The yellow tinge of the acid usually
met with in commerce, may depend either upon the
presence of iron, vegetable extract, or a small portion
of chlorine.

ACIDUM NITRICUM. L.E.D. *Nitric Acid.*
Aqua Fortis.

QUALITIES. A limpid liquid of the sp. gr. 1·500,
a fluid-ounce of which is equal to about 11 drachms 1
scruple by weight, and ought to saturate of pure limestone an ounce; it emits white fumes of a suffocating
odour. *Taste*, extremely acrid; it is highly corrosive,
and tinges the skin indelibly yellow. CHEMICAL

COMPOSITION. When of the sp. gr. 1·500, it contains 74·895 per cent. of dry acid (whose ultimate elements are one portion of nitrogen and five of oxygen) the compliment 25·105 parts is water, it ought therefore to be termed *Hydro*-nitric acid. It is decomposed with violent action by all combustibles, and when mixed with volatile oils, it causes their inflammation. It boils at 210, and when its specific gravity is below 1·4, it is strengthened, when stronger than 1·45 it is weakened by ebullition. USES. It is employed only as a pharmaceutical agent. ADULTERATIONS. *Sulphuric acid* may be detected by a precipitate being produced on the addition of nitrate of barytes; in the application however of this test, Mr Hume has shewn that unless the acid be diluted, a precipitate will occur, although sulphuric acid should not be present, a circumstance which depends upon the nitrate yielding its water, and becoming insoluble. *Muriatic acid* is discovered by nitrate of silver affording a precipitate at first white, but becoming coloured by exposure to light; the nitric acid ought to be perfectly colourless, and to preserve it in such a state it must be closely stopped, and kept in a dark place, or it will soon be converted into the nitrous kind.

ACIDUM NITRICUM DILUTUM. L.
Acidum Nitrosum Dilutum. E.D.

Dilute Nitric Acid.

It is much to be regretted that the proportion of water directed for the dilution of this acid, varies considerably in the different pharmacopœias; that prepared according to the Edinburgh, Dublin, and former London formulæ, being in strength to that of the pre-

sent Pharmacopœia of London, as 4 to 1. Dose *m* x
to xl. This acid is a very powerful antiphlogistic
remedy; it has been much extolled in diseases of the
liver, and in syphilis. Mr. Pearson however observes
that we ought not to rely upon it in any form of lues
venerea, although it may be often serviceable in re-
straining the progress of the disease when an impaired
constitution, or other circumstances, render the exhibition of mercury improper; when sufficiently dilute,
it forms an excellent lotion for old indolent ulcers.

ACIDUM NITROSUM. E.D. *Nitrous Acid.*

Qualities. A liquid emitting fumes of a flame
red colour, and of a very pungent and remarkable
odour. The acid is either blue, green, straw coloured,
clear orange-yellow, or deep orange-yellow, according
to the proportion of nitrous acid gas * with which it
is charged. Chemical Composition. This acid is
improperly denominated *Nitrous*, for it is nitric acid,
holding nitrous acid gas loosely combined; by dilution
this last constituent is disengaged, and the acid after
passing through a succession of different colours, becomes pure nitric acid; the application of a gentle
heat effects the same changes.

ACIDUM SULPHURICUM. L.E.D. Sulphuric
acid.
Oil of Vitriol, Vitriolic Acid.

Qualities. *Form,* a thick liquid of an oily consistence, sp. gr. 1·85. a fluid-ounce weighs a fraction
of a grain more than fourteen drachms. *Colour* none,

---

* *Nitrous acid gas* is a combination of nitrous gas and oxygen.

but it acquires a brown tinge from the smallest por‑
tion of carbonaceous matter; mere exposure to the
air is sufficient for this purpose, in consequence of the
acid disorganizing and carbonating the vegetable and
animal matter suspended in the atmosphere; it is there‑
fore evident that bottles in which it is preserved ought
not to have stoppers of cork, but those of glass. CHE‑
MICAL COMPOSITION. Like the other mineral acids,
it has never been obtained in an insulated state, with‑
out water, it is therefore *Hydro*-sulphuric acid ;
according to Davy, the composition of the strongest
acid may be thus expressed : sulphur 30, oxygen 45,
water 17. It has a very powerful affinity for water,
and produces when mixed with it a very considerable
heat; exposed to the atmosphere it imbibes at least
seven times its own weight of water, and so rapidly as
to double its weight in a month; when of the sp. gr.
1·85, it rises in vapour at about 550°, and distills un‑
altered, whereas weaker acids by being boiled lose
water, and are brought to that degree of concentra‑
tion; when diluted with 12 or 13 per cent of water,
an acid results of the sp. gr. 1·780, and in this state of
dilution it boils at 435°, and freezes sooner than water;
a knowledge of this curious fact suggests to the pru‑
dent chemist an important precaution; Mr. Parkes,
in his Chemical Essays, vol. ii. relates the occurrence
of a terrible accident which happened in consequence
of this circumstance not having been attended to ;—
" Carboy after carboy burst by the expansion of the
acid in the act of freezing, and had not the packed
carboys that remained been immediately immersed in
tepid water, not a single one would have escaped the
general wreck."
ADULTERATIONS. The ordinary acid of the shops
contains in general 3 or 4 per cent of saline matter,

which consists of about two-thirds of sulphate of potass,
and one-third of sulphate of lead. Dr. Ure observes,
that even more is occasionally found, in consequence
of the employment of nitre, to remove the brown colour given to the acid by carbonaceous matter; the
amount of adulterations, he observes, may be readily
determined by evaporating a definite weight of the
acid in a small capsule of platinum; these impurities
however in a medical point are immaterial; since they
are at once separated by dilution, but in a commercial
sense they deserve attention, as their presence considerably encreases the specific gravity of the acid;
indeed Dr. Ure is of opinion that genuine commercial
acid should never exceed 1·8485, and that any density
beyond this is the effect of saline contamination.
(*Journal of Science and the Arts, No. 7.*)

ACIDUM SULPHURICUM DILUTUM. L.E.D.
Dilute Sulphuric Acid.

By the dilution of this acid two objects are accomplished,—the acid is purified, and its dose more easily
apportioned. It is a circumstance of regret that the
strength of this preparation should so materially vary
in the different Pharmacopœias, as the annexed table
will exhibit.

Pharm:	Proportions by weight		Proportions by measure		Relative Strength & Dose	Specific Gravity
	Acid	Water	Acid	Water	Minims.	
P.L. 1810.	1	5½	1	9½	10	1·110
E.D.	1	7	1	12½	13	1·090
P.L. 1787.	1	8	1	14½	15	1·070

After the acid is diluted, the sediment should be carefully removed; the water employed for the purpose ought to be distilled, for, although it should be in its purest natural state, it will nevertheless contain impregnations capable of affecting the acid. Uses. In addition to the antiseptic and refrigerant virtues which it possesses, in common with the other mineral acids, it has astringent properties which render it a most valuable medicine, especially in weakness and relaxation of the digestive organs, in colliquative sweats, and in internal hæmorragy; on the same account, when sufficiently dilute, it has been successfully used as a collyrium, in the atonic stages of ophthalmia, and as an injection in protracted gonorrhæa. Dose m x to xl. To prevent it from injuring the enamel of the teeth it may be sucked through a quill, and the mouth should be carefully washed after each dose. *See Form.* 95. OFFICINAL PREPARATIONS. *Acidum Sulphuricum Aromaticum.** E. *Infusum Rosæ.* L.

ADEPS PRÆPARATA. L. ADEPS SUI SCROFÆ, *vulgo* Axungia Porcina. E. ADEPS SUILLUS PRÆ-PARATUS. D.

Prepared Hog's Lard. Fat.

QUALITIES. *Consistence* soft, or nearly semifluid. *Odour and Taste* none; at 97° it melts. CHEMICAL COMPOSITION. It is a very pure animal fat, the ultimate elements of which are oxygen, hydrogen, and carbon, in unknown proportions. SOLUBILITY. It is insoluble in water, and alcohol: with the alkalies

---

* *Elixir of Vitriol.* The Preparation sold under this name is the *Acid: Sulph: Aromat: E* and is imperfectly Ætherial in its nature. It is a grateful medicine A spurious article is often sold under this name, which is nothing but the diluted acid, coloured by the addition of a tincture.

it unites, and forms soaps. INCOMPATIBLE SUB-
STANCES. *Extracts, Spirituous Preparations, Tinctures,*
and *Infusions,* are incapable of uniting perfectly with
lard, without some intermedium; the following substances, on the contrary, are capable of contracting
with it a most intimate union. 1. *All dry powders,*
whether of a vegetable or mineral nature. 2. *Fixed
and Volatile Oils.* 3. *Balsams.* 4. *Camphor.* 5.
Soaps. It is principally employed in the formation
of ointments, plasters, and liniments.

ÆRUGO. L.D. $\left(\begin{array}{c}\text{Sub-acetas Cupri}\\ \textit{Impura}\end{array}\right)$ SUB-ACETIS
CUPRI. E.

Verdigris.

QUALITIES. *Form* a dry mass composed of minute
crystals, not deliquescent; *Colour* bluish-green. CHE-
MICAL COMPOSITION. Several constituents enter into
its composition, viz. Acetate and sub-acetate of copper, carbonate of copper, and copper, partly metallic,
and partly oxidized; it contains also the stalks of
grapes and other extraneous substances. SOLUBILITY.
Boiling water dissolves it in part, and produces in it
a chemical change, by transforming one portion of the
sub-acetate into the soluble acetate, and another into
an oxyd of copper, which is precipitated; with cold
water this substance demeans itself differently, the
acetate is dissolved by it, whilst that portion which is
in the state of *sub* salt remains suspended in the form
of a fine green powder. Vinegar converts all the
Ærugo into a soluble acetate, this liquid ought therefore never to be employed for favouring vomiting in
cases where an overdose has been swallowed, for the
reasons stated in the *Introductory Essay, page 4.*
Sulphuric acid poured on powdered *verdegris* decom-

poses it with effervescence, and vapours of acetic acid are disengaged. It appears from the experiments and observations of Duval and Orfila, that sugar exercises a chemical action on it, by which its solubility is diminished, and that on this account it acts as a specific against its poisonous effects　Uses　It is so uncertain and violent in its operation that it is rarely employed, except externally, * when it acts as a powerful detergent, and mild escharotic; and, in the form of ointment, is a valuable application for many cutaneous affections, especially the aggravated kinds of Tetter. OFFICINAL PREPARATIONS. *Ærugo Præparata*, D　*Linimentum Æruginis.* L.D.

ÆTHER SULPHURICUS RECTIFICATUS. L.

Rectified Sulphuric Æther.

QUALITIES. A colourless liquid of sp: gr: 739. *Odour* pungent and fragrant; it is highly volatile, and when perfectly free from alcohol it boils at 98°; it is extremely inflammable, a circumstance which should be remembered when it is poured from one vessel to another by candle light. CHEMICAL COMPOSITION. When pure, it consists of oxygen, hydrogen, and carbon; the rectified ether however still contains some water and alcohol, as Lovitz obtained an ether of ·632. SOLUBILITY. One part requires for its solution ten of water; with alcohol and ammonia it unites in every proportion. SOLVENT POWERS. It is one of the most powerful solvents known in vegetable chemistry, as it dissolves balsams, resins, gum-resins, wax, camphor,

---

* DR. SMFLLOME's OINTMENT FOR THE EYES. It consists of half a drachm of Verdegris finely powdered and rubbed with oil, and then mixed with an ounce of yellow Basilicon, *Ceratum Resinæ*, P.L.

extractive, &c.; it takes up about a twentieth of its weight of sulphur, but it exerts no solvent power upon the fixed alkalies. FORMS OF EXHIBITION. In any liquid vehicle, if in decoctions or infusions, they should be previously cooled. *See Formula* 108, 110, 111. MEDICAL USES. It is highly valuable as a diffusible stimulant, narcotic, and antispasmodic. DOSE. fȝss to fȝij, which, in order to produce the full effect of the remedy, must be repeated at short intervals. Ether independent of such virtues, has another valuable property consequent upon its rapid evaporation, that of producing cold and dryness; it is therefore when externally applied, and allowed to evaporate, a most powerful refrigerant, and has proved valuable in scalds or burns, in facilitating the reduction of strangulated hernia, and in diminishing excessive circulation in the brain; if however it be so confined, that its rapid evaporation is prevented, a very opposite effect is produced, and it proves stimulant, rubefacient, and even vesicatory. With regard to the other property incidental to it, that of producing dryness, I am not aware that it has hitherto been applied to any pharmaceutical purpose; the factmay be satisfactorily shewn by a very simple experiment, by rincing with ether a phial, to the interior of which drops of water obstinately adhere, and then exposing it to a current of air, it will be completely dry in a few minutes. It may be noticed in this place that a mixture of sulphuric and muriatic ethers evaporates instantaneously, and produces a degree of cold considerably below 0 of Farenheit. ADULTERATIONS and IMPURITIES. Its specific gravity affords the best indication of its purity; *Sulphuric acid* may be detected by a precipitation on the addition of a solution of barytes, and by its reddening the colour of litmus; *Alcohol*, by its forming

with phosphorus a milky instead of a limpid solution
M. Gay Lussac has observed that when kept for a
considerable time, without disturbance, it undergoes
spontaneous decomposition, and that acetic acid, perhaps some alcohol, and a particular oil, are produced
from it.

ALCOHOL. L.D. *Alcohol, Ardent Spirit.*

Qualities. A transparent, and colourless liquid
of the specific gravity ·815.; it does not become solid
by any known diminution of temperature; it boils
at 176°. and if water be added, its boiling point is
proportionably raised; hence, says Dr. Henry, the
temperature at which it boils is not a bad test of its
strength; it is combustible, and burns with a blue
flame, leaving no residue. Chemical Composition.
Alcohol, in a state of complete purity, consists of carbon, hydrogen, and oxygen, in proportions not hitherto
determined with accuracy; this preparation however
contains 7 per cent of water; Lovitz and Saussure succeeded in obtaining it at a specific gravity of ·791,
which may be considered as nearly pure. Alcohol
unites chemically with water; and caloric is evolved
during this union; the quantity of alcohol and water
in mixtures of different specific gravities, may be
learned from Mr. Gilpin's tables, *Philosophical Transactions*, 1794, or *Nicholson's Journal*, 4to. *vol.* 1.
The Edinburgh Pharmacopœia has no process for the
preparation of alcohol, but it most incorrectly assigns
the title to that which is the " Rectified Spirit " of
the other Colleges. Solvent Powers. Alcohol
dissolves soap; vegetable extract; sugar; oxalic,
camphoric, tartaric, gallic, and benzoic acids; volatile
oils; resins, and balsams; it combines also with sul-

phur, and the pure fixed alkalies, but not with their carbonates : for its other habitudes, and applications, see *Spiritus Rectificatus.*

ALLII RADIX. L.E.D.   Allium Sativum.

Garlic.

QUALITIES. This bulbous root has, when recent, a fœtid smell, and acrid taste, which are extracted by watery infusion ; by decoction they are nearly lost; by expression, the root furnishes almost one-fourth of its weight of a limpid juice, and by distillation, an odorous acrid essential oil is procured, and the exist-ence of sulphur may be detected. Garlic has a con-siderable analogy to squill, and onion, and like them, exerts a diuretic, diaphoretic, expectorant, and stimu-lant operation ; it is however but rarely used in mo-dern practice, as it possesses no superiority over re-medies less nauseous and objectionable ; the bruised root, externally applied, is highly stimulant, and ru-befacient. OFFICINAL PREPARATION. *Syrupus Allii.* D.

ALOES EXTRACTUM. *Aloes.*

There are three species met with in the shops, viz.

1. ALöE SPICATA. L. Socotorina, D. ⎰ Socotorine Aloes
   PERFOLIATA. E.   ⎱ Cape Aloes

2. ALöE VULGARIS. L. Hepatica. E.D. ⎰ Common or
                                       ⎱ Barbadoes Aloes

3. ALöE CABALINA. Fetid, Cabaline, ⎰ Employed only
   or Horse Aloes.   ⎱ by Farriers

QUALITIES. The above varieties of aloes differ in their purity, and likewise in their sensible qualities; the *Socotorine* is the purest, it is in sma l pieces of a reddis brown colour; the *Barbadoes* is in large masses, of a lighter colour, and having an odour much stronger and less pleasant; the *Cabaline* is still more impure, and less powerful. All the kinds are characterized by an intensely bitter taste, which in the *Socotorine*, is accompanied by an aromatic flavour. CHEMICAL COMPOSITION. In this there appears to be some obscurity; M. Braconnot *(Ann. Chim. tom. 68.)* conceives it to be a substance, *sui generis*, which he terms " *bitter resin*," whilst others regard it as composed of resin, gum, and extractive, the proportions of which are supposed to vary in the different species, but that their peculiar virtues reside in the extractive part. SOLUBILITY. It is to the slowness with which aloes undergoes solution in the *primæ viæ*, that it is indebted for the medicinal properties which distinguish this substance; by boiling water it is dissolved, but on cooling a precipitation ensues, and by long decoction, it becomes quite inert; weak acids dissolve it more abundantly than water, but proof spirit is the most perfect solvent : its solubility is increased by the addition of alkaline salts, and soaps, but by such a combination aloes undergoes a material change in its medicinal properties; the bitterness is diminished, its purgative effects impaired, and it ceases to operate specifically upon the large intestines, a fact so far valuable, as it enables us, in certain cases, to obviate its irritating action upon the rectum. MEDICAL USE. Aloes is a bitter stimulating purgative, emptying the large intestines, without making the stools thin; it likewise warms the habit, quickens the circulation, and promotes the uterine and hemorrhoidal fluxes. DOSE

g. v. to xv. No greater effect is produced by a large dose than from one comparatively moderate. FORMS OF EXHIBITION. The form of pill should be preferred on account of its extreme bitterness, as well as being, for the reasons above mentioned, the one most likely to fulfil the intention of its exhibition, for in addition to what has been stated (*Introductory Essay*, *page 20*) on the important influence of solubility, it may be here observed that since aloes does not undergo solution in the stomach, it is admirably adapted for the basis of remedies intended to obviate constitutional costiveness, for in our endeavours to supply the deficiencies of nature by the resources of art, we should at least attempt to imitate the modes of her operation; the natural stimulus of the intestines, the bile, is poured into them below the stomach, and whenever it regurgitates into that organ it produces disease; so it happens with our cathartic medicines, unless we so modify their solubility, that their operation cannot commence until after their passage through the stomach, we shall find that we only encrease the evil we are endeavouring to obviate, and that in addition to the torpor of the intestinal canal we shall induce the stomach to participate in the disease, or excite a morbid fretfulness in that organ, which will be attended with the most distressing symptoms.* *See Formulæ* 16, 17,

* ANDERSON'S PILLS consist of Aloes with a proportion of Jalap, and Oil of Aniseed

HOOPER'S PILLS.—Pil Aloës cum Myrrha (*Pil. Rufi*) Sulphate of Iron, and Canella Bark.

DIXON'S ANTIBILIOUS PILLS.—Aloes, Scammony, Rhubarb, and Tartarized Antimony.

SPEEDIMAN'S PILLS.—Aloes, Myrrh, Rhubarb, Extract of Camomile, and some Essential Oil of Camomile.

DINNER PILLS—LADY WEBSTER'S, or LADY CRESPIGNY'S PILL.— These popular Pills are the " *Pilulæ Stomachicæ*," vulgo, " *Pilulæ ante*

18. Aloes in combination with assafœtida, furnishes an eligible purgative in the dyspepsia of old persons. OFFICINAL PREPARATIONS. *Pulv: Aloes comp:* L. *Pil: Alöes cum Myrrha.* L.E.D. *Pil: Alöes comp. Pil: Alöes cum Assafœtida.* E. *Pil: Alöes cum Colo-cynthide.* E. *Pil: Cambogiœ comp: (a.h?)* L. *Pil: Rhei comp: (d)* E. *Pil: Scammon: cum Aloe.* D. *Decoctum Aloes comp:* L. *Extractum Alöes purificatum.* L.D. *Extractum Colocyntyidis comp:* L.D *Tinct. Alöes.* L.E.D. *Tinct: Alöes comp:* L.E.D *Tinct: Alöes Ætherea.* E. *Tinct: Benzoin: comp: (d)* L.E.D. *Tinct: Rhei et Aloes.* E. *Vinum Alöes.* L.E.D. ADULTERATIONS. It is frequently adulterated with common resin, but the fraud more generally committed is that of mixing with, or substituting the inferior species for the *Socotorine,* but the *Barbadoes Aloes* may, independent of its want of aromatic flavour, be distinguished from the *Socotorine* by a simple test, for the latter dissolves entirely in boiling water, and alcohol, whereas the former, when treated in a similar manner, leaves a considerable residue ; sometimes the *Horse Aloes* is made to appear so bright and pure, as not to be easily distinguished by the eye even from the *Socotorine,* but its rank odour, of which no art can divest it, will readily betray the fraud.

cibum " of the Codex Medicamentarius Parisiensis. Editio Quinta A.D. 1758. *viz.* ℞ Aloes optimæ ℨvj, Mastiches, et Rosarum rubrarum āā ℨij, Syrupi de Absinthio q, s, ut fiat massa, — the mass is divided into Pills of 3 grains each. The operation of this Pill is to produce a copious and bulky evacuation, and in this respect, experience has fully established its value. It is difficult to explain the *modus operandi* of the *Mastiche,* unless we suppose that it depends upon its dividing the particles of the Aloes, and thereby modifying its solubility.

ALUMEN. (*Super-sulphas Aluminæ*) Sulphas
         (*et Potassæ.*   ) Aluminæ E.

Alumen. D.   *Alum.*

QUALITIES. *Form* octohedral crystals, whose
sides are equilateral triangles; they are slightly efflorescent. *Taste,* sweet, rough, and acidulous. CHE-
MICAL COMPOSITION. It is a triple, or sometimes a
quadruple salt, with excess of acid, consisting of sulphuric acid and alumina, with potass, or ammonia, or
frequently both of them; the nature of the alkali
however does not in the least appear to affect the properties of alum. SOLUBILITY. A fluidounce of cold
water dissolves 30 grains, but if boiling four drachms;
it is insoluble in alcohol. INCOMPATIBLE SUB-
STANCES. *Alkalies* and *alkaline salts,* after neutralizing the excess of acid, precipitate the alumine. It
is also decomposed by *carbonate* and *muriate of ammonia, carbonate of magnesia,* and *tartrate of potass,
lime water, superacetate of lead,* and *the salts of mercury,* as well as by many vegetable and animal substances, especially *galls* and *kino.* It is on this account very injudicious to combine alum with any
vegetable astringent with a view to encrease its
virtues, thus the " *Pulvis Sulphatis Aluminæ compositus* " of the Edinburgh college, is less powerful
than any of the ingredients of which it is composed;
and the addition of alum to the decoction of bark,
undoubtedly diminishes its efficacy as an astringent
injection. MEDICAL USES. Alum is internally a
powerful astringent, in hæmorrhages and inordinate
fluxes, and is externally useful for repellent and astringent lotions, and collyria. DOSE, gr. x; in large
doses it is liable to excite nausea, and to constipate
the bowels. FORMS OF EXHIBITION. In solution,

or in substance, made into pills with extract; it is sometimes given with advantage in the form of whey (*Alum-whey. Serum Aluminosum*) made by boiling ℥ij in a pint of milk, and then straining, the dose of which is a wine glass full. By briskly agitating a drachm of alum with the white of an egg, a coagulum is formed (*Alum curd*) which is serviceable in some species of ophthalmia, when applied between two pieces of thin linen rag. As alum is not decomposed by sulphate of lime, hard water may be safely used for its solution. Alum has the effect of retarding, and in some instances of preventing, the acetous fermentation in vegetables, thus when added to common *paste* it prevents its becoming sour ; animal substances, as *glue*, are preserved by it in a similar manner. It has also the property of clearing turbid water, wine, and spirituous liquors, for which purpose it is extensively employed. OFFICINAL PREPARATIONS. *Liquor Alum : co.* L. *Pulv : Alum : co.* E.

ALUMEN EXSICCATUM, L. Ustum. D. *Dried Alum.* By the action of heat alum undergoes watery fusion, yields its water of crystallization, and loses more than one third of its weight; if the heat be too intense, or long continued, it is deprived of a great part of its acid. It has been recommended, in doses of a scruple, in cholic, when it has been said to operate gently upon the bowels, and to relieve the pain; I have myself experienced this good effect when the cholic has been produced by the action of lead : the preparation however is principally used as an external application, having a degree of escharotic power, but it should be remembered that, as it owes such power to an excess of acid, unless it be carefully prepared, it must be inefficient. It ought to redden syrup of violets.

ALUMEN RUPEUM. *Roche* or *Rock Alum.* This variety was originally brought from Roccha, formerly called Edessa, in Syria, in fragments about the size of an almond, covered with an efflorescence of a pale rose colour; that however which is now sold under this name is common English alum, artificially coloured. It is unimportant.

ALUMEN ROMANUM. *Roman Alum*, is in irregular octohedral masses, powdery on the surface it is the purest kind, and contains no ammonia in its composition.

AMMONIACUM. L.E.D. (*Heracleum Gummiferum*)
Ammoniac.

QUALITIES. *Form*, Masses composed of fragments, or tears, yellow on the surface, and white within; *Taste*, a nauseous sweet, followed by a bitter flavour; *Odour*, faint but not unpleasant. CHEMICAL COMPOSITION. Gum-resin, gluten, and some volatile matter. SOLUBILITY; it is partly soluble in water, vinegar, alcohol, æther, and the solutions of the alkalies; when triturated with water a milky liquor is formed, which is a solution of gum holding the resin in suspension, and if the yolk of an egg be employed the mixture is more permanent; water appears to be its proper solvent. USES. Stimulant, antispasmodic, and expectorant : in large doses gently purgative and sometimes diuretic; after the exhibition of smart purgatives, in combination with rhubarb, it proves valuable in mesenteric affections b correcting the viscid secretion of the intestines. FORMS OF EXHIBITION. In solution, see *Mist: Ammoniac*, and in pills with bitter extracts, myrrh, and other gum-resins; if rubbed with camphor a mass is at once produced very

suitable for pills; vinegar renders it soft, and adapt
it for plasters (*Form:* 104). Dose, grs. x to xxx.
Officinal Preparations. *Mist: Ammoniac:* L.D.
Pil: Scillœ co: L.E. *(a.)   Emplast: Ammoniac.* L.
Emplast: Gummos: E.   *Emplast: Ammoniac: cum
Hydrargyro.* L.   Adulterations. Two varieties
are met with in the market, that in tears, *guttœ ammoniaci*, which ought to be white, clear, and dry; and
that in lumps, *lapis ammoniaci*, which sells for one
third the price of the former, being very impure, and
generally adulterated with common resin, from which
it may be purified by softening the mass in a bladder
which is immersed in boiling water, and straining it
while fluid.

AMMONIÆ SUBCARBONAS. L.   Carbonas
Ammoniæ. E.D.
Sub-Carbonate of Ammonia.

Qualities. *Form,* white, semi-transparent masses,
which on exposure to air effloresce; *Odour,* pungent
and peculiar; *Taste,* acrid but cooling.   Chemical
Composition It will be found to vary materially in
its composition according to the temperature employed
for its preparation; the quantity of alkali varying
from 20 to 50 per cent.   Mr. Phillips states that this
salt, as usually prepared, contains about half its weight
of carbonic acid, and that its composition may be expressed as follows, carbonic acid 50, ammonia 39,
water 11.   Solubility   According to Duncan it is
soluble in twice its weight of cold water; Mr. Phillips
states four times; the mean of these will be found
nearly correct.   Its solubility however is increased
by increase of temperature, but when dissolved in

boiling water it effervesces, and undergoes a partial decomposition; it is quite insoluble in alcohol, and hence on the addition of spirit to a strong solution a dense coagulum is produced. INCOMPATIBLE SUBSTANCES. It is decomposed by *acids, fixed alkalies* and their *carbonates, lime, magnesia, alum, supertartrate of potass,* and all the *acidulous salts, sulphate of magnesia, acetate, sub-muriate,* and *oxy-muriate of mercury, super-acetate of lead, tartarized iron,* and the *sulphates of iron and zinc.* If it be added to decoctions and infusions they must be previously cooled. FORMS OF EXHIBITION. Since by exposure to air its virtues are impaired, it ought not to be kept in powdered mixtures; in the form of pill it is preserved much longer, especially if it be combined with some vegetable extract. USES. It is stimulant, antispasmodic, diaphoretic, powerfully antacid, exceeding in this respect the fixed alkalies, and in large doses it is emetic; It is also useful in syncope and hysteria, as *smelling salts,* and for making saline draughts, see *Acid: Citricum:* DOSE, grs. v to ℈j; to produce emesis, 3ss. See *Form.* 20, 101, 102. OFFICINAL PREPARATIONS. *Liquor Ammoniæ sub-carbonatis,* L. *Liquor Ammoniæ acetatis,* (f) L. E.D. *Cuprum Ammoniatum,* (f) L.E.D. ADULTERATIONS. This salt ought to be entirely volatilized by heat; if any thing remain it may be considered impure; it ought also to be free from all fetor; should this not be the case it may be corrected by subliming it in conjunction with powdered charcoal; there is at present a large quantity of this impure article in the market, which has been manufactured from the residue sold by the gas light companies. When long exposed to the air, the excess of ammonia, upon which its odour depends, escapes, and an inodorous neutral carbonate remains.

AMMONIÆ MURIAS. L. E. Sal Ammoniacum. D. vulgo, *Sal Ammoniac.*

QUALITIES. *Form,* dense, striated concavo-convex cakes, which arc persistent in the air ; or crystallized conical masses ; in this latter form it generally contains other salts, especially muriate of lime, which render it deliquescent. *Taste* bitter, acrid, and cool. CHEMICAL COMPOSITION. In consequence of the present unsettled opinions respecting the nature of muriatic acid, and ammonia, and the changes which they undergo by combination with each other, the composition of this salt is involved in much obscurity. According to Dr. Thomson, it consists of equal volumes of muriatic acid gas and ammoniacal gas, although he has subsequently observed that from the peculiar properties of the substance, it may be a compound of *Chlorine* and *Ammonium* (the hypothetical base of ammonia). Unlike all the other ammoniacal salts, it does not undergo decomposition by heat. SOLUBILITY. f℥ j of water at 60° dissolves about two drachms and a half; at 212°, it dissolves its own weight ; it is also soluble in $4\frac{1}{2}$ parts of alcohol; its solution in water is accompanied by considerable reduction of temperature. INCOMPATIBLE SUBSTANCES. The sulphuric and nitric acids unite with the ammonia, and disengage the muriatic acid, whilst ammonia is disengaged by the action of potass and its carbonate, carbonate of soda, lime, magnesia, &c. which combine with its muriatic acid ; with oxymuriate of mercury it combines and encreases its solubility, see *Hydrarg: Oxy-murias.* When united with super-acetate of lead, it decomposes it, and a muriate of lead is precipitated. It is obvious also that nitrate of silver, and all the metallic salts whose bases form insoluble compounds with muriatjc acid, are incompatible with it. Uses, rarely employed as an internal remedy, externally it is employed in lotions, either for the cold produced during its solution, in which case it should be applied as soon as the salt is dissolved, or for the stimulus of the salt, on which principle it acts as a powerful discutient in indolent tumours (*Form.* 86). It also constitutes an ingredient in a very useful plaster, in which it undergoes chemical decomposition ; this plaster consists of *Soap* ℥j, *lead plaster,* ℥ij, liquify them together, and add of *muriate of ammonia* ℈ss. The alkali of the soap enters into combination with the muriatic acid of the muriate of ammonia, and forms thereby muriate of potass, or soda, and ammoniacal gas (on which the virtue of the plaster depends) is slowly but abundantly liberated, acting as a powerful stimulant and rubefacient ; it should be applied immediately after it is formed, and be renewed every twenty-four hours, otherwise the intention is lost. (*Pharmacopœia Chirurgica.*) I have often applied this plaster with evident advantage to the chest in pulmonary affections, and I wish to recommend it to the attention of practitioners. Officinal Preparations. *Ammoniæ Sub-carbonas* (g.) L.E.D. *Liquor : Ammoniæ* (g). L. *Aqua Ammoniæ.* E.D. *Hydrarg : præcip: alb :* (f.) L. *Alcohol ammoniatum,* (g.) E.D. *Ferrum Ammoniat :* (f). L.E.D. Adulterations. This salt, if pure, may be entirely volatilized by a low heat ; the *sulphate of ammonia* however, as it is also volatile, cannot be discovered except by the muriate of barytes, which will indicate its presence by a copious precipitate.

AMYGDALÆ DULCES. ⎰ Varieties of ⎱ Sweet &
                  ⎱ "Amygdalus ⎰ Bitter
AMYGDALÆ AMARÆ. ⎰ Communis." ⎱ Almonds

QUALITIES The *sweet almond* is inodorous, and
has a sweet, bland taste; the *bitter almond*, when
triturated with water, has the odour of the peach, and
a pleasant bitter flavour. CHEMICAL COMPOSITION.
Boullay has lately confirmed the analogy which Proust
had stated to exist between the emulsion of sweet
almonds and human milk, viz. the former consists of
sweet oil 54, albumen 24, sugar 6, gum 3, with traces
of acetic acid; the indigestible property of the almond
depends upon its albuminous matter. The *bitter
almond* in addition to those constituents, contains
hydro-cyanic acid, (Prussic acid), and a peculiar volatile oil, upon which its narcotic properties depend,
but these deleterious elements are so modified by the
natural state of combination in which they exist with
sweet oil and albumen, that they may be eaten without inconvenience. Both sorts of almonds yield by
expression a large quantity of fixed oil, which is perfectly mild. See *Oleum Amygdal.* The water distilled from the bitter almond, when strongly impregnated, has been found to exert a deleterious action on
the human body, and to prove fatal to many animals.
The leaves of the peach tree, the pips of apples, and
the kernels of fruit, all contain hydro-cyanic acid,
but the vegetable most efficient on account of its presence, is the *cherry laurel*, the distilled water and oil
of which, is the most destructive of all narcotic poisons.
See *Orfila on Poisons.* Consistent with theory, the
watery extract of laurel is harmless, a fact easily explained, since the narcotic acid is entirely volatilized
before the fluid can assume the consistence of an extract. To counteract the poisonous effects of prussic

acid, Orfila recommends, after full vomiting has been
excited, the exhibition of three or four spoonsfull of
oil of turpentine, in the infusion of coffee, at intervals
of half an hour. M. Virey conceives that sulphate of
iron in solution is the best antidote, he having observed that the salt restored a cow that was nearly
killed by the essential oil of bitter almonds. M. Majendie has lately published some essays on the use of
prussic acid in pulmonary consumption ; there is
however nothing new in its application in such cases,
for Linnæus informs us that distilled laurel water
was frequently used in Holland in pulmonary consumption. *(Amœnitat: Academ: vol.* 4, *p.* 40.) SOLU-
BILITY. By trituration with water a milky mixture
is produced, *(an emulsion),* for which purpose the
sweet almonds should be previously freed from their
cuticle, *(blanched),* and this ought to be performed
by infusing them in tepid water, for when hot it
separates a portion of their oil, as is evident from
their being thus rendered yellow, and the emulsion
is therefore more liable to ferment, and be decomposed. ʒij of almonds saturate about fℨvj of water ;
since however this extemporaneous preparation is te-
dious and inconvenient, the London Pharmacopœia
very judiciously directs a confection to be ready prepared, ʒj of which, when triturated with fℨj of water,
immediately forms an elegant emulsion, *See Mistura
Amygdal.* Almonds form a useful intermedium for
suspending in water many substances, which are of
themselves not miscible with it, as camphor, and several of the gum-resins ; they also assist in the pulverization of refractory substances, as ipecacuan, &c.
OFFICINAL PREPARATIONS. *Confectio Amygdalarum.* L. *Emulsio Camphorœ* (i) E. *Emulsio Acaciæ
Arab:* E.D. AMYGDALÆ PLACENTA. *Almond Cake*

is the substance left after the expression of the oil, which, when ground, forms ALMOND POWDER, so generally used for washing the hands.

AMYLUM. L.E.D. $\left(\begin{array}{c}\text{Triticum Hybernum}\\ \text{Amylum.}\end{array}\right)$ Starch.

QUALITIES. *Form,* white columnar masses ; *Odour* and *Taste,* none. CHEMICAL COMPOSITION. Fecula is one of the proximate principles of vegetable matter, and *Starch* is the fecula of wheat.* SOLUBILITY. It is soluble in boiling water, forming with it a semi-transparent, insipid, inodorous and gelatinous paste, very susceptible of mouldiness, but which is retarded by the addition of alum ; it is insoluble, but falls to powder in coll water; nor is it dissolved by alcohol or ether; although potass dissolves starch, yet the solution of it is not disturbed by potass, carbonate of potass, nor ammonia, but an alcoholic solution of potass produces a precipitate ; acetate of lead, and infusion of galls occasion also precipitates. USES. As a demulcent it is generally employed as a vehicle for the exhibition of opium in the form of enema. The ordinary blue starch is coloured by a solution of smalt

* The fecula of various grains is employed as articles of diet for th. sick, e. g. SAGO, prepared from the pith of the *Cycas Circinalis,* its granular form is imparted to it by passing it, when half dry, through a coarse sieve. SALO , from the *Orchis Mascula.* TAPIOCA from the root of the *Jatropa Manihot.* By expressing the root of this plant, the juice of which is extremely acrid, and baking the cake that is left, an alimentary substance is prepared called CASSAVA, the peculiar merit of which, like tapioca, is to swell and soften in water, and thus to form an excellent pudding. ARROW ROOT from the *Maranta Arundinacea.* The arrow root however, usually sold, is the fecula of potatoes, 100 lbs. of which will yield about 10 lbs. of fecula, and it is worthy of remark that for this purpose frozen potatoes answer as well as those not poiled by the frost.

and alum, and is unfit for medicinal use; formerly it
was tinged yellow with saffron or turmeric, but this
went out of fashion on the execution of the famous
midwife Mrs. Collier, who was hanged in a ruff
starched with that colour. (*Gray's Supplement.*)—OF-
FICINAL PREPARATIONS. *Mucilago Amyli.* L.E.D.
Pulvis Tragacanth : comp : (a) L. *Pil: Hydrargyri
(k)* E. *Trochisci Gummos :* E.

It has been lately ascertained that *Iodine* is a delicate test of the presence of starch; if a drop or two
of a solution of this substance in alcohol be added to
an aqueous solution of starch, a blue compound is
formed which eventually precipitates. Iodine may
therefore be employed for ascertaining the goodness
of starch, a test which is very important, for much of
what is sold under the name of starch, does not possess its peculiar characters.

ANETHI SEMINA. L.E. (*Anethum Graveolens*
                       Semina.)
                 Dill Seed.

These seeds when dry have an aromatic sweetish
odour, and a warm pungent taste, qualities which
reside in an essential oil, and which is extracted
by distillation with water and by digestion with alcohol; the bruised seeds yield their flavour to boiling
water by simple infusion. The seeds are but rarely
used; the distilled water is a valuable carminative for
children.

ANISI SEMINA. L.E.D. (*Pimpinella Anisum*)
                        (*Semina.*)

Anise Seeds.

Like the dill seeds, warm and carminative; water
extracts very little of their flavour; rectified spirit
the whole. It may be remarked in this place that the
value of aniseed, as well as all those seeds which yield
essential oil by distillation, may be estimated by their
specific gravity, the heaviest yielding the largest proportion of oil: a chondrometer employed by corn-
chandlers might be very conveniently applied to such
a purpose. The seeds imported from Spain, which
are smaller than the others, contain most oil, and are
to be preferred.

ANTHEMIDIS FLORES. L.E. (*Anthemis Nobilis.*)

Chamomili Flores. *Chamomile Flowers.*

QUALITIES. The odour of the flowers is strong
and fragrant; *Taste* bitter and aromatic, with a slight
degree of warmth. CHEMICAL COMPOSITION. The
active principles are essential oil, resin. and bitter extractive. SOLUBILITY. Both water and alcohol take
up the active parts of the flowers; hot water, by infusion, dissolves nearly one fourth of their weight,
but boiling dissipates the essential oil, on which account they should never form an ingredient in a decoction. USES. The flowers given in substance are
said to have cured intermittents; they are however
but rarely used; externally they are applied in fo-
mentations. See *Infusum Anthemidis.* OFFICINAL
PREPARATIONS. *Decoctum Anthemidis nobilis.* E.D.
Infusum Anthemidis. L. *Extractum Anthemidis,* L.E.

Oleum Anthemidis. L. * There is a great variety in
the quality and price of chamomile flowers, those
which are large and whitish are to be preferred as the
freshest; by keeping they become invalid, and are
deprived of their aromatic principle, and essential oil.
They are always inferior in wet seasons. The double
flowered varieties are also less powerful than the
single kind, since the qualities reside in the disc florets.

ANTIMONII OXYDUM. L.
Oxide of Antimony.

This substance differs as well in medicinal influence,
as in chemical composition, from that which was designated by the same name in the former pharmacopæia
of London, and is a much more dangerous and violent
preparation. Mr. Phillips has justly observed that
the activity of the oxides of Antimony is diminished in
proportion to the quantity of oxygen which they contain; the present preparation is a *protoxide,* containing 20 per cent of oxygen. Since it has no claims on
account of its value as a remedy, or on that of its
utility for the preparation of other antimonial compounds, it might, and ought to be abandoned.

ANTIMONII SULPHURETUM. L.
Sulphuret of Antimony.

QUALITIES. This article appears in the market in
conical loaves, which are dark grey externally, but
possess, internally, a striated structure, and considerable brilliancy; the Edinburgh and Dublin colleges
direct this substance to be levigated with water, and

* CHAMOMILE DROPS. The nostrum sold under this name is a spirit
flavoured with the essential oil of Chamomile.

kept in the state of powder; it should however never
be purchased in that form, as it is not unfrequently
adulterated with sulphuret of lead, whereas it cannot
contain such admixture when its form is characteris-
tically crystalline and striated. CHEMICAL COMPO-
SITION. Antimony 100, Sulphur 35·572. From the
time of Basil Valentine to the present, this preparation
has been known in the market by the name of *Antimony*, a name which it is evident can only with propriety be applied to the pure metal. SOLUBILITY.
It is insoluble in water and alcohol ; since however it
is slightly acted upon by vegetable acids, cups were
formerly made of it, which imparted to wine that stood
in them for some time, an emetic quality. USES. It
is principally employed for the preparation of the other
antimonial combinations, for which purpose it is more
eligible than the metal itself, as being less contaminated with metallic impurities. Its medicinal energies depend altogether upon the state of the stomach,
and must therefore be extremely uncertain ; when it
meets with any acid in the stomach, it acts with
extreme violence, a circumstance which requires precaution. In times of remote antiquity it was used by
females as a black pigment, for staining the eye-lashes ;
it is at present given to horses, mixed with their food,
to make their coats smooth. OFFICINAL PREPARA-
TIONS. Dr. Black constructed a table representing a
view of all the preparations whose basis was antimony ;
many of these however have fallen into disuse, and the
nomenclature of all is changed. The following arrangement of the medicines prepared from the sulphuret of
antimony,* is presented to us by Mr. Thomson, in his

---

* The Sulphuret of Antimony is an ingredient in SPILSBURY's DROPS.
See *Hydrargyri Oxymurias.* Dr. Duncan also observes that it seems to
constitute a quack remedy which has acquired some reputation in Ireland for the cure of cancer, where it is used as an external application
to the sore.

London Dispensatory. 1. By TRITURATION, *Sulphuretum Antimonii Præparatum.* E.D. 2. By THE ACTION OF HEAT WITH PHOSPHATE OF LIME, (oxidized) *Pulvis Antimonialis.* L.D. *Oxidum Antimonii cum Phosphate Calcis.* E. 3. By THE ACTION OF ALKALIES, (oxidized), *Antimonii Sulphuretum Præcipitatum.* L.E. *Sulphur Antimoniatum Fuscum.* D. 4. By THE ACTION OF ACIDS, (oxidized), *Antimonii Oxydum.* L. *Oxydum Antimonii Nitro-muriaticum.* D. *Antimonium Tartarizatum.* L. *Tartris - Antimonii, Olim Tartarus Emeticus.* E. *Tartarum-Antimoniatum,* sive *Emeticum* D. *Liquor Antimonii Tartarizati.* L. *Vinum Tartritis Antimonii.* E.

ADULTERATIONS. The importance of employing this article in a state of great purity, for the preparation of so many active and valuable medicines, is obvious. It ought to be entirely volatalized by a red heat; *Lead* is discovered by its imparting to the antimony a foliated, instead of a striated texture, and from not being vaporizable; *Arsenic* by the garlic odour emitted when thrown upon live coals, or by the numerous tests mentioned under the history of that article; *Manganese* and *Iron,* from not being vaporizable, and from other tests.

ANTIMONII SULPHURETUM PRÆCIPITATUM. L.E.
Sulphur Antimoniatum Fuscum. D.
Precipitated Sulphuret of Antimony.

QUALITIES. *Form,* a brilliant orange coloured powder; *Taste,* slightly styptic, but inodorous. CHEMICAL COMPOSITION. Very complicated attractions are exerted during the preparation of this substance; the result of which is an hydro-sulphuret of Oxide of Antimony, with excess of sulphur. SOLUBILITY. It is quite insoluble in water. USES. According to the dose, it is diaphoretic, cathartic, or emetic; it is, however, less certain than many other preparations, and, unless in combination with mercury for cutaneous affections, is not very often employed. INCOMPATIBLE SUBSTANCES. All acids, and acidulous salts, encrease its emetic properties; when therefore acid is suspected to prevail in the primæ viæ, it should be combined with soap, magnesia, (*Form :* 64) or aromatic confection ; on the contrary, the confection of roses, and vehicles containing acids, should be carefully avoided. FORM OF EXHIBITION. Pills. DOSE, grs. I to V. OFFICINAL PREPARATIONS. *Pilula Hydrargyri Sub-Muriatis (e.)* L. ADULTERATIONS. It is often sophisticated with chalk, and other extraneous matter; it ought not to effervesce with acids, it should be entirely vaporizable by heat, and its colour should be bright orange.

ANTIMONIUM TARTARIZATUM. L. Tartris Antimonii E. Tartarum Antimoniatum. D.

Tartar Emetic.

QUALITIES. *Form,* crystals whose primitive form is the regular tetrahedron, although it assumes a variety of secondary forms. *Colour,* white. *Odour,* none. *Taste,* slightly styptic and metallic : on exposure to the air, the crystals slightly effloresce ; thrown upon burning coals, they become black, and afford metallic antimony. CHEMICAL COMPOSITION. This is involved in much doubt and obscurity ; it is stated

in the various dispensatories to be a triple salt, consisting of tartaric acid, oxide of antimony, and potass,
and which therefore, says Mr. Thomson, on the principles of the reformed nomenclature, ought to be
termed a *tartrate of antimony and potass.* The truth
of these views, however, is extremely questionable.
I am inclined to believe with Gay Lussac, that in the
various metalline compounds, of which supertartrate of
potass is an ingredient, this latter substance acts the
part of a simple acid, an opinion which receives much
support from the great solvent property of cream of
tartar, and from the striking fact, that it is even capable of dissolving various oxides which are insoluble in
tartaric acid, of which the protoxide of antimony is an
example. According then to this view, tartar emetic
is a salt composed of bi-tartrate *(super-tartrate)* of
potass, which acts the parts of an acid, and protoxide
of antimony: from the experiments of Mr. Phillips,
it would appear that 100 parts of the bi-tartrate will
dissolve 70 of the protoxide. In this state of doubt it
must be admitted that no name can be more appropriate than *Antimonium Tartarizatum.* SOLUBILITY.
Much discrepancy of opinion exists upon this subject,
owing probably to the variation and incidental impurities to which this salt is liable. Dr. Duncan, who
selected very pure specimens for examination, states
that it is soluble in three times its weight of water at
212°, and in fifteen at 60°. This solution, when the
salt is pure, is perfectly clear and transparent, but if
long kept, unless a considerable portion of spirit be
added, it undergoes decomposition; a precipitate
indeed sometimes takes place very rapidly, but this is
generally tartrate of lime, an incidental impurity,
derived from the super-tartrate of potass. INCOM-
PATIBLE SUBSTANCES. *Mineral Acids, Alkalies and*

their Carbonates, and many of the Metals, Soaps, Hydro-Sulphurets, and many infusions and decoctions of bitter and astringent Vegetables, e. g. f℥j. of the decoction of yellow bark is capable of completely decomposing ℈j of this salt, and of rendering it inert. Berthollet has accordingly recommended the immediate exhibition of this decoction when an overdose of the salt has been taken. Infusion and tincture of galls throw down curdled and inert precipitates of a dirty white colour, inclining to yellow. Rhubarb is equally incompatible. The extract of this substance therefore never ought to be employed in forming pills of tartar emetic. The *Alkaline Sulphates,* provided they be perfectly neutral, produce no disturbance in solutions of *tartar emetic,* and therefore cannot be considered incompatible with them; if there be any excess of acid, as in *alum, bi-sulphate of potass,* &c. then its decomposition is effected, and a white insoluble sulphate of antimony is precipitated. It appears therefore that the famous " Emeto-purgative" of the French school, consisting of sulphate of soda, and tartarized antimony in solution, is by no means the unchemical mixture which some have considered it to be, and that it really produces its effects from the operation of its original ingredients, and not from that of any new compounds, *(Sulphate of Antimony, Tartrate of Soda, and Sulphate of Potass)* which have been erroneously supposed to result. FORMS OF EXHIBITION. Solution is its best form, see *Liquor Antimonii Tartariz.* DOSE. It either vomits, purges, or sweats, according to the quantity exhibited, thus grs. ¼ will, if the skin be kept warm, promote a diaphoresis, gr. ½ will procure some stools first, and sweating afterwards, and gr. j will generally vomit and then purge, and lastly sweat the patient; in very

minute doses, as grs. $\frac{1}{10}$ or $\frac{1}{12}$ combined with squill
and ammoniacum, it acts as an expectorant, (see
Formula 1, 2, 3, 8, 60. It is decidedly the most manageable, and the least uncertain of all the antimonial
preparations, and the practitioner would probably
have but little to regret, were all the other combinations of this metal discarded from our pharmacopæias.
Tartar Emetic, when triturated with lard, in the proportion of ℥iss or ℥ij to ℥j of the latter, forms a very
powerful rubefacient, occasioning a pustular eruption
on the skin, and proving very serviceable in deep
seated inflammations. OFFICINAL PREPARATIONS.
grs. j is contained in f℥ss of *Liquor Antimonii Tart:*
L. and *Vinum Tartratis Antimonii.* E.* ADULTE-
RATIONS. It should be always purchased in its crystalline form; a solution of it, in distilled water, ought
to furnish a copious gold coloured precipitate, with
sulphuret of ammonia; a precipitate, soluble in nitric
acid, with acetate of lead; and a white, and extremely
thick precipitate, dissolving with facility in pure nitric
acid, with lime water. If the crystals deliquesce, the
presence of other salts may be inferred.

AQUA. Water.

Water, from its extensive powers as a solvent, never
occurs in a state of absolute purity, although the
nature, and degree of its contamination, must necessarily vary according to circumstances and situation.
It is generally found holding earthy matter in a state
of mechanical suspension, or saline, and other bodies
in chemical solution. The usual varieties of common
water are classed and defined by Celsus, and modern

* NORRIS's DROPS. A spirituous solution of Tartarized Antimony.

chemists have not found any reason to reject the arrangement. " *Aqua levissima pluvialis est ; deinde fontana, tum ex flumine, tum ex puteo ; posthœc ex nive, aut glacie ; gravior his ex lacu ; gravissima ex palude.*"

1. RAIN WATER. *Aqua Pulvialis*, when col‐ lected in the open fields, is certainly the purest natural water, and consequently of the least specific gravity ; the bodies which it holds in solution, are carbonic acid, a minute portion of carbonate of lime, with traces of muriate of lime.

2. SPRING WATER. *Aqua Fontana*, in addition to the substances detected in rain water, generally contains a small proportion of muriate of soda, and frequently other salts ; the larger springs are purer than smaller ones, and those which occur in primitive countries, and in siliceous rocks, or beds of gravel, necessarily contain the least impregnation. An im‐ portant practical distinction has been founded upon the fact, that the water of some springs dissolve soap, whilst that of others decompose, and curdle it ; the former has been termed *soft*, the latter *hard* water ; soft water is a more powerful solvent of all vegetable matters, and is consequently to be preferred for do‐ mestic, as well as medicinal purposes.

3. RIVER WATER. *Aqua ex Flumine*, being de‐ rived from the conflux of numerous springs and rain water, generally possesses considerable purity ; that the proportion of its saline ingredients should be small is easily explained by the precipitation which must necessarily take place from the union of different solutions ; it is, however, liable to hold in suspension particles of earthy matter, which impair its trans‐ parency.

4. WELL WATER. *Aqua ex Puteo*, is essentially the same as spring water, being derived from the
same source; it is, however, more liable to impurity
from its stagnation, or slow infiltration ; hence our old
wells furnish much purer water than those which are
more recent, as the soluble particles are gradually
washed away.

5. SNOW WATER. *Aqua ex Nive*, has been supposed to be unwholesome, and in particular, to produce a disease in the throat, but it does not appear
upon what principle its insalubrity can depend ; the
prejudice however is a very ancient one, for Hippocrates observes, that snow or ice water is unwholesome, in consequence of its finer particles being
evaporated, and lost during its solution : it appears to
differ only from rain water in being destitute of air,
to which water is certainly indebted for its briskness,
and perhaps many of its good effects upon animals and
vegetables. The same observations apply to *Ice
Water*.

6. LAKE WATER. *Aqua ex Lacu*, is a collection
of rain, spring, and river waters, contaminated with
various animal and vegetable bodies, which, from its
stagnant nature, have undergone putrefaction in it.

7. MARSH WATER. *Aqua ex Palude*, being the
most stagnant is the most impure of all water, and is
generally loaded with decomposing vegetable matter.

To what extent the impurities of water are capable
of influencing their salubrity, has been a subject of
interesting enquiry from the age of Hippocrates to
the present day. To many of these natural contaminations, too much importance has been certainly
attached ; it is an affected refinement to suppose that
the presence of minute portions of such earthy and

calcareous salts, as generally occur in solution, can impart any noxious quality to water;* whilst on the contrary, animal and vegetable impurities, or earthy bodies in a state of mechanical suspension, cannot fail to prove injurious, and must be regarded as the true " SCELERA AQUARUM." Guided by false analogies many have supposed that they recognised the origin of all calcareous diseases in the earthy impurities of water; the researches however of chemistry have removed this delusion, by demonstrating that the substances found in water never enter into the composition of urinary calculi. Metallic and other accidental contaminations are necessarily highly injurious, and the water in which their presence is suspected, should be submitted to the most careful examination.

For the purification and preservation of water numerous methods have been adopted; the mechanical impurities may be removed by filtration, which is performed through porous stones, or alternate layers of sand or charcoal; muddy water may be also cleared by adding a few grains of alum to each pint,† and in that proportion, the water is not rendered in the least disagreeable: when water has contracted a putrid

* I take this opportunity of observing that I have made analyses of several of those springs in Cornwall, which have from time immemorial enjoyed a reputation in the neighbourhood for curing diseases, amongst which were the waters of Holy-well, so named from its supposed virtues, and those of Permiscen Bay, equally extolled for their medicinal qualities. But I have only been able to detect minute quantities of carbonate of lime, derived from infiltration through banks of calcareous sand. *See Transactions of the Royal Geological Society of Cornwall.*

† I am informed by a respectable chemist in this town, that he sells a large quantity of alum for this very purpose, as well as to publicans for the sake of clearing their spirituous liquors; for the same end, we are told, thas the wine merchants in Paris put into each cask of wine as much as a pound of alum.

smell, it may be rendered sweet by agitating it with a
small portion of magnesia. Dr. Black observes that
nitrate of silver, which is one of the most antiseptic
substances known, will preserve water from putrefaction for ever, and that it may at any time be separated
therefrom in a few minutes, by adding a small lump of
common salt; this fact in itself is curious, but the
experiment is too hazardous to recommend. As that
peculiar property of water which is termed *hardness*,
generally depends upon the presence of *sulphate of
lime*, the addition of an alkaline carbonate twenty-
four hours previous to its being used, will be found
to restore it, or if it should depend upon *super-car-
bonate of lime*, long ebullition, without any addition,
will be found sufficient for its cure.

Water when kept for a long time in casks, especially
on long voyages, is partially decomposed, and a volume
of carbureted hydrogen is evolved, imparting to such
water the peculiar smell and taste which characterise
it; this decomposition may in a great degree be obviated by charring the interior of the water casks.
In Pharmacy it ought to be remembered that whenever
common water is employed it should not be *hard;*
filtered rain water may be recommended as the most
eligible on such occasions.

AQUA DISTILLATA. L. E. D.
Distilled Water.

Qualities. *Taste*, vapid, from the absence of air;
and slightly empyreumatic, in consequence probably
of the presence of a small quantity of extractive
matter, which has undergone partial decomposition.
a fluid-ounce weighs 454½ grains. Medicinal Use.

I

In extemporaneous prescriptions, distilled water should be always ordered whenever the formula contain any of the following substances :—*Acidum Sulphuricum, Acidum Citricum ; Antimonium Tartarizatum ; Argenti Nitras ; Cuprum Ammoniatum ; Ferrum Tartarizatum ; Hydrargyri Oxy-murias ; Liquor Ammoniæ ; Liquor Plumbi Acetatis ; Liquor Potassæ ; Plumbi Super-Acetas ; Solutio Muriatis Barytæ ; Vinum Ferri ; Zinci Sulphas ; Ferri Sulphas.* Distilled water ought also to be employed in preparations where much water is evaporated, as in the formation of extracts, since the residual matter of common water will remain mixed with the product of the process, and uselessly add to its bulk, or even in some cases, produce in it chemical changes ; unless however. under such circumstances, common water purified by filtration should be ordered, as the air which it contains imparts to it a pleasant and sprightly flavour ; in making infusions or decoctions, it is very important that the water should be free from those impurities which impart to it *hardness*, and which render it a far less powerful solvent of vegetable matter, nor indeed can resinous substances be mixed with such water, even when assisted by a mucilaginous medium ; on which account, in prescribing emulsions, it may perhaps be prudent to direct the employment of distilled water. Tests of its Purity. Its transparency ought not to be disturbed by the addition of nitrate of silver, or muriate of barytes.

AQUA MARINA. Sea Water.

Until the late able researches of Dr. Murray, we possessed but an imperfect knowledge of the composi-

tion of sea water, it is not therefore surprising that
the analysis performed by different chemists should be
found to be so materially at variance ; the true cause
of such discordance is now easily understood, for it
appears, that in the examination of a mineral water
or any compound saline solution, the substances obtained fiom it are not necessarily the original ingredients, but frequently the products of new combinations established by the operation of analysis, and that
consequently the nature of the results obtained may
vary according to the modes in which such analysis
has been conducted, or even according to the degree
of dilution in which the saline substances exist.* The

* The law which determines such combinations has been investigated
with singular ingenuity and success by Dr. Murray, (*Transactions of the
Royal Society of Edinburgh*, 1816). Berthollet had already established
the important fact, that combinations are often determined by the force
of cohesion, in such a manner, that in principles acting on each other,
those on which this force operates most powerfully, in relation to the
fluid which is the medium of action, are combined together ; hence from
a knowledge of the solubility of the compounds which substances form,
we may predict what combinations will be established when they act
on each other, *those always combining which form the least soluble compounds.*
(See Introductory Essay, page 33). It is for the extension of these
views, and for the useful application of them that we are indebted to
Dr. Murray, who justly observes that if the force of cohesion can so
far modify chemical attraction, as to establish among compound salts
dissolved in any medium, those combinations whence the least soluble
compounds are formed, we are entitled to conclude that the reverse of
this force, i. e. the power of a solvent, may produce the opposite effects,
or cause the very reverse of these combinations to be established, so
that in a concentrated medium the least soluble will be formed, and in
a dilute one, the more soluble compounds will be established, hence
follows the simple rule by which the actual state in which saline bodies
exist in a solution may be determined, viz. *that in any fluid containing the
elements of compound salts the binary compounds existing in it will be generally
those which are most soluble in that fluid, and the reverse combinations will only be
established by its concentration favouring the influence of cohesion.* It appears
that by simply evaporating a saline solution we may produce changes

elements of the salts contained in a pint of sea water
are, *Lime* 2·9, *Magnesia* 14·8, *Soda* 96·3, *Sulphuric
Acid* 14·4, *Muriatic Acid* 97.7. total 226·1 grains, and
supposing these elements to be combined in the modes
which Dr. Murray's views appear to establish, the
saline contents of a pint of sea water may be expressed
as follows, *Muriate of Soda* 159·3, *Muriate of Magnesia* 35·5, *Muriate of Lime* 5.7, *Sulphaté of Soda*
25·6 grains, total 226·1 grains; besides such saline
contents, it is contaminated with various animal and
vegetable bodies, in consequence of which it becomes,

in its composition, and obtain products which never existed in its
original state of dilution; thus suppose *muriate of magnesia* and *sulphate of
soda* to be dissolved in water, as is actually the case in the water of the
ocean, and the solution to be concentrated by evaporation from heat;
the combinations of *sulphate af magnesia*, and *muriate of soda*, being on the
whole less soluble in water, this circumstance of inferior solubility, or
the force of cohesion thus operating, actually determines the formation
of these compounds, and the production of sulphate of magnesia from
the bittern is to be explained upon this principle. Since it appears
therefore that the influence of solubility is most important, temperature,
to whose dominion it is under all circumstances subject, must necessarily be alike powerful; let us exemplify this fact by the action of
the very salts under consideration: it has been just stated that *muriate
of magnesia* and *sulphate of soda*, decompose each other in a *concentrated*
solution at a high temperature, producing muriate of soda, and sulphate of magnesia, but at temperatures below 32°. the reverse actually
takes place, muriate of soda and sulphate of magnesia reacting, and
being converted into sulphate of soda and muriate of magnesia; a fact
evidently owing to the relation of the solubility of these salts to temperature. Muriate of soda has its solubility scarcely altered, either by
heat or cold, sulphate of soda is, in these respects, completely the reverse, hence at an elevated temperature, muriate of soda is the least,
and sulphate of soda the most soluble salt, whilst at low temperatures, the reverse of this happens. All the circumstances of this investigation are most interesting, the medical practitioner will at once
perceive its importance, as enabling him to appreciate the real nature
of saline solutions, and even in many instances, to preserve their
identity. See *Aquæ Minerales.*

when long kept, highly offensive. MEDICAL USE.
As a cathartic a pint is the ordinary dose, which
should be taken in the morning, at two doses, with an
interval of half an hour between each; this quantity
contains half an ounce of purgative salt, of which
about three fourths are muriate of soda, but it is
much more active than a similar portion of any artificial combination. In procuring sea water for medicinal purposes, there is a precaution, the importance
of which experience has suggested to me, that it be
not hastily drank on the beach, before the particles of
sand, with which under such circumstances it is generally mixed, are allowed to subside; from the neglect of
this precaution I have witnessed serious consequences.
The most important advantages of sea water are derived from its external use as a bath.

AQUÆ DISTILLATÆ. L.D.   AQUÆ STILLA-
TITIÆ. E.
Distilled Waters.

These are water impregnated with the essential oils
of vegetables, and are principally designed as grateful
vehicles for the exhibition of more active remedies;
ample directions for preparing them are given in the
several Pharmacopœias, and if they be rectified by
redistillation they may be kept for several years; the
usual mode of preserving them is by adding spirit,
which has also the incidental advantage of preventing
them from being frozen, during the winter season.
Some recommend a film of the essential oil to be diffused over the water's surface. They may be extemporaneously prepared by adding to water what have
been called *Essences,* which consist of essential oil

and alcohol, or by rubbing any essential oil with ten times its weight of sugar, or, what answers still better, of magnesia ; when however they are so prepared they never retain their transparency. The properties of each water may be learnt by referring to the vegetable from which it is distilled.

AQUÆ MINERALES. Mineral Waters.

Although all waters that flow from the earth, are, as they contain mineral bodies in solution, strictly speaking, *mineral* waters; yet this term is especially applied to such only as are distinguished from spring, lake, river, or other water, by a peculiarity in colour, taste, smell, or any obvious properties, or by the medicinal effects which they produce, or are known to be capable of producing.

To the medical practitioner the history of these waters is most interesting and instructive, involving highly important subjects of chemical and physiological inquiry. These waters are without doubt indebted for their medicinal virtues to the operation of the substances which they hold dissolved, but this is so materially aided by the peculiar state of dilution in which they exist, as well as by the mere bulk, and temperature of the water itself, as to render extremely doubtful the success of every attempt to concentrate their powers by evaporation. To what extent dilution may modify the chemical condition of saline solutions has been satisfactorily demonstrated by the researches of Dr. Murray (See *Aqua Marina*), and to what degree an encrease in the solubility of any remedy may influence its medicinal properties has been considered

at some length, in the Introductory Esay of this work,
(*page* 19). It is certain that, in general, soluble salts
are capable of exerting a much more powerful effect
upon the animal economy, than those which are insoluble; on which account, the earthy muriates, especially that of lime, are amongst the most active ingredients of mineral waters. Although chemical analysis has frequently from its own imperfection, failed
in ascertaining their presence, it seems probable that
muriate of lime, and *sulphate of soda*, exist in all those
springs that furnish, by the usual methods of examination, *sulphate of lime*, and *muriate of soda;* for the
same reasons it is equally probable, that iron, which
in certain waters has been supposed, from the analysis,
to exist as a *carbonate*, is in its native solution a true
muriate; this is undoubtedly the fact with respect to
the Bath waters. Is it then surprising, that medical
practitioners should hitherto have failed in their attempts to emulate, by artificial arrangements, the
medicinal efficacy of active mineral springs? For the
investigation of the true composition of mineral waters
the researches of Dr. Murray furnish a simple and
elegant formula. *Determine by precipitants the weight*
of the acids and bases, suppose them united in such a
manner that they shall form the most soluble salts; and
these salts will constitute the true saline constituents of
the water under examination.

Mineral waters admit of being divided into four
classes, viz.

1. ACIDULOUS; owing their properties chiefly to
carbonic acid ; they are tonic and diuretic, and in
large doses produce a transient exhilaration ; the most
celebrated are *Pyrmont, Seltzer, Spa, Carlsbad* and
Scarborough.

2. CHALYBEATE; containing iron in the form of *sulphate*, *carbonate*, or *muriate*; they have a styptic, inky taste; *Hartfell* near *Moffat*, *Peterhead*, *Tunbridge*, *Brighton*, *Cheltenham*, *Bath*, *Lemington Priors*, *Castle Horneck*, near *Penzance*, &c.

3. SULPHUREOUS WATERS, derive their character from a sulphurretted hydrogen, either uncombined or united with lime, or an alkali, *Enghien*, *Aix la Chapelle*, *Harrowgate*, *Moffat*.

4. SALINE; mostly purgative, and are advantageously employed in those hypochondriacal and visceral diseases that require continued, and moderate relaxation of the bowels, *Cheltenham*, *Lemington*, *Seidlitz*, and all brackish waters.

Some springs, as those of *Bath*, *Matlock*, and *Buxton*, owe their virtues rather to temperature than to any other cause, and others, as *Malvern*, to the diluent power alone of the water.

ARGENTI NITRAS. L. Nitras Argenti. E.D

Fused Nitrate of Silver, olim, *Lunar Caustic*.

QUALITIES. Fused nitrate of silver is in small cylinders of a dark grey colour, and presenting, when broken across, a crystalline structure. *Odour*, none; *Taste*, intensely bitter, austere, and metallic; it tinges the skin indelibly black; when perfectly free from copper, it is not deliquescent. CHEMICAL COMPOSITION; oxide of silver 70. nitric acid 30. SOLUBILITY. In an equal weight of water, at 60°. it is also soluble in alcohol. INCOMPATIBLE SUBSTANCES. *Fixed alkalies* and *alkaline earths*, the *muriatic*, *sulphuric*, and *tartaric* acids, and all the salts which

contain them ; *Soaps, arsenic, hydro-sulphurets,
astringent vegetable infusions, undistilled waters.* The
solutions of nitrate of silver are not disturbed by ammonia, the *ammoniaco-nitrate* being very soluble ;
nitrate of silver tinges the skin. and hair black, and
has been frequently employed for the latter purpose ; *
it likewise forms the basis of permanent ink.† MEDI-
CAL USE. Tonic, antispasmodic, and escharotic ; it
is said to prove efficacious in epilepsy, but during a
trial for several years in the Westminster hospital, I
never could discover its virtues ; many of the cases in
which it has been supposed to have been successful,
probably derived advantage from the purgative medicines which were simultaneously administered. It is
principally useful as an external application, and may
be considered as the strongest and most manageable
caustic that we possess, whilst in solution it acts as
a useful stimulant to indolent ulcers. FORMS OF EX-
IIIBITION. For internal use in pills made with crumb
of bread, with the addition of some sugar, to prevent
the mass from becoming too hard. DOSE, gr $\frac{1}{8}$, gradually increased to gr. j. ADULTERATIONS. *Copper*
may be always suspected, when it deliquesces, and is
to be immediately detected by its solution assuming a
blue colour, when supersaturated by ammonia. The
sticks should be preserved in closely stopped phials,
and covered with soft and dry paper.—ANTIDOTE.

---

* For the same purpose the French employ a pomatum prepared with
the oxide of bismuth, and it is said to answer the intention.

† PERMANENT INK FOR MARKING LINEN. This preparation is a
solution of nitrate of silver, thickened with *sap green*, or *cochineal*. The
Preparing Liquid, with which the linen to be marked is previously wetted,
is a solution of soda, boiled with gum, or some animal mucilage. It is
a curious circumstance that if *potass* be used for this purpose, the marking ink will run.

When this substance has been taken in excess, muriate
of soda is its true antidote; indeed so completely does
it decompose, and separate it from water, that if a
saturated solution of nitrate of silver be filtered through
common salt, it may be afterwards drank with impunity. This circumstance alone, would of necessity
render nitrate of silver a very uncertain remedy.

ARMORACIÆ RADIX. L. E. $\left(\begin{array}{c}\textit{Cochlearia}\\\textit{Armoracia}\end{array}\right)$

Raphanus Rusticanus, D. *Horse Radish Root.*

QUALITIES. *Taste* hot and acrid; *Odour* pungent.
CHEMICAL COMPOSITION. All its virtues depend
upon an essential oil. SOLUBILITY. Both water and
alcohol extract its active principles, but they are dissipated by decoction. MEDICAL USES. As a stimulant in paralysis it is often useful; Sydenham found
it successful in dropsies which were consequent on
intermittent fevers; Cullen recommends a syrup made
with the infusion of horse radish, to remove that species of hoarseness which depends upon local relaxation;
Dr. Withering extolls an infusion of this root in milk
as a cosmetic both safe and effectual. INCOMPATIBLE
SUBSTANCES. *Alkaline Carbonates*: *Oxy-muriate of
Mercury; Nitrate of Silver;* the *Infusion of Galls,*
and of *Yellow Cinchona Bark,* produce precipitates
with the infusion of this root. FORMS OF EXHIBI-
TION. In substance scraped or swallowed whole, or
in infusion. DOSE of the substance ʒj, of an infusion
fʒij. OFFICINAL PREPARATIONS. *Infusum Armoraciæ comp:* L. *Spiritus Armoraciæ comp:* L. D.

ARSENICI OXYDUM. L. Oxydum Arsenici.
E. Arsenicum. D. *White Arsenic*, vulgo *Arsenic*.

QUALITIES.—*Form*, shining, semivitreous lumps,
breaking with a conchoidal fracture, and when reduced
to powder, bearing some resemblance to white sugar;
Taste, acrid and corrosive, leaving an impression of
sweetness. *Specific gravity* 5·, it is volatilized at the
temperature of 383 *Fah* : and in the state of vapour is
quite inodorous, although it is asserted in many chemical works of authority to yield a smell like that of
garlic; the fact is that the alliaceous or garlic-like
smell is wholly confined to *metallic* arsenic in a state
of vapour, and whenever the arsenious acid yields this
odour, we may infer that its decomposition has taken
place; this happens when it is projected upon ignited
charcoal, or when heated in contact with those metallic
bodies which readily unite with oxygen, as *Antimony*
and *Tin*. It is stated by Orfila and other chemists,
that if it be projected upon heated copper the alliaceous odour is evolved; this however takes place
only when the copper is in a state of ignition, at which
temperature its affinity for oxygen enables it to reduce
the arsenious acid, for I find by experiment that if a
few grains of this substance be heated on a plate of
copper, by means of a spirit lamp or blowpipe, no
odour is perceptible, for the whole of the acid is dissipated before the copper can acquire a sufficiently
exalted temperature to deoxidize it. If the arsenious
acid be heated on a plate of zinc, the smell is not
evolved until the metal is in the state of fusion ; if
instead of these metals we employ in our experiments
those of gold, silver, or platina, no alliaceous smell
whatever is produced, at any temperature. It is probable that arsenical vapours which yield this peculiar

odour are less noxious than those which are inodorous, but I am not aware that the knowledge of
this fact can be applied to any purpose of practical
importance. CHEMICAL COMPOSITION. This substance possesses many of the essential habitudes of an
acid, as for instance, that of combining with the pure
alkalies to saturation; it is therefore very properly
denominated *Arsenious Acid.* It may be farther acidified by distilling it with nitrous acid, and the compound which results is a white concrete substance
termed *Arsenic Acid*; from experiments on the quantity of oxygen absorbed by metallic arsenic, during its
conversion into these two compounds, instituted by
Proust and Davy, it appears that the *arsenious* acid
consists of about 25 of oxygen and 75 of metal, and the
arsenic acid of 33 of oxygen, and 67 of metal, or the
quantity of metal being the same, that the oxygen in
the latter compound is to that in the former nearly as
three to two. SOLUBILITY. We have but lately
been set right upon this point, Klaproth has shewn
that it requires for its solution 400 parts of water at
60°, and only 13 at 212°, and moreover, that if 100
parts of water be boiled on the arsenious acid, and
suffered to cool, it will retain three grains in solution,
and deposit the remainder in tetrahedrous crystals;
this fact shews the importance of employing boiling
water in every chemical examination of substances
supposed to contain arsenious acid. It is soluble in
alcohol and oils; with lime water it produces a white
precipitate of *arsenite of lime*, which is soluble in an
excess of arsenious acid; with magnesia it forms a
soluble *arsenite*, which proves very virulent. The
poisonous effects of arsenious acid are so amply detailed
in medical works, that it would be superfluous to
dwell upon them in this place; it may, however be

interesting and useful to record an account of the
pernicious influence of arsenical fumes upon orga-
nized beings, as I have been enabled to ascertain in
the copper smelting works of Cornwall and Wales;
this influence is very apparent in the condition both of
the animals and vegetables in the vicinity; horses and
cows commonly lose their hoofs, and the latter are
often to be seen in the neighbouring pastures crawling
on their knees and not unfrequently suffering from
a cancerous affection in their rumps, whilst the milch
cows, in addition to these miseries, are soon deprived
of their milk; the men employed in the works are
more healthy than we could *a priori* have supposed
possible; the antidote upon which they all rely with
confidence, whenever they are infested with more than
an ordinary portion of arsenical vapour, is *sweet oil,*
and an annual sum is allowed by the proprietors in
order that it may be constantly supplied; this opinion
is not solitary, for Tachenius relates that the poisonous
effects, such as convulsions, gripes, and bloody stools,
with which he was seized from exposure to the fumes
of arsenic, were relieved by milk and oil.

It deserves notice that the smelters are occasionally
affected with a cancerous disease in the scrotum, similar to that which infests chimney-sweepers, and it is
singular that Stahl in describing the putrescent tendency in the bodies of those who die from this poison,
mentions in particular the gangrenous appearance of
these parts. It is a very extraordinary fact that previous to the establishment of the copper works in
Cornwall the marshes in their vicinity were continually
exciting intermittent fever, whereas since that period
a case of ague has not occurred in the neighbourhood;
I have heard it remarked by the men in the works,
that the smoke *kills* all fevers. The fact is here

stated without any other comment than that the agri
cultural improvements which have taken place in the
district are not sufficient to afford any clue to the explanation of the circumstance. MEDICAL USES.
Much has been said upon this subject, and the propriety and safety of its exhibition has been often
questioned ; there can be no doubt but that the greatest circumspection is required in the practitioner who
administers it, and it ought not, in my opinion, to
be employed until other remedies have failed; that
it is capable of accumulating in the system is very
evident, and this, in certain habits, may predispose
the patient to serious diseases ; the form in which it is
most manageable and least dangerous, is that of solution. See *Liquor Arsenicalis.* Some practitioners
have exhibited it in substance, made into pills, by
rubbing one grain with ten of sugar, and then beating
the mixture with a sufficient quantity of crumb of
bread, to form ten pills, one of which is a dose. The
Chinese and other oriental nations form the sulphuret
of arsenic (*realgar*) into medical cups, and use lemon
juice, after it has stood some hours in them, by way of
cathartic. As an external application, arsenic has
long been extolled in the cure of cancers.*

---

* PLUNKETT's OINTMENT, consists of arsenious acid, sulphur, and
the.powdered flowers of the *Ranunculus Flammulá*, and *Cotula Fætida,*
levigated and made into a paste with the white of an egg.

PATE ARSENICALE. This favourite remedy of the French surgeons
consists of 70 parts of cinnabar, 22 of *sanguis draconis*, and 8 of arsenious
acid, made into paste with saliva, at the time of applying it. This combination, observes a periodical writer, is similar, with the exception of
the ashes of the soles of old shoes, to that recommended by Father
Cosmo, under the name of " *Pulvis Anti-carcinomatosa.*"

SINGLETON'S EYE SALVE, or GOLDEN OINTMENT. Under this name
is sold a preparation which consists of sulphuret of arsenic (*orpiment*)

ARS

ADULTERATIONS. It is frequently sophisticated
with chalk, gypsum, or sulphate of barytes; the fraud
is instantly detected by its not being entirely volatilized by heat, or by any insoluble residuum occurring
in preparing the *Liquor Arsenicalis*, according to the
directions of the pharmacopæia. To many the adulteration of so active a substance may seem unimportant, but in consequence of its being thus rendered a
medicine of variable activity, it is one of the most dangerous frauds which can be committed; a very unpleasant circumstance lately occurred from such a
cause in one of our public institutions: arsenic had
been obtained from the shop of a respectable chemist,
who had not usually supplied the establishment, for
the purpose of preparing the arsenical solution; the
article happened to be less adulterated than that which
had been previously employed; the solution however
was prepared in the usual way, and the usual dose
was continued; the patients were soon seized with
violent pains in the bowels, and the cause was not
detected until by an examination of the bottle the
usual sediment was not discovered.

ANTIDOTES. Late researches have shewn that *sulphuret of potass*, on which physicians have placed so
much reliance, merits no confidence. The great indication to be fulfilled in all cases of poisoning is to excite vomiting, and to administer liquids, which are the
least liable to act as solvents of the acrid matter, on
which account lime water presents itself as a very appropriate fluid.

with lard, or spermaceti ointment. The *Unguentum Hydrargyri Nitrico
Oxydi* of the London College, is also sold under the same title.
In Paris Arsenic forms the basis of several blistering cerates. Such
applications cannot be safe.

1. *By its reduction to a metallic form.* Mix a portion of the suspected powder with three times its
weight of *black flux* (consisting of finely powdered
charcoal one part, dry carbonate of potass, two parts)
put the mixture into a thin glass tube, hermetically
closed at one end, about eight inches in length, and
one fourth of an inch in diameter; should any of the
powder adhere to the sides of the tube, it must be
carefully brushed off with a feather, so that the inner
surface of its upper part may be perfectly clean and
dry; the closed end of the tube, by way of security,
may be thinly coated with a mixture of pipe clay and
sand, but this operation is not absolutely necessary;
the open extremity is to be loosely plugged with a
piece of paper; the coated end must be now heated
on a chaffing dish of red hot coals, when the arsenic,
if present, will sublime, and be found lining with a
brilliant metallic crust the upper part of the tube; a
portion of this reduced metal, if it be arsenic, will,
when laid on heated iron, exhale in dense fumes which
are characterised by a strong smell of garlic.

It merits particular notice, that in reducing by the
above process the arsenious acid to the state of metal,
the presence of potass in the flux is very essential, since
it forms immediately an *arsenite of potass*, and thereby
fixes the arsenious acid, and prevents it from being
volatilized before the temperature is sufficiently high
to enable the charcoal to decompose it; an ignorance
of this fact has not unfrequently proved a source of
disappointment and fallacy.

Another method of identifying *white arsenic* by
metallization, is to form at the moment of its reduc-

tion, an alloy with copper, this is easily effected in the
following manner,—Mix the suspected powder with
black flux, as in the former experiment, and place
the mixture between two polished plates of copper,
bind them tightly together by iron wire, and expose
them to a low red heat; if the included substance
contained arsenic, a white stain will be left on the
surface of the copper, which is an alloy of the two
metals. If in this, as in the former experiment, charcoal be employed without the addition of a fixed alkali, the result may, for the reason which it is need-
less to repeat, prove unsatisfactory.

2. By the Application of certain Reagents,
or Tests, to its Solutions.

A great and important question has arisen in medical jurisprudence, whether any chemical proofs of
the presence of *white arsenic*, short of its actual reduction to the state of metal, can be depended upon, or
ought to be received as evidence in the courts of criminal law. After a full experimental investigation of
the subject, and an impartial review of all the facts
which bear upon the question, the author feels no
hesitation in declaring it to be his conviction, that
white arsenic may be detected without any fear of
fallacy, by a proper application of certain tests, and
that the contrary opinion, is entirely founded in error, and unsupported by experiment, as will more
fully appear in the sequel.

(A) *Fused Nitrate of Silver*, or *Lunar Caustic*. For
this test we are indebted to Mr. Hume of London,
who first gave it to the public in the Philosophical
Magazine for May, 1809, vol. xxxiii. His method of

K

applying it is as follows : Into a clean Florence flask
introduce two or three grains of the suspected powder, to which add about eight ounces of rain or distilled water, and heat the solution until it begins to
boil, then, while it boils, frequently shake the flask,
and add to the hot solution a grain or two of sub-carbonate of potass, agitating the whole to make the
mixture uniform. Pour into a wine glass about two
table spoonsfull of the solution, and touch the surface
of the fluid with a stick of lunar caustic. If arsenic
be present, a beautiful yellow precipitate will instantly
proceed from the point of contact, and settle towards
the bottom of the glass as a flocculent and copious
precipitate.

By this test the 60th part of a grain may be satisfactorily recognised in two ounces of water. The
presence of some alkali is essential to the success of
the experiment, since arsenious acid is unable by the
operation of simple affinity to decompose the nitrate
of silver.* The validity of this test has been questioned on the following grounds, which shall be fairly
examined in order.

*The alkaline phosphates are found to produce preci-
pitates with silver, analogous in colour and appearance
to the arsenite of silver.* This is undoubtedly the case
when the experiment is performed in the manner just
stated, but there are other reagents which will immediately distinguish these bodies; I have also shewn

---

* If any trifling opacity occur in a simple solution of arsenic, when
assayed by the nitrate of silver, it may be considered as the effects of
some casual impurities; this is further demonstrated by bringing over the
surface of the arsenical liquid, a piece of blotting paper, or a stopper,
moistened with a solution of ammonia, when there will instantly form
a copious yellow precipitate of arsenite of silver.

that there is a mode of so modifying the application
of the silver test itself, that no error or doubt can
arise in the use of it, from the presence of phosphoric
salts.† My method consists in conducting the trial
on writing paper, instead of in glasses, thus—drop
the suspected fluid on a piece of white paper, making
with it a broad line ; along this line a stick of lunar
caustic is to be slowly drawn several times successively, when a streak is produced of a colour resembling that known by the name of *Indian Yellow;* and
this is equally produced by the presence of arsenic
and that of an alkaline phosphate, but the one from
arsenic is rough, curdy, and flocculent, as if effected
by a crayon, that from a phosphate homogeneous and
uniform, resembling a water colour laid smoothly on
with a brush ; a more important, and distinctive peculiarity soon succeeds, in less than two minutes the
phosphoric yellow fades into a *sad green,* and becomes
gradually darker, and ultimately, quite black ; the
arsenical yellow, on the other hand, remains permanent, or nearly so, for some time, when it becomes
brown. In performing the experiment the sun-shine
should be avoided, or the transitions of the colour
will take place too rapidly. It would be prudent also
for the inexperienced operator to perform a similar
experiment on fluids known to contain arsenic, and a
phosphoric salt, as a standard of comparison. In this
way the nitrate of siver, without the intervention of
any other test, is fully capable of removing every
ambiguity, and of furnishing a distinguishing mark of
difference between the chemical action of arsenic and
the phosphates. Mr. Hume states that he has repeated
this experiment to his entire satisfaction,* and that,

† Annals of Philosophy, vol. IC. p. 60.
* London Medical and Pyhsical Journal, January 1818.

in a late unfortunate case of poisoniug, he derived
considerable information by its application.   The
laborious author of the London Dispensatory accepts
it as an excellent test, but observes that it is rendered
more luminous by brushing the streak lightly over
with liquid ammonia, immediately after the application of the caustic, when, if arsenic be present, a
bright queen's yellow is produced which remains permanent for nearly an hour; but that when the lunar
caustic produces a white-yellow before the ammonia
is applied, we may infer the presence of some alkaline phosphate, rather than that of arsenic.   One of
the great advantages of this test is the very small
quantity that is required for examination; it would be
well therefore for the operator to perform the experiment in both ways on a separate paper.

    *The Muriates produce precipitates with silver so
copious and flocculent, as to overcome every indication
which the presence of arsenic would otherwise afford.*
Dr. Marcet proposes to obviate this difficulty, by
adding to the fluid to be examined dilute nitric acid,
and then cautiously to apply the nitrate of silver until the precipitation ceases, in this way the muriatic
acid will be entirely removed, whilst the arsenic, if
it be present, will remain in solution, and may be
rendered evident by the affusion of ammonia, which
will instantly produce the yellow precipitate in its
characteristic form.   This mode however it must be
confessed appears complicated, and requires some
chemical address for its accomplishment; it should be
also known that the yellow precipitate thus produced,
is not always permanent, for it is soluble in the nitrate of ammonia formed during the process.   Under
these circumstances, it is surely preferable to precipitate at once from the suspected fluid all the sub-

stances which nitrate of silver can affect, and then to expose the mixed and ambiguous precipitate, so obtained, to a low heat in a glass tube, when the arsenious acid will be immediately separated by sublimation ; in this way the presence of muriates may even in certain cases, be serviceable, especially if the quantity of arsenic be minute, for by encreasing the bulk of the precipitate we shall decrease the difficulty of its examination. By this process also I should propose to meet the embarrassments which are stated to arise from the influence of various animal and vegetable substances, as milk, broth, wine, &c. so frequently present in the suspected liquid, and which are known to alter the character of the arsenical indications.

It has been stated that in consequence of the inability of arsenious acid to decompose nitrate of silver by simple elective attraction, the presence of alkali becomes indispensable in the examination, for which purpose Dr. Marcet has suggested the superior advantages which will attend the use of ammonia in cases where the arsenic has not been previously combined with a fixed alkali, since it does not, when added singly, decompose nitrate of silver, a circumstance which in using the fixed alkalies is very liable to occasion fallacy. This led Mr. Hume to form, at once, a triple compound, an *ammoniaco-nitrate of silver,** which is

* The following is the formula for its preparation. Dissolve ten grains of lunar caustic in ten times its weight of distilled water, to this add, *guttatim*, liquid ammonia, until a precipitate is formed ; continue cautiously to add the ammonia, repeatedly agitating the mixture until the precipitate is nearly redissolved. The object of allowing a small portion to remain undissolved is to guard against an excess of ammonia. Wherever the test is used, the liquid to which it is added ought to be quite cold.

a triumph in the art of analysis, for whilst it obviates
the necessity of ascertaining the proportion of alkali
required in each experiment,* it possesses the valuable property of not in the least disturbing the phosphate of soda.

(B) *Sulphate of Copper.* Like the preceding test
this requires also, for its success, that the arsenious
acid should be combined with some alkali, in which
case, by the operation of double elective attraction,
an arsenite of copper is thrown down of a very striking
and characteristic colour, being that of the well-known
pigment called *Scheele's green*; if arsenic be not present in the liquid so assayed, and a fixed alkali has
been employed, the result will be a delicate *sky blue*,
instead of the *grass green* precipitate.

Mr. Hume recommends the employment of ammonia, in preference to the fixed alkalies, for the reasons stated under the consideration of the silver test,
and he proposes to form, by a similar process, an *Am-
moniaco-Sulphate of Copper*, in using which however
care must be taken that it be not too highly concentrated, for in that state it will not-produce precipitation. Much controversy has taken place on the subject of sulphate of copper as a test for arsenic, and it
has been stated with more confidence than truth that
a *decoction of onions* has the property of imparting to
the copper precipitate, which is produced by a fixed
alkali, a colour and appearance analogous to that
which is occasioned by arsenic. This opinion was
boldly advanced and supported on a most important
trial at the Lent assizes for Cornwall in 1817.

* This is very important, for an excess of ammonia redissolves the
yellow precipitate, and therefore defeats the object of the test. The
fixed alkalies, in excess, have not such a property.

Since this event an opportunity * has occurred which

* The great impression made upon the public mind in Cornwall by the above trial, produced a disposition to regard the cause of every sudden death with more than usual jealousy.

In consequence of a report having arisen that a young woman had died after an illness of forty-eight hours, and been hastily buried at Madron, the magistrates of that district issued their warrant for the disinterment of the body, and requested my attendance at the examination. It appeared upon dissection that the immediate cause of death was inflammation of the intestines; the stomach was found to contain a considerable portion of liquid, which was carefully collected and examined; no solid matter could be discovered in it. It appeared to consist principally of the remains of a quantity of pennyroyal tea, which had been the last thing administered to the deceased; this was divided into several portions, and placed in separate wine glasses, and submitted, in the presence of the sheriff and other gentlemen, to a series of experiments, amongst which the following may be particularized, as bearing upon the question at issue.

1st. A few drops of a solution of sub-carbonate of potass were added to the liquid, in one of the glasses, when its colour, which was before of a light hazel, was instantly deepened into a reddish yellow; the sulphate of copper was then applied, when a precipitate fell down, which every one present immediately pronounced to be of a *vivid green* hue, but on pouring off the supernatant liquid, and transferring the precipitate on white paper, it assumed a blue colour, without the least tinge of green; the explanation of the phenomenon, and the fallacy to which it gave rise, was obvious; the yellow colour imparted to the liquid by the alkali, was the effect of that body upon vegetable extract, and will generally take place on adding it to the infusions of vegetable substances.

2nd. To another portion of the liquid, the ammoniaco-nitrate of silver was added; a slight turbidness arose, but no yellow precipitate occurred.

3rd. After adding a fixed alkali, the surface of the liquid was touched with a stick of lunar caustic, but no yellow precipitate was produced.

4th. The liquid was next assayed in a watch glass, for a *phosphate of soda*, by endeavouring to form a triple salt with magnesia and ammonia, as suggested by Dr. Wollaston; the result proved that *phosphate of soda* was not present. It is unnecessary to pursue the relation of the experiments; I conceive that sufficient evidence has been adduced to establish the truth of the explanation. I have frequently repeated the first experiment, substituting for the gastric infusion, a decoction of onions, and with similar results.

has enabled me to examine this alleged fact, by a fair
and appropriate series of experiments, the result of
which satisfactorily proved that the opinion was
grounded on an optical fallacy, arising from the *blue*
precipitate assuming a *green* colour, in consequence
of having been viewed through a yellow medium;
the phosphoric salts may also, under similar circumstances, be mistaken for arsenic, for the intense blue
colour of the phosphate of copper will thus necessarily appear green. This instance of optical fallacy
is not solitary, *corrosive sublimate* has been said to
possess the character of an acid because it turns the
syrup of violets green, whereas this change is to be
attributed to the combination of the yellow hue of
the sublimate with the blue colour of the violet.

Whenever therefore such a source of fallacy can
be suspected, the operator would do well to repeat
his experiment on white paper, in the manner I have
before proposed, and the results which are obtained
in glasses should always be examined by day light,
and viewed by reflected, and not by transmitted light.

There are several other tests by which arsenic may
be identified. The process described in the Dublin
Pharmacopœia for the preparation of *Arsenias Kali*,
the arseniate, or rather super-arseniate of potass,
which has been long known under the name of " the
arsenical salt of Macquer," has been strongly advised
as a collateral proof; it consists in decomposing the
nitrate of potass by the arsenious acid, but since this
problem requires that the suspected poison should be
in a solid and palpable form, it is impossible to examine its pretensions to our confidence, without being
reminded of the story so often told to us in our
infancy, of catching a bird by laying salt upon its tail

It is necessary to observe in this place that the *arse-niate*, like the *arsenite of potass*, or that of *ammonia*, is obedient to the silver test, but that instead of the yellow precipitate, which is produced by the latter salt, we obtain by the former, a red, or brick-coloured one.

In taking an impartial review of all the evidence which the investigation of this subject can furnish, it must appear to the most fastidious that the silver and copper tests above described are capable, under proper management, of furnishing striking and infallible indications, and that in most cases, they will be. equally conclusive, and in some even more satisfactory in their results, than the metallic reproduction upon which such stress has been laid, and for this obvious reason, that unless the quantity of metal be considerable, its metallic splendour and appearance is often very ambiguous and questionable ; it has to my knowledge happened to a medical person, by no means deficient in chemical address, to ascribe to the presence of arsenic that which was no other than a film of very finely divided charcoal ; in this state of doubt the last resource was to ascertain whether it yielded, or not, upon being heated, an alliaceous odour ; surely an unprejudiced judge would prefer the evidence of sight as furnished by the arsenical tests, to that of smell, as afforded in this last experiment. No one will attempt to deny that it is the duty of the medical practitioner who is called upon to decide so important a question as the presence of arsenic, to prosecute by experiment every point which admits the least doubt ; he should also remember that in a criminal case, he has not only to satisfy his own conscience, but that he is bound, as far as he is able,

to convince the public mind of the accuracy and
truth of his researches, and he fails in his duty if
he omits, through any false principle of humanity,
to express the strong conviction which the success of
such experiments must necessarily have produced in
his mind. The application of chemical reagents on
solutions suspected to contain arsenic, throws no obstacle whatever in the way of the metallic reduction
of that body, but, on the contrary, it furnishes pre-
paratory steps in the process, since the precipitates
which are produced may be collected, and easily decomposed, as before stated.

ASARI FOLIA L.E.D. $\left(Asarum\ Europœum\right)$
Asarabacca Leaves.

QUALITIES. The leaves, when recent, are nauseous,
bitter, and acrimonious ; properties which are impaired by keeping. CHEMICAL COMPOSITION, a peculiar
acrid principle, not well understood. SOLUBILITY,
water by infusion extracts its sensible properties, but
they are lost by decoction. USES. As an errhine;
Dr. Cullen has remarked that they form the most
useful species of this genus of local stimulants. DOSE,
gr. iij to v. repeated every night until the full effect
is produced. OFFICINAL PREP. *Pulvis Asari compositus.* E.D.

ASSAFŒTIDA. L.E.D. $\left(\begin{array}{l}\text{Ferula Assafœtida}\\ Gummi\ Resina.\end{array}\right)$

QUALITIES. *Form,* small irregular masses, adhering together, of a variegated texture, and contain-

ing many little shining tears of a whitish, reddish, or violet hue. *Taste,* bitter and sub-acrid. *Odour,* fœtid and alliaceous, but this latter property is very much impaired by age. Chemical Composition. Gum (or according to Brugnatelli, *extractive*) 60, resin 30, and essential oil 10 parts. Solubility. It yields all its virtues to alcohol and ether; if triturated with water it forms a milky mixture, but which is not permanent, unless some intermede be employed for the suspension of the gum-resin; for this purpose egg may be added, in the proportion of one yolk to a drachm of assafœtida, or a permanent mixture may be effected by carefully triturating the gum resin with double its weight of mucilage. If ʒvj of assafœtida be triturated with ʒss of camphor, a mass results of a proper consistence for a plaster; if triturated with carbonate of ammonia, it is easily reduced to powder, but undergoes no other change. Forms of Exhibition : in mixture or in pills. Dose, gr. v to ℈j. *Form* : 111. Properties, stimulant, antispasmodic, expectorant, and anthelmintic; in cases of flatulent cholic, it has, in the form of enema, acted like a charm. Officinal Prep : *Mist: Assafœtid:* L.D. *Tinct: Assafœtid:* L.E.D. *Spir: Ammoniæ fœtid:* (a) L.E.D. *Tinct: Castorei comp:* (a) E. *Pil: Aloes cum Assafœtid:* (d) E. *Pil: Galbani comp:* (a) L. *Enema Fœtid:* D. Impurities. Its characteristic odour should be powerful, and when broken, its fracture ought to exhibit a bluish-red appearance. It ought not to be brittle.

BALSAMUM PERUVIANUM. L.E.D.
(Myroxylon Peruiferum).

Peruvian Balsam.

QUALITIES. *Form,* a viscid liquid of a reddish brown colour. *Odour,* fragrant and aromatic. *Taste,* hot and bitter. CHEMICAL COMPOSITION. Resin, volatile oil, and benzoic acid; it is therefore a true *balsam*; the term was formerly applied to every vegetable resin having a strong scent, and the fluidity of treacle, and which was supposed to possess many medicinal virtues; it is now restricted to those resins which contain the benzoic acid in their composition, of which there are only three, viz. the Balsams of *Peru, Tolu,* and *Benzoin.* SOLUBILITY, water when boiled upon it dissolves only a portion of benzoic acid; ether is its most complete solvent; alcohol dissolves it completely, but the quantity of this menstruum must be considerable. PROPERTIES, stimulant, and tonic, on which account in certain chronic affections of the lungs, it has been found a serviceable expectorant; Sydenham gave it in pthisis, but wherever any inflammatory action is to be apprehended Dr. Fothergill wisely cautions us against its use. FORMS OF EXHIBITION, diffused in water by means of mucilage, or made into pills with any vegetable powder. DOSE, gr. v to ʒj. ADULTERATIONS, a mixture of resin and some volatile oil with benzoin, is often sold for Peruvian Balsam, and the fraud is not easily detected, and is probably of but little importance.

BALSAMUM TOLUTANUM. L.E.D.
(Toluifera Balsamum)

Balsam of Tolu.

QUALITIES. *Form,* a thick tenacious liquid becoming concrete by age, in which state it is usually found in the shops. *Taste,* warm and sweetish. *Odour,* extremely fragrant, resembling that of lemons. CHEMICAL COMPOSITION. Volatile oil, resin, and benzoic acid. SOLUBILITY. It is soluble in alcohol, forming a tincture which is rendered milky by water, but no precipitate falls. When dissolved in the smallest quantity of a solution of potass, its odour is changed into one that resembles clove pink. FORMS OF EXHIBTION. It may be suspended in water by means of mucilage, or yolk of egg, but is rarely employed except on account of its agreeable flavour;* its virtues are similar to those of the balsam of Peru. OFFICINAL PREP: *Tinct: Benzoini comp:* L.E.D. *Tinct: Toluiferi Balsam:* E.D. *Syrup: Tolutan:* L.

BELLADONNÆ FOLIA, L.E.D.
(Atropa. Belladonna)

Deadly Nightshade.

QUALITIES. The leaves are inodorous. *Taste,* slightly nauseous, sweetish, and subacrid; their peculiar properties are not lost by drying. CHEMICAL COMPOSITION. Vauquelin found that the leaves contained a substance analogous to albumen, salts with a base of potass, and a bitter principle on which its

---

* TOLU LOZENGES. Sugar 8 oz. Cream of Tartar 1 oz. Starch 2 drachms. Tinct : Toluiferæ Balsami E. one fluiddrachm, mucilage of Gum Tragacanth q. s.

narcotic properties depended. SOLUBILITY, water is the most powerful solvent of its active matter. USES, it is a powerful sedative and narcotic, both as an internal medicine and as an external application. FORMS OF EXHIBITION; every part of the plant is poisonous, and the berries from their beautiful appearance have often tempted the unwary; the leaves however furnish the most convenient form of exhibition; externally, they may be used as a poultice, internally, one grain of the dry leaves powdered, and gradually encreased to 10 or 12 grains, or the leaves may be infused in boiling water in the proportion of four grains to two fluid-ounces, which may be given as a dose. A little of this infusion, dropped into the eye, permanently dilates the pupil, for which intention it has been successfully applied previous to the operation of the cataract. The extract of this plant, since its active principle is fixed, ought to possess activity, but, as it occurs in commerce, it is found to be very uncertain and variable, a circumstance which entirely depends upon the manner in which it has been prepared. An overdose of belladonna produces the most distressing and alarming symptoms, and so paralising is its influence, that vomiting can be hardly excited by the strongest doses of tartarized antimony; in such cases, vinegar will be found the best antidote, after the exhibition of which, emetics are more likely to perform their duty. OFFICINAL PREP: *Extract: Belladonnæ*. L. *Succus spissatus Atropæ Belladonnæ.* E.

BENZOINUM. L.E. Benzoe. D. (Styrax Benzoin) vulgo, *Benjamin.*

QUALITIES. *Form*, brittle masses, composed of white and brownish, or yellowish, fragments; *Odour*, fragrant; *Taste*, scarcely perceptible. When heated, it exhales benzoic acid in the form of crystals. CHE-MICAL COMPOSITION. Resin, and a large proportion of benzoic acid. SOLUBILITY. It is readily dissolved by alcohol and ether, and is again separated from them by water; solutions of lime, and the fixed alkalies separate the benzoic acid from it, which can afterwards be recovered from such solutions by the addition of an acid. USES: it is considered expectorant, and was formerly used in asthma, and other pulmonary affections; it has however fallen into disuse, and is now principally employed in perfumery, and odoriferous fumigations. * OFFICINAL PREP: *Acidum Benzoinum.* L.E.D. *Tinct: Benzoini comp:†* L.E.D. IMPURITIES; it is found in the market in various degrees of purity, the best is yellowish, studded with white spots; the worst is full of dross, and very dark or black.

* FUMIGATING PASTILLES. *Benzoin* generally constitutes the chief ingredient in these compositions, to which may be added any variety of odoriferous substances; the following formula may be offered as a specimen: ℞ Benzoin ʒj, *Cascarilla* ʒss, *Myrrh* Ꝺj, *Olei nuc: moschat:* *ol: Caryophyll:* āā gr.x.*potassæ nitratis* ʒss, *carb: ligni* ʒvj, *mucilag: gum:* *Trag.* q. s.

† VIRGIN's MILK. A spirituous solution of Benzoin mixed with about twenty parts of *rose water*, forms a cosmetic long known by this name. Under the same title also a very different preparation is sold, *vid. Liquor Plumbi acetatis.*

FRIAR'S BALSAM, WADE's DROPS, JESUIT'S DROPS. These preparations are nothing more than the *Tinctura Benzoini composita.*

PECTORAL BALSAM OF HONEY. Is the tincture of *Benzoin,* or that of *Tolu.*

ESSENCE OF COLTSFOOT. This preparation consists of equal parts of the *Balsam of Tolu,* and the *Compound Tincture of Benzoin,* to which is added double the quantity of *rectified Spirit of Wine;* and this forsooth is a *Pectoral for Coughs!* If a patient with a pulmonary affection recovers during the use of such a remedy, would not the recovery be more properly designated an ESCAPE than a CURE?

CALAMI RADIX. L. Acori Calami Radix. *E.*
Acorus. D. (Acorus Calamus) *Sweet Flag Root.*

QUALITIES. This root is full of joints, crooked,
and flattened on the sides, internally of a white colour, and loose spongy texture. *Odour,* fragrant and
aromatic. *Taste,* bitter and pungent, qualities which
are improved by exsiccation. CHEMICAL COMPOSI-
TION. The principles in which its qualities reside
appear to be essential oil, and bitter extractive; the
root likewise contains fecula, which is copiously precipitated from its infusion by acetate and super-acetate of lead. Watery infusion extracts all its virtues,
but decoction impairs them. Spirit is also an appropriate solvent. USES. It is not employed so frequently as it deserves; it would be a useful addition to many of the compound infusions of vegetable
stomachics. DOSE. A cupfull of the infusion made
by adding ʒvj of the dried root to f℥xij of boiling
water.

CALUMBÆ RADIX. L. (*Plantæ adhuc*)
(*Anonymæ*)
Colomba Radix E.   Colomba D.

Calumba Root.

QUALITIES. *Form;* the dried root imported into
this country is in transverse sections; the bark is
thick, and easily detached; the wood is spongy and
yellowish; the pieces are frequently perforated, evidently by worms. *Odour,* slightly aromatic. *Taste,*
bitter, and somewhat acrid. CHEMICAL COMPOSI-
TION; Cinchonin, bitter resin, and starch, in addition
to which, M. Planche has found a peculiar animal-

like substance. SOLUBILITY. Boiling water takes
up about one-third of its weight, but proof spirit appears to be its most perfect menstruum. INCOMPATIBLE SUBSTANCES. No change is occasioned in the
infusion by the solutions of nitrate of silver, sulphate
of iron, muriate of mercury, or tartarized antimony;
but precipitates are produced by the *infusion of galls
and yellow Cinchona bark,* by *acetate and superacetate
of lead; oxy-muriate of mercury;* and *lime-water.*
The infusion very soon spoils. DOSE of the powdered
root gr. xv to ʒss; of the infusion f℥iss to f℥ij. USES.
It is one of the most valuable tonics and stomachics
which we possess. It seems to be superior to many
others, from not possessing astringent, and stimulant
powers, on which account it is singularly eligible in
certain pulmonary and mesenteric affections; it may
be given in combination with chalybeates, aromatics,
saline purgatives, or with rhubarb, as circumstances
may require. OFFICINAL PREPARATIONS. *Infus:
Calumbæ.* L. *Tinct: Calumbæ.* L.E.D. It becomes
worm-eaten by age, and, in that condition, should be
rejected. Those pieces which have the brightest colour, and the greatest specific gravity, are the best.
The root of *white briony,* tinged yellow with the tincture of Calumba, has been fraudulently substituted
for this root.

CAMBOGIA. L. (*Stalagmitis.*) Gambogia. E.D.
 Gamboge.   (*Cambogioides.*)

QUALITIES. *Form.* Lumps of a solid consistence,
breaking with a vitreous fracture; *Odour* none; *Colour* deep yellow, bordering on red, and becoming,
when moistened, a brilliant light yellow. *Taste*
slightly acrid, but which is not experienced unless it

L

be allowed to remain long in the mouth. CHEMICAL
COMPOSITION. One part of gum, and four parts of a
brittle resin; but this knowledge throws no light on
the nature of its cathartic property. SOLUBILITY.
When triturated with water two thirds of its substance
are speedily dissolved, and a turbid solution results;
alcohol dissolves nine tenths, and forms a yellow
transparent tincture, which is rendered turbid by
the addition of water; sulphuric ether dissolves six
tenths of the substance; it is also soluble in alkaline
solutions, and the resulting compound is not rendered
turbid by water, but is instantly decomposed by acids,
and the precipitate so produced is of an extremely
brilliant yellow colour, and soluble in an excess of
acid. INCOMPATIBLE SUBSTANCES. No bodies appear to produce in gamboge such a chemical change,
as to destroy the chemical properties which distinguish
it, but by a mechanical admixture, its solubility, and
consequently its operation, may be materially modified; see *Introductory Essay, page* 21. Dr. Cullen
found that the inconvenience arising from its too rapid solubility, and sudden impression upon the stomach, might be obviated by diminishing the dose, and
repeating it at short intervals as directed in *Form:*
26. FORMS OF EXHIBITION. No form is more judicious than that of pill. DOSE, gr. 2 to gr. 6. USES.
It is a powerful drastic cathartic, and hydragogue,
very liable to excite vomiting, and from this peculiar
action upon the stomach it has been frequently employed with success in the expulsion of teniæ (Form:
121.) and it accordingly enters as an ingredient into
many of the compositions which are sold for the cure
of tape worms. OFFICINAL PREP: *Pil: Cambogiæ
camp:* L. There is a considerable difference in the

degree of purity in which this substance occurs in the market; it should be estimated by its clearness and brilliancy.

CAMPHORA. L.E.D. (*Laurus Camphora**)
Camphor.

QUALITIES. *Form*, a white brittle substance, unctuous to the touch, but possessing at the same time a degree of ductility which prevents its being easily pulverised, unless a few drops of spirit be previously added. *Odour* peculiar, fragrant, and penetrating. *Taste* bitter, pungent, and aromatic. *Specific gravity* ·9887, it therefore swims on water; it is so volatile that during warm weather a considerable proportion will evaporate, especially if at the same time the atmosphere be rather moist.† It is readily ignited, and burns with a brilliant flame and much smoke. CHEMICAL COMPOSITION. It is a proximate vegetable

* Although the Camphor of commerce is generally furnished by the *Laurus Camphora*, yet it is abundantly yielded by many other plants. It is said that what is imported from Sumatra is the product of the *Dryobolans Camphora*. It is also contained in the roots of the *Cinnamon, Cassia,* and *Sassafras laurels*, and in those of *Galangale, Zedoary*, and *Ginger*; in *Cardamom seeds* and *Long Pepper*. The essential oils of *Lavender, Sage, Thyme, Peppermint, Rosemary,* and those of many other labiate plants yield camphor by distillation. Camphor may be also artificially formed by driving a stream of muriatic acid gas through oil of turpentine; this factitious product however, is to be distinguished from native camphor in not being soluble in weak nitric acid, and also in not being precipitated by water from its solution in strong nitric acid.

† It is a curious fact that the conversion of volatile substances into a gaseous state is always facilitated by the presence of water in the atmosphere; this is strikingly exemplified by the greater rapidity with which limestone is burnt, and reduced to quick lime, in moist weather, and by the assistance which is rendered, in a dry season, by placing a pan of water in the ash-pit. This is one cause of medicines so soon losing their virtues when kept in a humid atmosphere, as on the sea coast.

principle, resembling the essential oils in many of its
habitudes, and it will probably be found hereafter to
be a compound of an essential oil with some vegetable
acid. SOLUBILITY ; water may be said to dissolve
about a nine hundreth part of its weight, or f℥j rather more than gr ½, but its solvent power is considerably increased by the addition of carbonic acid gas ;
camphor is also rendered more soluble by trituration
with magnesia ; it is soluble in an equal weight of
alcohol, but is again separated by the addition of
water ; it is also dissolved by oils, both fixed and
volatile,* especially if their temperature be a little
raised, and by sulphuric and other ethers, but strong
acetic acid may be said to be its most powerful solvent. By repeatedly distilling it with nitric acid it is
converted into *Camphoric acid*, an acid distinguished
by peculiar properties, and composing, with alkalies
and earths, a class of salts called *Camphorates*, but
which do not possess any medicinal value. The alkalies do not produce any effect upon camphor. IN-
COMPATIBLE SUBSTANCES. It is not affected by any
substance with which we can combine it FORMS OF
EXHIBITION. It is preferable in the form of mixture,
since it is very liable in the solid state to excite nausea, and from swimming on the contents of the stomach, to occasion pain at its upper orifice. If a
larger dose be required than that which water can
dissolve, an additional proportion may be suspended
by means of sugar, almonds, egg, or mucilage, for
which purpose three times its weight of gum arabic
is required. Camphor has also the property of uniting
with gum-resins, and of converting them into soft,

* AN ODONTALGIC REMEDY in great repute consists of a solution of
camphor in oil of turpentine, a fluidounce of which will dissolve two
drachms.

and uniform masses; hence they may sometimes be conveniently applied for diffusing it in water; it may be formed into pill masses by stiff mucilage, fœtid gums, or by a confection. MEDICINAL USE. In moderate doses it exhilarates without raising the pulse, and gives a tendency to diaphoresis ; and under certain conditions of the body, when opium fails, it promotes sleep. As its effects are transient, its dose should be repeated at short intervals. FORMULÆ 10, 48, 53, 59, 103, 109, 112, 115, 119, 125. Camphor is said to correct the bad effects of opium, mezereon, lyttæ, and the drastic purgatives, and diuretics. DOSE gr. ij to ℈j. In excessive doses it occasions anxiety, vomiting, syncope, and delirium ; these violent effects are best counteracted by opium. OFFICINAL PREPARATIONS. *Mistura Camphoræ.* L.D. *Emulsio Camphorata.* E. *Spiritus Camphoræ* L.E.D. *Tinctura Camphoræ comp:* L.E.D. *Acidum Acetosum Camphoratum.* E.D. *Linimentum Camphoræ.* L.E.D. *Liniment: Camphoræ comp:* L. *Liniment: Saponis. (d)* L.E.D.* ADULTERATIONS. It has been stated that pure camphor may be known by placing it upon hot bread, when it will turn moist, whereas an adulterated specimen becomes dry—with what can it be adulterated?

CANELLÆ CORTEX. L.E.D. (*Canella Alba*)
(*Cortex*)

Canella Bark.

Wild Cinnamon.

QUALITIES. *Form.* It occurs in quilled and flat pieces; the former are of a whitish yellow colour, considerably thicker than cinnamon, the latter, which are probably the bark of the larger branches, or of

---

* For the different empirical Liniments, see Article SOAP.

the stem of the tree, are yellow on the outside, and pale brown within. *Odour* resembling that of cloves. *Taste* warm, pungent, and slightly bitter. CHEMICAL COMPOSITION. Its virtues depend upon an essential oil, and a bitter resin. SOLUBILITY. Water extracts only the bitterness, but proof spirit both the bitterness and aroma. MEDICAL USES. As a warm stimulant to the stomach, and as a corrigent to other medicines. In America it is considered as a powerful antiscorbutic. DOSE of the powdered bark gr x to ʒss. OFFICINAL PREP. *Tinc. Gentian. comp. (a, c)* E. *Vinum Aloes, (a, c)* L. D. *Pulv. Aloes cum canella, (c)* D.

CAPSICI BACCÆ. L. E. D.   (Capsicum)
  Berries of the Capsicum.   (Annuum.)

QUALITIES. *Form.* Pods, long, pointed and pendulous; *Colour,* when ripe, a bright orange red. *Odour* aromatic and pungent. *Taste* extremely acrimonious and fiery. SOLUBILITY. Its qualities are partially extracted by water, but more completely by ether and spirit. CHEMICAL COMPOSITION. Cinchonin, a resin in which its acrimony appears to reside, and mucilage. INCOMPATIBLE SUBSTANCES. The infusions of capsicum are disturbed by *Infusion of Galls; Nitrate of Silver; Oxy-muriate of Mercury; Acetate of Lead; the Sulphates of Iron, Copper and Zinc; Ammonia, Carbonate of Potass and Alum,* but not by sulphuric, nitric, or muriatic acid. MEDICAL USES. It is a most powerful stimulant to the stomach, and is unaccompanied with any narcotic effect; as a gargle in cynanche maligna, and in relaxed states of the throat it furnishes a valuable remedy; combined with purgatives, it proves serviceable in dyspepsia; *see*

Formula 16. FORMS OF EXHIBITION. It may be given, made into pills with crumb of bread, or in the form of tincture, diluted with water; for the purpose of a gargle, a simple infusion in the proportion of gr j to f℥j of boiling water, or f℥vj of the tincture to f℥viij of the *Infusum Rosæ*, may be directed. DOSE, of the substance grvj to x, of the tincture f℥j to f℥ij in an aqueous vehicle. OFF: PREP: *Tinct: Capsici.* L. D.

Cayenne Pepper is an indiscriminate mixture of the powder of the dried pods of several species of capsicum, but especially of the Capsicum *baccatum*, (Bird pepper.)

ADULTERATIONS. Cayenne pepper is generally mixed with *muriate of soda*, which disposes it to deliquesce. *Red Lead* may be detected by digesting it in acetic acid, and adding to the solution sulphuret of ammonia, which will produce, if any lead be present, a dark coloured precipitate; or the fraud may be discovered by boiling some of the suspected pepper in vinegar, and after filtering the solution adding to it sulphate of soda, when a white precipitate will be formed, which, after being dried and exposed to heat, and mixed with a little charcoal, will yield a metallic globule of lead.

CARBO LIGNI. L. E. D. *Charcoal.*

QUALITIES. It is a black, inodorous, insipid, brittle substance; when newly prepared it possesses the property of absorbing very considerable quantities of the different gases; it is also capable of destroying the smell and taste of a variety of vegetable and animal substances, especially of mucilages, oils, and of matter in which *extractive* abounds. The use of charring the interior of water casks, and of wrapping charcoal in cloths that have acquired a bad smell, depends upon this property; for the same reason it furnishes a very excellent tooth powder,* for which purpose, that which is obtained from the shell of the cocoa nut is to be preferred. None of the fluid menstrua with which we are acquainted have any action whatever as solvents upon carbon.† MEDICAL USES. It is antiseptic, and has been administered, internally, to correct the putrid eructations which sometimes attend dyspepsia, but in order to produce this effect it should be newly prepared, or such as has been preserved from the access of air, for it operates by absorbing the putrid gas, as well as by checking the decomposition of the undigested element. DOSE, grs x to ʒj. It has been lately asserted to possess powers as an antidote to arsenic; if this be true, its action can only be mechanical, by absorbing, like a sponge, the arsenical solution; and thereby defending the coats of the stomach from its virulence.‡ Charcoal, when mixed with boiled bread, forms a very valuable poultice for foul and gangrenous sores.

Charcoal is prepared for the purposes of medicine and the arts, from a variety of substances, viz.

* LARDNER'S PREPARED CHARCOAL consists of cretaceous powder, or chalk finely powdered, rendered grey by the addition of charcoal, or ivory black.

† A CONCENTRATED SOLUTION OF CHARCOAL is sold for cleaning the teeth.

‡ I apprehend that this property will explain how charcoal acts as a test for arsenic, which was discovered by Mr. Thomson. See London Dispensatory, second edition, page 58. "Into the suspected solution stir a moderate quantity of charcoal powder; allow it to settle, then pour off the supernatant liquid, and when the powder which remains is dry, sprinkle some of it on a hot poker, when, if the solution contained arsenic, the odour of garlic will be rendered sensible,

Burnt Sponge, *Spongia Usta.* L. Consists of charcoal, with portions of phosphate, and carbonate of lime, and subcarbonate of soda; it has been highly commended in bronchocele and scrophulous complaints, in the form of an electuary, or in that of a lozenge.

Vegetable Æthiops. *Pulvis Quercus marinæ.* From the *fucus vesiculosus,* or bladder wrack, used as the preceding.

Ivory Black. *Ebur ustum.* From ivory shavings burned; used as a dentrifice and a pigment, but bone black is usually sold for it.

Lamp Black. *Fuligo Lampadum.* By burning esinous bodies, as the refuse of pitch, in furnaces of a peculiar construction.

Wood Soot. *Fuligo ligni,* collected from chimnies under which wood is burnt. It contains sulphate of ammonia, which imparts to it its characteristic bitterness. It has been considered antispasmodic, and a tincture was formerly prepared of it.

CARDAMOMI SEMINA. L. D. (Elettaria Cardamomum.)
Amomum Repens. E. *Cardamom Seeds.*

Qualities. *Odour,* aromatic and agreeable; *Taste,* warm and pungent, but, unlike the peppers, they do not immoderately heat the stomach. Solubility. Water, alcohol and æther extract their virtues; the two latter most completely, and the result is transparent, whereas the watery infusion is turbid, and mucilaginous. Chemical Composition. Fecula, mucilage, and essential oil. Medical Uses. They are carminative and stomachic, and prove grateful

adjuncts to bitter infusions; they are principally em-
ployed to give warmth to other remedies. Dose of
the powder, gr vj to ℈j. Officinal Prep: *Extract:
Colocynth: comp: (c)* L.D. *Tinct: Cardamomi,* L.E.D.
Tinct: Cardamom: comp: L. D. *Tinct: Cinnamomi,
co. (a)* L. E. *Tinct. Gentian,* co. *(d)* L. *Tinct.
Rhei, (c)* L. E. D. *Tinct. Rhei cum Aloe, (c)* E.
Tinct. Sennœ, (c) L. D. *Spir. Ether. Aromat. (a)*
L. *Vinum Aloes socot, (c)* E. *Confect. Aromat. (a)*
L. *Pulv. Cinnamom co. (a)* L. E. D. *Pil. Scillilicœ,
(d)* E. *Infus. Sennœ,* D *(c)*.

Cardamom seeds should be kept within their husks,
or their virtues will soon be considerably impaired;
they are frequently mixed with *grains of paradise,*
which are much hotter and more spicy, and less aromatic in their flavour.

CARICÆ FRUCTUS. L.D. Fici Caricæ Fructus, E.

The preserved Fruit of the Fig.

Qualities of the dried fig are too well known to
require description. The fig consists almost entirely
of mucilage and sugar. Uses. It has been already
stated that the most ancient cataplasm on record was
made of figs, (2 Kings chap. xx. 7.) they are employed
medicinally in many demulcent decoctions, as *Decoctum Hordei comp.* L. D. They are gently aperient;
it is curious to learn that they constituted the chief
part of the food of the ancient Athletœ.

CARYOPHYLLI. L.

(Eugenia Caryophyllata. *The unopened flowers dried.*)
Caryophilli Aromatici Germen, E.
Caryophylli aromat. Calyx, D.

Cloves.

Cloves are the unexpanded flowers, or flower-buds, of the clove tree, which are first obtained when the tree is six years old; they are gathered in October and November, before they open, and when are they still green, and are dried in the sun, after having been exposed to smoke, at a heat of 120°, till they assume a brown hue. It is a curious fact that the flowers when fully developed are quite inodorous, and that the real fruit is not in the least aromatic. QUALITIES. *Form,* that of a nail, consisting of a globular head, formed of the four petals of the corrolla, and four leaves of the calyx not yet expanded; and a germen situated below nearly cylindrical, and scarcely an inch in length. *Odour,* strong, fragrant, and aromatic. *Taste,* acrid, aromatic and permanent.

SOLUBILITY. Water extracts their odour, but little of their taste; alcohol and ether take up both completely. MEDICAL USES. They are more stimulant than any of the other aromatics; they are sometimes given alone, but more generally as a corrigent to other medicines. OFFICINAL PREP. *Infusum Caryophyllorum,* L. *Spir. Lavand. co.* D. FRAUDS. The Dutch frequently mix the best cloves with those from which the oil has been drawn.

CARYOPHYLLI OLEUM. This essential oil, in consequence of the resinous matter which it holds in solution, has a specific gravity of 1.020, and consequently sinks in water. When the oil has a hot fiery

taste, and a great depth of colour, it is adulterated.
It is imported from the spice islands. On account of
its stimulant properties, it is added to griping extracts,
or used as a local application in the tooth ache.
Vauquelin obtained from the leaves of the *Agatho-
phyllum ravensara* an essential oil, in every respect
similar to that of cloves.

CASCARILLÆ CORTEX. L. D. (Croton Cascarilla.)

Croton Eleutheria E.

Cascarilla Bark.

Qualities. *Form,* curled pieces, or rolled up
into short quills; its fracture is smooth and close, of
a dark brown colour; *Odour* light and agreeable;
when burning, it emits a smell resembling that of
musk, which at once distinguishes it from all other
barks *Taste* moderately bitter, with some aromatic
warmth. Chemical Composition. Mucilage, extractive, resin, volatile oil, and a large proportion of
woody fibre. Solubility. Its active constituents
are partially extracted by alcohol and water, and
completely by proof spirit. Medical Uses. Carminative and tonic; it is an excellent adjunct to
cinchona, rendering it by its aromatic qualities, more
agreeable to the stomach, and increasing its powers.
It is valuable in dyspepsia, and flatulent cholic, in
dysentery and diarrhœa, and in the gangrenous thrush
peculiar to children. Forms of Exhibition. It is
most efficacious in substance; it may however be
given in the form of infusion, or tincture. Decoction
dissipates its aromatic principle; the extract therefore
merely acts as a simple bitter. (*Formulæ* 96, 99.)

Dose of the powder, grs xij to ʒss. Officinal
Preparations. *Infus. Cascarill.* L. *Tinc. Cascarill.*
L. D. *Extract. Cascarill.* D.

CASSIÆ PULPA. L. E. D. (Cassia Fistula,)
  Cassia Pulp.   (*Lomentorum Pulpa.*)

The fruit is a cylindrical pod, scarcely an inch in
diameter, but a foot or more in length; the exterior
is a hard brown bark; the interior is divided into
numerous transverse cells, each of which contains an
oval seed, imbedded in a soft black pulp. Qualities.
Odour faint and rather sickly. *Taste* sweet and mucilaginous. Solubility. Nearly the whole of the
pulp is dissolved by water, partially by alcohol and
sulphuric ether. Chemical Composition. Sugar,
gelatine, gluten, gum, and a small portion of resin,
extractive, and some colouring matter. Uses. It is
gently laxative, and is adapted for children and very
delicate women, but it should be always given in
combination with manna, or some other laxative, or
it is apt to induce nausea, flatulence and griping.
Officinal Preparations. *Confectio Sennæ* L.
There are two kinds of this drug in the market; that
from the West Indies, the pods of which are generally
large, rough, thick rinded, and contain a nauseous
pulp; and that from the East Indies, which is to be
preferred, and which is distinguished by smaller and
smoother pods, and by their containing a much blacker
pulp. The pulp ought not to have a harsh flavour,
which arises from the fruit having been gathered
before it was ripe, nor ought it to be sour, which it is
very apt to become upon keeping.

---

* Essence of Coffee. The Cassia pulp is said to form the basis
of this article.

CASTOREUM, L. E. D. (Castor Fiber, (Roscicus))
         Castor.   (*Concretum sui generis.*)

This substance is secreted by the beaver, in bags
near the rectum.* QUALITIES. *Odour,* strong and
aromatic. *Taste* bitter, sub-acrid, and nauseous. *Colour*
reddish brown. CHEMICAL COMPOSITION. Volatile
oil, resin, mucilage, extractive, iron, and small portions
of the carbonates of potass, lime and ammonia. Lau-
gier also detected the presence of benzoic acid.
SOLUBILITY. Its active matter is dissolved by alcohol,
proof spirit, and partially by water ; the tincture made
with alcohol is the least nauseous, and the most efficacious; the spirit of ammonia is also an excellent
menstruum, and in many cases improves its virtues.
FORMS OF EXHIBITION. It may be given in substance, as a bolus, or in the form of tincture, but its
exhibition in the form of extract or decoction is chemically incorrect. DOSE, grs x to ℈j, and in clysters
to ℥j. MEDICAL USES. It is antispasmodic, and
seems to act more particularly on the uterine system.
It certainly proves beneficial as an adjunct to antihysteric combinations. OFFICINAL PREF. Tinct.
Castorei.† L. E. D. ADULTERATIONS. It is sometimes counterfeited by a mixture of dried blood, gum
ammoniacum, and a little real castor, stuffed into the
scrotum of a goat; the fraud is detected by comparing
the smell and taste with those of real castor ; and by
the deficiency of the sebaceous follicles, which are
always attached to genuine specimens. There are
two kinds in the market, the Russian, and Canadian,

* The ancients erroneously considered them as the testicles of the
beaver.

† BATEMAN's PECTORAL DROPS consist principally of the Tincture
of Castor, with portions of camphor and opium, flavoured by anise
seeds, and coloured by cochineal.

the former however, which is the best, has become
extremely scarce; it may be distinguished from the
latter, by being larger, rounder, heavier, and less corrugated on the outside.

CATAPLASMATA. *Poultices.*

Cataplasms are generally extemporaneous preparations, and are calculated to fulfil several different indications, viz. 1, as STIMULANTS. *Cataplasma Sinapis,*
L. D. 2, ANTISEPTICS. *Cataplasma Fermenti.* L.
A powerfully antiseptic cataplasm may be made by
stirring finely powdered charcoal into a common
linseed meal poultice. 3, SEDATIVES. The most
efficient of which are composed of *Conium, Digitalis*
or *Hyoscyamus.* 4, EMOLLIENTS. For which purpose
the common farinaceous poultice is the most eligible.
The consistence of a cataplasm ought to be sufficiently
tenacious to prevent its spreading farther than is
designed, and yet not so hard as to occasion any
mechanical irritation.

Every substance, whether liquid or solid, may
become an ingredient in this species of composition;
in adapting them however for this purpose, some
share of chemical knowledge will be found necessary,
notwithstanding that the direction of them is more
generally entrusted to the nurse than to the medical
practitioner. For example, care must be taken not
to reduce into pulp, by decoction, substances that
contain volatile principles; and in preparing active
liquids to be added to linseed meal, so as to produce
a proper consistence, we must always be directed by
their chemical composition.

CATECHU EXTRACTUM, L. E. D.

(Acacia Catechu, *Extractum.*) Catechu. olim.

Terra Japonica.   Japan Earth.

Qualities. There are two varieties of catechu
in the market, tne one of a light yellowish, the other
of a chocolate colour; they differ only in the latter
having a more austere and bitter taste. Chemical
Composition. Tannin, gallic acid, a peculiar extractive matter, mucilage, and earthy impurities.
Solubility. It is almost totally dissolved both by
water and spirit. Incompatible Substances. Its
astringency is destroyed by alkaline salts; and precipitates are produced by metallic salts, especially by
those of iron. Medical Uses. It is a most valuable astringent. Forms of Exhibition. In infusion, tincture, or powder. *(Form. 88, 90.)* In the
form of a lozenge, from its gradual solution, it may
be very advantageously applied in relaxed states of
the uvula and fauces; I have found this remedy successful in cases where the *sulphate of zinc* was inefficient. From its great astringency it also forms an
excellent dentrifice, especially when the gums are
spongy; for this purpose I have employed equal parts
of powdered catechu, and peruvian bark, with one
fourth the quantity of the powder of myrrh. Dose, grs.
x to Ʒj. Officinal Prep. *Infus. Catechu. Tinct.
Catechu.* L. E. D. *Electuarium Mimosæ Catechu,* E.D.

CERA. L. E. D. *Wax.*

It is admitted into the list of the Materia Medica
under two forms, viz.

1. CERA FLAVA. *Yellow, or Unbleached Wax.*

QUALITIES. *Odour* faintly honey like; it is brittle, yet soft; when chewed, it does not, if pure, adhere to the teeth; it melts at 142°, and burns entirely away. CHEMICAL COMPOSITION. It is the honeycomb of the bee, melted with boiling water, pressed through cloth bags, and ultimately cast into round cakes for the market. Whether it be an animal product, or a vegetable substance merely collected by the bee, has been a question of dispute; the former opinion is probably correct, although wax is certainly produced as a secretion by many plants. The yellow wax contains a portion of pollen which imparts to it its colour, and increases its fusibility. SOLUBILITY. It is insoluble in water, and in cold alcohol, or ether, but it is soluble in boiling alcohol and ether, in fixed oils, and in alkalies. USES. It is chiefly employed in the composition of external applications. ADULTERATIONS. *Earth* or *peas-meal*, may be suspected when the cake is very brittle, and the colour inclines to grey; *Resin* is detected by putting it in cold alcohol, which will dissolve the resinous part without acting on the wax. *Tallow* is discovered by the greater softness and unctuosity of the cake, and by its suffocating smell when melted; when this latter substance is employed, turmeric is added to disguise its paleness.

2. CERA ALBA. *White, Bleached, or Virgin's Wax.*

QUALITIES. This substance differs only from the former, in being colourless, harder, heavier, and less fusible. USES. It is said to be demulcent, and very useful in dysentery, but it is rarely used. FORMS OF EXHIBITION. It may be formed into a mixture by melting it with one third of its weight of soap, and then gradually adding to it any mucilaginous liquid. ADULTERATIONS. *White lead* may be detected, by

melting the wax in water, when the oxide will fall to
the bottom of the vessel; *tallow* may be suspected,
when the cake wants its usual translucency.

CERATA, L. E.   Cerates.

These compositions are characterized by a degree
of consistence, intermediate between that of plasters,
and that of ointments.   As this consistence is derived
from the wax which they contain, they very properly
derive from it the generic appellation of cerates.
OFFICINAL PREP.   *Ceratum Simplex*, L.   *Cerat.
Calaminæ*. L.   *(C. Carbonatis Zinci Impuri. E.   Unguent. Calaminare. D.)*   These preparations have
been long known under the name of *Turner's Cerate ;*
they form the basis of many extemporaneous cerates,
in some of which, nitric oxide of mercury, and in
others, the liquor of acetate of lead, are introduced.
Cerat. Cetacei. L.   *(C. Simplex*. E.)   *Cerat. Lyttæ*, L.
(Spermaceti cerate six, powdered flies one part.) As it
is intended to promote a purulent discharge from a
blistered surface, it may be reduced in strength according to circumstances.   *Cerat. Plumbi Superacetatis*. L.
Cerat. Plumbi comp. L.   This is *Goulard's* Cerate.
Cerat Resinæ L.   *(Unguent. Resinosum. E.   Unguent.
Resinæ albæ. D.)   Cerat. Sabinæ*. L.   *(Ung. Sabinæ*. D.)
It is intended to keep up a purulent discharge from a
blistered surface; in practice however it is often found
to fail, from the difficulty of obtaining it good, since
the acrid principle of the plant is injured by long
boiling, and by being previously dried; the ointment
also loses its virtues by exposure to the air.   There
are besides many magistral,* or extemporaneous

---

* KIRKLAND's NEUTRAL CERATE.   Is formed by melting together
℥viij of Lead Plaster with f℥iv of olive oil, into which are to be stirred
℥iv of prepared chalk; when the mixture is sufficiently cooled, f℥iv of
acetic acid, and ℈iij of pulverized super-acetate of lead are to be added,
and the whole is to be stirred, until nearly cold.

cerates of great value in surgical practice, for an account of which, consult a useful little manual, entitled " *Pharmacopœia Chirurgica.*"

CETACEUM. L. ⎛Physeter Macrocephalus,⎞
Spermaceti. E. D. ⎝ *Concretum sui generis.* ⎠

Spermaceti.

QUALITIES. *Form,* flakes, which are unctuous, friable, and white. *Odour* and *taste* scarcely perceptible. *Sp. Grav.* 9.433. It melts at 112°. CHEMICAL COMPOSITION. It is a peculiar modification of fatty matter. SOLUBILITY. It is insoluble.in water, and cold alcohol, but soluble in hot alcohol, ether, and oil of turpentine, but it concretes again as the fluids cool ; in the fixed oils it is completely soluble. The alkaline carbonates do not affect it, but it is partially dissolved in the pure alkalies, and with hot ammonia it forms an emulsion which is not decomposed on cooling. USES. It is demulcent and emollient, but it possesses no advantages over the bland oils. FORMS OF EXHIBITION. It may be suspended in water by means of mucilage, or yolk of egg. (*Formulæ* 76, 78, 79.) OFFICINAL PREP. *Ceratum Simplex.* E. *Ceratum Cetacei* L. *Unguent. Cetacei.* L. D. From exposure to hot air, it becomes rancid ; but it may be again purified, by being washed in a warm solution of potass.

CINCHONA. L. E. D. *Bark. Peruvian Bark.*
Jesuit's Bark.

Notwithstanding the labours of the Spanish botanists, the history of this important genus is still in-

M 2

volved in considerable perplexity, and owing to the mixture of the barks of several species,* and their importation into Europe under one common name, it is extremely difficult to reconcile the contradictory opinions which exist upon the subject, nor indeed would such an investigation be consistent with the plan and objects of this work. Under the trivial name *officinalis*, Linnæus confounded no less than four distinct species of chinchona, and under the same denomination the British Pharmacopœias, for a long period, placed as varieties the three barks known in the shops; this error indeed is still maintained in the Dublin Pharmacopœia, but the London and Edinburgh colleges have at length adopted the arrangement of Mutis, a celebrated botanist, who has resided in South America, and held the official situation of Director of the exportation of bark for nearly forty years, viz.

CINCHONÆ CORDIFOLIÆ† CORTEX. L. E. Cortex Peruvianus. D. Heart-leaved Cinchona Bark, commonly called *Yellow* bark.

CINCHONÆ LANCIFOLIÆ CORTEX. L. E. Cortex Peruvianus. D. Lance-leaved Cinchona Bark, common *Quilled* bark.—*Pale* bark.

CINCHONÆ OBLONGIFOLIÆ CORTEX. L. E. Cortex Peruvianus. D. Oblong-leaved Cinchona Bark, called *Red* bark.

* There are no less than twenty-five distinct species of Cinchona, independent of any additions which we may owe to the zeal of Humboldt and Bonpland; and Mr. A. T. Thomson, in his London Dispensatory states that in a large collection of dried specimens, of the genus Cinchona, in his possession, collected in 1805, both near Loxa and Santa Fé, he finds many species which are not mentioned in the works of any Spanish botanist.

† Mr. A. T. Thomson regards this as the species which yields the common *pale* bark of the shops, and states, upon the authority of Mutis and Zea, that the Cinchona *Lancifolia* yields the *Yellow* bark.

QUALITIES. The *odour* and *taste* of these three species are essentially the same, although they differ in intensity. They are all bitter, sub-astringent and aromatic, but the flavour of the *Yellow* bark is incomparably the most bitter, although less austere and astringent, whilst the red bark has a taste much less bitter, but more austere and nauseous than either of the other species. CHEMICAL COMPOSITION. No vegetable substance has been more frequently, or more ably submitted to analysis, and an attempt has even been made by Vauquelin, to establish a classification upon the different effects which reagents produce upon the different kinds of bark; but the intermixture of the barks, as they occur in commerce, throws insuperable obstacles in all our researches, and we are compelled to rest satisfied with general results. The following may be stated as the known constituents of cinchona. Cinchonin, (a peculiar vegetable principle characterized by its power of producing a precipitate with the infusion of nut-galls,) resin, extractive, gluten, tannin, a small portion of volatile oil, and some salts, whose base is lime, one of which is found only in *yellow* bark, and has been discovered to contain a peculiar vegetable acid, which Vauquelin denominated *kinic*, but which Dr. Duncan more properly calls *cinchonic* acid. In the *red* bark, Fourcroy detected also a portion of citric acid, some muriate of ammonia, and muriate of lime. Upon which of these principles the tonic and febrifuge virtues of bark depend, has not been satisfactorily explained. Deschamps attributes them to cinchonate of lime, and asserts that two doses of thirty-six grains each will cure any intermittent.* Westring considers

* ESSENTIAL SALT OF BARK. The preparation, sold under this empirical title, is an extract prepared by macerating the bruised substance of bark in cold water, and submitting the infusion to a very slow evaporation.

tannin as the active constituent, whilst M. Seguin
assigns all its virtues to the principle which precipitates
tannin, and which he mistook for gelatine. Fabroni
however concludes from his experiments that the
febrifuge property does not belong essentially and
individually to the astringent, the bitter, or any other
soluble principle, since the quantity of these encreases
by protracted ebullition, whilst the virtues of the
decoction evidently decrease. This argument however will not go far, when we learn that by long
boiling, important chemical changes are produced in
the liquid. In the midst of these difficulties, experience
interposes her aid, and demonstrates that the virtues
of bark must depend upon the combination of all its
principles, for no preparation however carefully made,
or scientifically combined, will equal, in efficacy, bark
in the state of powder; even the ligneous fibre,
which the chemist pronounces to be inert and useless,
may produce its share of benefit, by modifying the
solubility of the other ingredients, or by performing
some mechanical duty which we are at present unable
to appreciate. SOLUBILITY. Cold water extracts
its bitter taste, with some share of its odour; when
assisted by a moderate heat, the infusion is stronger,
but becomes turbid as it cools; the infusion cannot
be kept, even for a short time, without undergoing
decomposition, and being spoiled ; wine also extracts
the virtues of bark, and it is prevented by this substance from becoming sour, a fact which probably
depends upon the avidity with which bark combines
with oxygen, and which seems to throw some light
upon the cause of its antiseptic virtues. The colouring matter of wine is precipitated by bark, as it is by
charcoal, in the course of a few days. By decoction
the active matter of cinchona is, in a great degree,

extracted, but if the process be protracted beyond
eight or ten minutes, it undergoes a very important
chemical change ; it combines with oxygen, becomes
insoluble, and medicinally considered, it is rendered
inert; on this account, the extract is necessarily a
very inefficient preparation ; if we attempt to redis-
solve it, not more than one half is soluble in water.
Vinegar is a less powerful solvent than water; the
active matter of bark is rendered more soluble by the
addition of mineral acids, and by the earths and alkalies, these latter bodies deepen its colour ; *lime water*
has been recommended as a solvent, and it affords an
excellent form for children and dyspeptic patients;
for the same reason we obtain a stronger and perhaps
a more efficient preparation, by triturating it with
magnesia, previous to the process of infusion. Alcohol
is a very powerful solvent, but the great activity of
this menstruum so limits its dose that we are prevented
from exhibiting a sufficient quantity of the bark in
the form of tincture; it furnishes however an excellent
adjunct to other preparations.

INCOMPATIBLE SUBSTANCES. Precipitates are
produced by the *salts of iron, sulphate of zinc, nitrate
of silver, oxymuriate of mercury, tartarized antimony,
solutions of arsenic, &c.* Any considerable portion of
a tincture produces also a precipitation, which sometimes does not immediately take place, and the medicinal value of the bark is probably not impaired by
it ; as the infusions of *nut galls* and some other vegetable astringents precipitate the cinchonin from bark,
it becomes a question how far such liquids are medicinally compatible; saline additions, as *alum, muriate
of ammonia*, &c. have been frequently proposed, but
in many of such mixtures decompositions arise, which
must deceive us with regard to the expected effects.

FORMS OF EXHIBITION. No form is so efficient as that of powder, but where the stomach rejects it, it must be administered in *infusion* or *decoction;* with the addition of its *tincture.* (Formulæ 92, 95, 96, 97.) DOSE of the powder, gr. v to ʒij or more, of the infusion or decoction f℥ij. MEDICAL USES. It is powerfully tonic and antiseptic; it was introduced into practice for curing intermittent fevers, but since that period, it has been generally used in diseases of debility, in fevers of the typhoid type, and in gangrene. It was first conjectured to be useful in gout, by Sydenham; in acute rheumatism Dr. Haygarth has strongly recommended its exhibition : when however it is used in these diseases, the greatest attention ought to be paid to the state of the bowels, and purgatives should be occasionally interposed. OFFICINAL PREP. *Infus. Cinchonæ,* L. E. D. *Decoct. Cinchon.* L. E. D. *Extractum Cinchon.* L. E. *Extract. Cinchonæ resinosum.* L. D. *Tinct. Cinchonæ,* L. E. D. *Tinct. Cinchonæ comp.* L. E. D. ADULTERATIONS. The frauds committed under this head are most extensive; it is not only mixed with inferior barks, but frequently with genuine bark, the active constituents of which have been entirely extracted by decoction with water. In selecting cinchona bark, the following precautions may be useful, it should be dense, heavy and dry, not musty, nor spoiled by moisture; a decoction made of it should have a reddish colour when warm; but when cold, become paler, and deposit a brownish red sediment. When the bark is of a dark *colour* between red and yellow, it is either of a bad species, or it has not been well preserved. Its *taste* should be bitter, but not nauseous, nor very astringent, with a slight agreeable acidity; when chewed, it should not appear in threads, nor of much length ; the *odour* is not very strong, but when bark has been well cured, it is always perceptible, and the stronger it is, provided it be pleasant, the better may the bark be considered. In order to give bark the form of *quill*, the bark gatherers not unfrequently call in the aid of artificial heat, by which its virtues are deteriorated ; the fraud is detected by the colour being much darker, and upon splitting the bark, by the inside exhibiting stripes of a whitish sickly hue. In the form of powder, cinchona is always found more or less adulterated. During a late official inspection of the shops of apothecaries and druggists, the Censors repeatedly met with powdered cinchona having a harsh metallic taste, quite foreign to that which characterizes good bark. Much has been said of late concerning the probability of the genuine species of the cinchona tree becoming extinct ; in consequence of which some succedaneum has been anxiously sought for ; the bark of the broad leaved willow, *Salix Caprea*, has been proposed for this purpose. Vogel recommends the root of *Geum urbanum avens;* others propose that of the *Datisca canabina.*

The *Cinchona Caribœa* of the Edinburgh Pharmacopœia is said by Dr. Wright, to whom we are indebted for our knowledge of it, to have satisfactorily answered in all cases where the Peruvian bark was indicated.

CINNAMOMI CORTEX. L. E. D. (Laurus Cinnamomum.) *Cinnamon.*

All the qualities of cinnamon depend upon the presence of an *essential oil.* It is principally employed

to cover the taste of nauseous medicines. ADULTER-
ATIONS. It is sometimes intermixed with cinnamon
from which the oil has been drawn; the fraud is
detected by the weakness of the odour and taste of
the specimen; sometimes it is mixed with *cassia*, but
this is soon discovered, for cassia is thick and clumsy,
breaks short, and smooth, and has a remarkably slimy
taste, whereas the fracture of cinnamon is shivery,
and its flavour warm and clean. Cinnamon ought
not to leave a mawkish taste in the mouth, this circumstance denotes an inferior quality: there is an
inferior kind imported into Europe from China,
through the hands of private merchants; this is distinguished by being darker coloured, rougher, denser,
and by breaking shorter; the taste is also harsher,
more pungent, and ligneous, without the sweetness
of the Ceylon cinnamon. DOSE of the cinnamon in
powder is from grs. x to Ʒj. OFFICINAL PREP.
Aqua Cinnamomi, L. E. D. *Spir. Cinnamomi*, L. E. D.
Tinct. Cinnamom. L. E. D. *Tinct. Cinnamom. co.* L.
Pulv. Cinnamom. comp. L. E.

CINNAMOMI OLEUM. It is principally imported
from Ceylon: it has a whitish yellow colour, a pungent burning taste, and the peculiar fine flavour of
cinnamon in a very great degree. It should sink in
water, and be entirely soluble in alcohol. It is one
of the most powerful stimulants which we possess.
DOSE, *m* i to iij, on a lump of sugar.

COCCUS. L. E. (Coccus Cacti.) Coccinella. D.
Cochineal.

It is an insect imported from Mexico, and New
Spain, and has the appearance of a wrinkled berry,
or seed, of a deep mulberry colour, with a white

powder between the wrinkles. Uses. Its medicinal
virtues are now entirely discredited, and it is only
employed for the sake of its colouring matter, for the
purpose of a dye; it was known by the Phœnicians,
and was the *tolu* of the Jews. Its watery solution
is of a violet crimson, its alcoholic of a deep crimson,
and its alkaline of a purple hue; the colour of the
watery infusion is brightened by acids, cream of tartar,
and alum, and at the same time partly precipitated.
Incompatible Substances. The colouring matter
is decomposed by *sulphate of iron, sulphate of zinc,*
and *acetate of lead.* Officinal Prep. *Tinct. Cardamom. comp.* L. D. *Tinct. Cinchon. comp.* L. D.
Tinct. Gentian, comp. E. *Tinct. Cantharid.* D. Adulterations. It is invariably adulterated with pieces
of dough, formed in moulds, and coloured with cochineal. I understand that this fraud gives employment
to a very considerable number of women and children
in this metropolis. A cargo of the counterfeit article
was some time since exported, in order to obtain the
drawback; by throwing a suspected sample into water,
we shall dissolve the spurious ones, and ascertain the
extent of the adulteration.

COLCHICI RADIX. L. E. D. (Colchicum)
                           (Autumnale.)
The *Bulb* of the Meadow Saffron.

Qualities. When recent, it has scarcely any
odour, but its *taste* is bitter, hot and acrid. Chemical
Composition. Its properties reside in a milky juice,
and depend upon an essential oil; it contains also
extractive matter, which, when in solution, undergoes a chemical change, similar, I apprehend, to that
which takes place in the infusions of senna, and it

would appear with similar inconvenience. Sir Everard
Home ascertained that this deposit, in the vinous
infusion, excites nausea and griping, but that it may
be removed without destroying the efficacy of the
medicine. The virtues of this bulb are very variable,
according to the place of growth, and season of the
year. It should be gathered upon the first appearance
of its leaves in spring, for the bulb begins to decay
when the flower expands. In autumn it is quite
inert. It is also necessary to extract the virtues of
the bulb as soon as it is gathered, for although removed from the earth, the developing process of
vegetation continues, and the substance undergoes a
corresponding series of chemical changes, and finally
becomes as inert as if it had remained in the ground.
It is a problem of some importance to discover a
method of destroying the vegetable life of the bulb,
without, at the same time, injuring its virtues, for
I apprehend that a want of attention to the above
precaution frequently renders the vinous infusion inactive. The flower of the *meadow saffron* is very
poisonous to cattle. SOLUBILITY. Vinegar and
wine* are the best menstrua for extracting its active

* EAU MEDICINALE DE HUSSON. After various attempts to discover
the active ingredient of this Parisian remedy, it is at length determined
to be the *colchicum autumnale* which several ancient authors, under the
name of *hermodactyus*, have recommended in the cure of gout, as stated
in the historical preface to this work. The following is the receipt for
preparing this medicine. Take two ounces of the root of *colchicum*, cut
it into slices, macerate it in four fluid-ounces of proof spirit, and filter.
    Dr. WILSON'S TINCTURE FOR THE GOUT. This is merely an infusion
of *colchicum*, as Dr. Williams of Ipswich has satisfactorily shewn. Since
the discovery of colchicum being the active ingredient of the *eau
medicinale*, numerous empirical remedies have started up, containing the
principles of this plant in different forms.
    The expressed juice of the colchicum is used in Alsace to destroy
vermin in the hair: it is very acrid, and excoriates the parts to which
it is applied.

qualities; by decoction its essential oil is dissipated.
MEDICINAL USES. It has been much extolled on the
continent as a remedy in dropsy, especially in hydro-
thorax, and in humoral asthma; its operation however as a diuretic, is less certain than squill. As a
specific in gout its efficacy has been fully ascertained,
it allays pain, and cuts short the paroxysm. INCOM-
PATIBLE SUBSTANCES. In my opinion, acids, and
all oxygenating substances render the vinous infusion
drastic, on the contrary, alkalies render its principles
more soluble, and its operation more mild, but not
less efficacious. Magnesia may judiciously accompany
its exhibition. DOSE of the saturated vinous infusion,
the only form in which its successful operation can
be ensured, fʒss to fʒj, whenever the patient is in
pain. OFFICINAL PREP. *Acetum Colchici.* L.
Oxymel Colchici, D. *Syrupus Colchici Autumnalis*, E.

COLOCYNTHIDIS PULPA. L. E. D.

(Cucumis Colocynthis.)

Colocynth. *Bitter Cucumber.*

QUALITIES. The medullary part of this fruit,
which is alone made use of, is a light, white, spongy
body. *Taste* intensely bitter, and nauseous. *Odour*,
when dry, none. CHEMICAL COMPOSITION. Mucilage, resin, bitter extractive, and some gallic acid.
SOLUBILITY. Alcohol and water alike extract its
virtues, but the active principle resides both in the
portion soluble in water, and in that which is insoluble. MEDICINAL USES. It is a very powerful
drastic cathartic, and was employed by the ancients in
dropsical and lethargic diseases. Many attempts have
been made to mitigate its violence, which is best

effected by triturating it with gummy farinaceous substances, or the oily seeds; the watery decoction or infusion is much less severe, and has been recommended in worm cases, but it is rarely employed, except in combination with other purgatives. Mixed with paste, or other cements, it is used to keep away insects, which it does by its extreme bitterness. Dose, grs. iv to x. INCOMPATIBLE SUBSTANCES. The infusion is disturbed by *acetate*, and *super-acetate of lead; nitrate of silver; sulphate of iron*, and by the *fixed alkalies*. OFFICINAL PREP. *Extract. Colocynth.* L. *Extract. Colocynth. comp.* L. D. *Pil. Aloes cum Colocynth.* E. D. When the fruit is larger than a St. Michael's orange, and has black, acute pointed seeds, it is not good.

CONFECTIONES. L. *Confections.*

Under this title the London College comprehends the *conserves* and *electuaries* of its former Pharmacopœia, and of the present Edinburgh and Dublin Pharmacopœias; but in strict propriety, and for practical convenience, the distinction between *conserves* and *electuaries* ought to have been maintained. Saccharine matter enters into each of these compositions, but in different proportions, and for different objects. In conserves it is intended to preserve the virtues of recent vegetables; in electuaries, to impart convenience of form. See *Electuaria.*

CONFECTIO AMYGDALARUM. L. This preparation affords an expeditious mode of preparing the almond emulsion; it should be used in the proportion of a drachm to each fluid ounce of distilled water.

Confectio Aromatica. L. *Electuarium Aromaticum.* E. D. This is a very useful combination of
various aromatics, to which the London and Dublin
colleges have added a *carbonate of lime;* this circumstance makes the preparation a judicious constituent
for the exhibition of active salts, liable to be invalidated by the presence of acid in the stomach, but, at
the same time, it renders it incompatible with *acids,
antimonial wine,* &c. These observations do not, of
course, extend to the *aromatic electuary* of the Edinburgh pharmacopœia.

Confectio Opii. L. *Electuarium Opiatum.* E.
This is a combination of aromatics, with opium, intended as a substitute for the *Mithridate,* and *Theriaca*
of the old pharmacopœias. It is highly useful in
flatulent cholic, and diarrhœa, and in all cases where
a stimulant narcotic is indicated. One grain of opium
is contained in grs. 36 of the London, and in grs. 43
of the Edinburgh preparation.

Confectio Rosæ Caninæ, olim *Conserva Cynos-
bati.* Its acidity depends upon uncombined citric
acid, a circumstance which it is essential to remember
when we direct its use in combination. The hip, or
fruit of this plant, beat up with sugar, and mixed
with wine, is a very acceptable treat in the north of
Europe.

Confectio Rosæ Gallicæ. *Confection of the
Red Rose.* Principally used as a vehicle for more
active medicines.

Confectio Scammoneæ. L. D. It is a stimulating
cathartic, and may be given in the dose of ʒss to ʒj.

Confectio Sennæ. L. E. D. olim *Electuarium
Lenitivum.* It is gently laxative, and is an excellent
vehicle for the exhibition of more powerful cathartics.
(*Form.* 12.) When properly made, it is an elegant

preparation, not apt to ferment, nor to become acescent; the directions of the pharmacopœia are however rarely followed. Jalap blackened with walnut liquor, is frequently substituted for the more expensive article cassia; and the great bulk of it, sold in London, is little else than prunes, figs, and jalap. I understand that a considerable quantity is also manufactured in Staffordshire, into which unsound and spoilt apples enter as a principal ingredient. The preparation sold at Apothecaries Hall is certainly unique in excellence. Dose ʒij or more.

The above are the principal confections which are employed in modern practice, for, happily, the shops are at length disencumbered of those numerous insignificant conserves, unknown to the ancients, but which were ushered into use by the Arabian physicians, and which continued for so many years to disgrace our dispensatories, and to embarrass our practice. The French in their new Codex Medicamentarius, have limited their electuaries to a number not exceeding nine; they have however made up in complexity for deficiency in number; the *Electuarium de croco*, which is intended to answer the same ends as our confectio aromatica, has no less than twelve ingredients, although the force of the combination depends entirely upon carbonate of lime, cinnamon, and saffron, and so it is with the rest.

CONII FOLIA. L. E. (Conium) Cicuta. D.
  Hemlock.   (Maculatum.)

QUALITIES. The leaves when properly dried, have a strong, and narcotic odour, and a slightly bitter and nauseous taste; the fresh leaves contain not only the narcotic, but also the acrid principle;

by exsiccation, the latter is nearly lost, but the former undergoes no change; the medicinal properties of the leaves are therefore improved by the operation of drying. Chemical Composition. The medicinal activity of the plant resides in a resinous element, which may be obtained in an insulated form, by evaporating an ethereal tincture, made with the leaves, on the surface of water; it has a rich dark green colour, and contains the peculiar odour, and taste of hemlock, in perfection; half a grain, when taken, will produce vertigo and head-ache. It may be distinguished by the name of *Conein*. The watery extract of this plant can therefore possess but little power, a fact which Orfila has fully established by experiment. Solubility. Alcohol and ether extract its virtues. Incompatible Substances. Its energies are greatly diminished by vegetable acids; hence vinegar is its best antidote. Medical Uses. It is a powerful sedative, and has been deservedly commended for its powers in allaying morbid irritability : according to my own experience, in well directed doses, it is by far the most efficacious of all palliatives, for quieting pulmonary irritation. It has been extolled also in the cure of schirrus and cancer, and it will, without doubt, prove in such cases, a valuable resource, from its sedative influence. Forms of Exhibition. The dried leaves, powdered, and made into pills, *(Form.* 116, 118.) The powder ought to have a fine lively green colour. Dose, grs. iij gradually increased, until some effect is produced. Several different plants have been mistaken for, and employed in the place of hemlock, such as *Cicuta Virosa*, (the water hemlock.) *Æthusa Cynapium*, *Caucalis anthriscus*, and several species of *Chærophyllum*. Officinal Prep. *Extract. Conii* L. E. D.

N

CONTRAJERVÆ RADIX. L. E.

(Dorstenia Contrajerva Radix.)

Contrajerva Root.

The qualities of this plant are alike extracted by spirit and water; the watery decoction, however, is very mucilaginous; as it contains no astringent matter, the salts of iron do not affect it. DOSE of the powdered root, grs. v to ʒss, but it is rarely used. Has it any virtues? The Spanish Indians have long used it as an antidote to poisons; the Spanish word *contrahiérba* signifies antidote. OFFICINAL PREP. *Pulv. Contrajerv. co. L.*

COPAIBA, L. E. (Copaifera Officinalis.,

Balsamum Copaibæ. D.

Copaiba, Copaiva, or Capivi Balsam.

QUALITIES. *Consistence* that of oil, or a little thicker. *Colour,* pale golden yellow. *Odour,* fragrant and peculiar. *Taste,* aromatic, bitter, and sharp. *Spec. Grav.* 0.950. CHEMICAL COMPOSITION. It is improperly denominated a balsam, for it contains no benzoic acid, but consists of resin, and essential oil. SOLUBILITY. It is insoluble in water, but soluble in ten parts of alcohol, and in expressed and essential oils; with the pure alkalies it forms white saponaceous compounds, which are soluble in water, forming opaque emulsions. MEDICAL USES. Stimulant, diuretic, and laxative; it seems to act more powerfully on the urinary passages than any of the other resinous fluids, hence its use in gleets, and in fluor albus. Its use gives the urine an intensely bitter

taste, but not a violet smell, as the turpentines do.
FORMS OF EXHIBITION. Diffused in soft, or distilled
water, by yolk of egg, or by twice its weight of mucilage, f3ss to every f3j of water forms an elegant mixture, or it may be given dropped on sugar.

ADULTERATIONS. A considerable quantity sold in
London is entirely *factitious*. A curious trial took
place some time since, between the owner of certain
premises that were burnt down, and the Governors
of the Sun Fire Office, in consequence of the latter
refusing to indemnify the proprietor for his loss,
because the fire had been occasioned by his *making*
Balsam of Copaiba. This article is also adulterated
with mastiche and oil; M. Bucholz asserts that if it does
not dissolve in a mixture of four parts of pure alcohol,
and one of rectified ether, we may infer its adulteration;
rape oil is also frequently mixed with it, in which
case, if dropped into water, the drops will not retain
their spherical form, as they invariably will, if pure.

CORNUA. L. E. D. (Cervus Elaphas.)

Stag's, or Hart's Horn.

The horns of the stag differ only from bone, in containing less of the phosphate of lime, and a larger
proportion of gelatine; by boiling, they yield a clear,
transparent, and flavourless jelly, in quantity about
one fourth of the weight of the shavings employed:
to obtain which we should boil 3iv in f3vij of water,
until reduced to f3vj. ADULTERATIONS. This article
is often sophisticated with the shavings of mutton
bone; the fraud is detected by their greater degree of
brittleness. They were formerly so much used for the
preparation of ammonia, that it was commonly called
Salt, or Spirit of Hartshorn.

CRETA PRÆPARATA. L. D.

Carbonas Calcis Preparatus. E.   *Prepared Chalk.*

This is common chalk, the coarser particles of which have been removed by the mechanical operation of washing. It consists of carbonate of lime, with various earthy impurities. The Dublin pharmacopœia directs a chemical process, for obtaining a perfectly pure carbonate, (*Creta Præcipitata,*) but it appears to be an unnecessary refinement. MEDICAL USES. It is antacid and absorbent, on which account it is useful in acidities of the primæ viæ, and in diarrhœas, after the removing of all irritating matters, by previous evacuation. From its absorbent properties, it is a good external application to ulcers discharging a thin ichorous matter. DOSE, grs. x to ℈ij, or more. It is almost unnecessary to state, that it must not be combined with acidulous salts; I have however seen a formula for a powder, intended as an astringent, in which chalk and alum entered as ingredients. OFFICINAL PREP. *Hydrargyrus cum creta*, L. *Pulvis cretæ comp.* L.E. *Pulv. Opiatus*, E. *Mist Cretæ*, L. E. *Trochisci Carbonatis Calcis,* E. *ConfectioAromatica,* L. E.

CROCI STIGMATA, L. E. (Crocus) Crocus, D.
           Saffron.   (Sativus.)

QUALITIES. *Form,* cakes, consisting of the stigmata of the flower, closely pressed together. *Odour,* sweet, penetrating, and diffusive. *Taste,* warm and bitterish. *Colour,* a rich and deep orange red. CHEMICAL COMPOSITION. One hundred parts consist of sixty-two of extractive, the remaining parts are chiefly ligneous fibre, with small portions of resin and essential oil. Bouillon, Lagrange, and Vogel have examined this extractive matter very accurately, and from the circumstance of its watery infusion, assuming different colours when treated with different agents, they have named it *polychroite*. Thus chlorine and light destroy its colour, sulphuric acid changes it to indigo, which gradually becomes lilac, and nitric acid gives it a green hue. Solubility. It yields its colour and active ingredients to water, alcohol, proof spirit, wine, vinegar, and in a less degree to ether; the watery infusion, and the vinous tincture, soon grow sour, and lose their properties, and the solution in vinegar becomes quickly colourless. Med. Uses. It is now never employed but for the sake of its colour, or aromatic flavour, as an adjunct to other substances. It is much used in foreign cookery to colour rice, &c. Officinal Prep. *Syrup. Croci.* L. *Tinct. Croci sativi*, E. *Confect. Aromat.* L. D. *Pil. Aloes cum Myrrha.* L. *Tinct. Aloes comp.* L. E. D. *Tinct. Cinchonæ comp.* L. D. *Tinct. Rhei*, L. *Tinct. Rhei comp.* L. Adulterations. It is not unfrequently sophisticated with the fibres of smoked beef, or the petals of flowers, especially of the marigold, *(Calendula Officinalis,)* and of the safflower, *(Carthamus Tinctorius.)* The former of these fraudulent ingredients is indicated by the unpleasant odour which arises when the saffron is thrown upon live coals; the latter, by infusing the specimen in hot water, when the expanded stigmata may be easily distinguished from the other petals of substituted flowers; a deficiency of colour and odour in the infusion, indicates that a tincture or infusion has already been drawn from the saffron, and that it has been subsequently pressed again into a cake. In the market is to be found saffron from Sicily, France, and Spain, besides the English; that which is imported from Spain is generally spoiled with oil, in which it is dipt, with the intention of preserving it. The cake saffron, sold in some of the less respectable shops, consists of one part of saffron, and nine of marigold, made into a cake with oil, and then pressed, which is sold in considerable quantities for the use of birds, when in moult-

CUBEBÆ. (Piper Cubeba.) *Cubebs.*

This Indian spice formerly held a place in our materia medica, and entered into the composition of *mithridate* and *theriaca*, but being inferior in pungency and aromatic warmth to pepper, it fell into disuse. Lately, however, it has been ushered into surgical practice for the cure of gonorhœa, with all the extravagance of praise, which usually attends the revival of an old, or the introduction of a new, medicine. It has been pronounced to be a specific in this complaint, if taken in the early stages, in the dose of a desert spoonful three times a day, in a sufficient quantity of water. The Indians have been long acquainted with the influence which cubebs exerts upon these organs; thus Garcias, "*Apud Indos cubebarum in vino maceratarum est usus ad excitandam venerem.*" As the qualities of this spice does not reside in volatile elements, an extract, made with rectified spirit, will be found to possess the whole of its virtues. The French, in their new *Codex Medicamentarius*, have introduced the cubebs into their list of materia medica.

CUPRI SULPHAS. L. E. D. Sulphate of Copper.
vulgo Blue Vitriol. Blue Copperas.

QUALITIES. *Form.* Crystals, which are rhomboidal
prisms. *Colour,* a deep rich blue. *Taste,* harsh, acrid,
and stypstic; they slightly effloresce; when treated
with sulphuric acid, no effervescence occurs, a circumstance which at once distinguishes this salt from
Œrugo. CHEMICAL COMPOSITION. According to
the latest experiments, it is an *oxy-sulphate,* consisting
of one proportional of peroxide with two proportionals
of sulphuric acid, and when crystallized, it contains
ten proportionals of water; its beautiful colour depends
on this last ingredient. SOLUBILITY. It is soluble
in four parts of water at 60, and less than two at 212°;
the solution shews an excess of acid by reddening
litmus. In alcohol it is insoluble. INCOMPATIBLE
SUBSTANCES. *Alkalies and their carbonates; sub-
borate of soda; acetate of ammonia; tartrate of potass;
muriate of lime; nitrate of silver; acetate, and super-
acetate of lead; oxy-muriate of mercury; all astringent
vegetable infusions, and tinctures.* Iron immersed in
the solution, precipitates copper in a metallic form;
hence the exhibition of the filings of iron has been
proposed as an antidote.* MEDICAL USES. It is

* It may be here observed, that Copper, in its metallic form, exerts
no action upon the system. A most striking instance of this fact occurred, during my hospital practice, in the case of a young woman,
who swallowed six copper penny pieces, with a view of destroying
herself; she was attended by Dr. Maton and myself, in the Westminster
Hospital, for two years, for a disease which we considered visceral, but
which was evidently the effect of *mechanical* obstruction, occasioned by
the coin. After a lapse of five years, she voided them, and then confessed the cause of her protracted disease; during the whole course of
which, no symptom arose, which could in any way, be attributed to

emetic, from grs. ij to xv. tonic, gr ¹ ; it is, however, but rarely used internally; externally it is employed as an escharotic, and, in solution, as a stimulant to foul obstinate ulcers * OFFICINAL PREPARATIONS. *Solut. Cupri Sulphat. comp.* E. *Cuprum Ammoniatum (f.)* L. E. D.

the poisonous influence of copper. Mr. A. T. Thomson relates also two cases, of halfpence being swallowed by children, in one of which the copper coin remained six months in the intestines, and in the other two months. The filings of copper were formerly a favourite remedy in rheumatism, a drachm of which has been taken with impunity for a dose. It appears therefore that metallic copper does not undergo any change in the digestive organs, by which it is converted into a poison, notwithstanding the presence of substances, which, out of the body, would at once render it destructive, as we have too many cases to shew, from the careless use of copper utensils in cookery. It is, however, a very important fact, that copper cannot be dissolved while tin is coexistent in the mixture, hence the great use of tinning copper utensils; and farther, it is asserted, that untinned coppers are less liable to be injurious when pewter spoons are used for stirring, than when silver ones are employed for that purpose; the explanation of this fact is obvious. For the same reason, M. Proust has shewn that the tinning of kitchen utensils, which consists of equal parts of lead, cannot be dangerous from the presence of the latter metal, since it is sufficient that the lead should be combined with tin, in order to prevent it from being dissolved in any vegetable acid, for the tin, being more oxidable than the lead, is exclusively dissolved, and prevents the second from being attacked. In short, the lead cannot appropriate to itself an atom of oxygen, but the tin would carry it off in an instant.

* BATES's AQUA CAMPHORATA. Sulphate of copper is the base of this preparation, which was so strongly recommended by Mr. Ware. The following was his recipe : ℞ *Cupri Sulph. Boli Gallic, a. a.* gr. xv. *Camphoræ* gr. iv, *solve in aq. fervent.* ℥iv, *dilueque cum Aquæ Frigidæ,* oiv. *ut fiat Collyrium.*

CUPRUM AMMONIATUM. L. D.

Ammoniaretum Cupri. E. *Ammoniated Copper.*

Qualities. *Form*, a violet coloured mass, which, on exposure to air, becomes green, and is probably converted into a carbonate. *Taste*, styptic, and metalline. *Odour*, ammoniacal. Chemical Composition. It is a triple salt, a sub-sulphate of oxide and copper, and ammonia. The Edinburgh College is certainly incorrect in calling it an *ammoniuret.* Solubility, fℨj of water dissolves ℈j of this salt. Med. Uses. It is tonic, and antispasmodic. Dr. Cullen first proposed its exhibition in epilepsy, and it has frequently been employed with evident advantage in that disease. It has been also given in chorea, after a course of purgatives. Forms of Exhibition. It may be formed into pills, with bread; to which an addition of sugar has been recommended, to prevent them from becoming hard; but we must remember that recent experiments have shewn, that sugar has the power of counteracting the operation of copper. Dose, gr. ¼ cautiously encreased to grs. v. twice a day. Officinal Preparations. *Liquor Cupri Ammoniati.* L.

CUSPARIÆ CORTEX. L. (Cusparia febrifuga.)

Bonplandiæ Trifoliatæ Cortex. E.

Angustura, Cortex. D.

Cusparia, or Angustura Bark.

Qualities. *Form.* Pieces covered with a whitish wrinkled thin epidermis; the inner surface is smooth, of a brownish yellow colour. *Odour*, not strong, but peculiar. *Taste*, bitter, slightly aromatic, and permanent. CHEMICAL COMPOSITION. Cinchonin, resin, extractive, carbonate of ammonia, and essential oil. SOLUBILITY. Its active matter is taken up by cold, and hot water, and is not injured by long decoction, but the addition of alcohol precipitates part of the extractive. Alcohol dissolves its bitter and aromatic parts, but proof spirit appears to be its most complete menstruum. INCOMPATIBLE SUBSTANCES. *Sulphate of Iron; Sulphate of Copper; Oxy-muriate of Mercury; Nitrate of Silver; Tartarized Antimony; Acetate, and Super-acetate of Lead; Potass;* and perhaps the *Mineral Acids*, for they produce precipitates, as do also the *infusions of Galls*, and *Yellow Cinchona.* MED. USES. Stimulant and tonic, it does not, like cinchona, oppress the stomach, but imparts a degree of warmth, expels flatus, and encreases the appetite for food : with respect to its powers in the cure of intermittents, many doubts are entertained. FORMS OF EXHIBITION. In substance, infusion, decoction, tincture, or extract ; its nauseous taste is best disguised by cinnamon. DOSE of the powder, grs. v, to Ʒj ; of the infusion or decoction, f℥j ; in large doses all the forms are liable to excite nausea. OFFICINAL PREP. *Infusum Cuspariæ.* L. *Tinctura Bonplandiæ Tripoliatæ.* E. *Tinct. Angusturæ.* D. ADULTERATIONS. There is found in the market a particular bark, which has been called FINE ANGUSTURA, but which is of a different species, and is a very energetic poison. This bark is characterised by having its epidermis covered with a matter which has the appearance of rust of iron, and which, moreover, possesses certain chemical properties of this metal, for if water acidulated with muriatic acid be agitated in contact with its powder, it assumes a beautiful green colour, and affords, with an alkaline prussiate, (*Hydro-cyanate of Potass*) a Prussian blue precipitate.

DATURÆ STRAMONII HERBA. E. D. *The herbaceous part of the Thorn Apple.*

This plant contains gum, resin, carbonate of am- monia, and the narcotic principle. Its root, smoked in the manner of tobacco, has been much extolled as a remedy in the paroxysm of spasmodic asthma; it is, however, a dangerous application ; the same transient feelings of relief may be procured by smoking a mix- ture of opium and any aromatic herb. It is said to be sometimes used by the Turks instead of opium, and the Chinese infuse the seeds in beer. An extract, from the seeds, has been recommended in this country, as being less liable than other narcotics to affect the head. I have repeatedly tried its power in pthisis, but with no advantage.

DECOCTA. L. E. D. *Decoctions.*

These are solutions of the active principles of vege- tables, obtained by boiling them in water. To decide upon the expediency of this form of preparation, in each particular case, requires a knowledge of the chemical composition of the substance in question. In conducting the operation, the following rules must be observed.

1. *Those substances, only, should be decocted, whose medicinal powers reside in principles, which are soluble in water.*

2. *If the active principle be volatile, decoction must be an injurious process; and, if it consist of extractive matter, long boiling, by favouring its oxidizement, will render it insipid, insoluble, and inert.*

3. *The substances to be decocted should be previously bruised, or sliced, so as to expose an extended surface to the action of the water.*

4. *The substances should be completely covered with water, and the vessel be slightly closed, in order to prevent, as much as possible, the access of the air: the boiling should be continued without interruption, and gently.*

5. *In compound decoctions, it is sometimes convenient not to put in all the ingredients from the beginning, but in succession, according to their hardness, and the difficulty with which their virtues are extracted, and if any aromatic, or other substances containing volatile principles, or oxidizable matter, enter into the composition, the boiling decoction should be simply poured upon them, and covered up until cold.*

6. *The relative proportions of different vegetable substances to the water, must be regulated by their nature; the following general rule may be admitted; of roots, barks, or dried woods from ℥ij to ℥vj to every pint of water; of herbs, leaves, or flowers, half that quantity will suffice.*

7. *The decoction ought to be filtered through linen, while hot, as important portions of the dissolved matter are frequently deposited on cooling; care must be also taken that the filtre is not too fine, for it frequently happens, that the virtues of a decoction depend upon the presence of particles, which are suspended in a minutely divided state.*

8. *A decoction should be prepared in small quantities only, and never employed, especially in summer, forty-*

eight hours after it has been made. It should be considered as an extemporaneous preparation, introduced into the pharmacopœia for the purpose of convenience, and for the sake of abridging the labour of the physician.

It is very important that the water, employed for making decoctions, should be free from that quality which is denominated *hardness.*

The officinal decoctions may be classed into simple and compound preparations.

1. *Simple.*

DECOCTUM CINCHONÆ. See Cinchona. The codex of Paris directs a decoction of bark, " *Decoctum Kinæ Kinæ*," which is only half the strength of ours, but contains an addition of a small quantity of carbonate of potass.

DECOCTUM CYDONIÆ. The inner coats of the seeds of the Quince *(Pyrus Cydonia)* yield a very large proportion of mucilage, but, as hot water extracts from them also fecula and other principles, the decoction very soon decomposes. It has been strongly recommended as an application to erysipelatous surfaces. It is coagulated by *alcohol, acids,* and *metallic salts.*

DECOCTUM DIGITALIS. D. This is a very improper form for the exhibition of digitalis, being variable in strength.

DECOCTUM DULCAMARÆ. In making this decoction we must take care that the operation of boiling is not continued too long. See *Dulcamaræ Caules.* Dose from f℥ss to f℥j.

DECOCTUM LICHENIS. L.E.D. In this preparation we have the bitter principle of the plant united with its fecula. A portion of the former may be removed by macerating the lichen, and rejecting the first water. If ʒj of the mass be boiled for a quarter of an hour, in fʒoj of water, we shall obtain muci-lage, of a consistence similar to that composed of one part of gum arabic, and three of water. Its exhibi-tion requires the same precaution as that of *Mucilago Acaciæ*. Dose; a wine glass full occasionally.

DECOCTUM PAPAVERIS. L. In making this decoc-tion the whole of the capsule should be bruised, in order to obtain its mucilage and anodyne principle; the seeds should be also retained, as they yield a por-tion of bland oil, which encreases the emollient qua-lity of the decoction. A large quantity of fixed oil is constantly in the market, which is derived from the seeds of the poppy. This decoction is a useful fomentation in painful swellings, &c.

DECOCTUM QUERCUS. L.E. Decoction is the usual form in which *Oak Bark* is exhibited, since all its active principles are soluble in water. Its astrin-gent virtues depend upon gallic acid, tannin, and extractive. The decoction is disturbed by the fol-lowing substances, *the infusion of yellow cinchona ; acetate,* and *super-acetate of lead ; solutions of isin-glass ;* the *preparations of iron ; oxy-muriate of mer-cury,* and *sulphate of zinc ;* all *alkaline substance* de-stroy its astringency, and are consequently incompa-tible with it. It is principally useful as a local astringent, in the forms of gargle, injection, or lotion. Its internal exhibition in obstinate diarrahœas, and alvine hemorrhages, has also proved highly benefi-cial.

DECOCTUM SARSAPARILLÆ. L.E.D. See Sarsa-parilla. The only salts which occasion precipitates in this decoction are, *nitrate of mercury,* and *super-acetate of lead ;* and *lime water.*

DECOCTUM VERATRI. Stimulant and acrid; internally, it is cathartic, but too violent to be safely exhibited; it is useful as a lotion in scabies, and other cutaneous eruptions.

2. Compound Decoctions.

DECOCTUM ALOES COMPOSITUM. It resembles the well known *Beaume de vie,* and is a scientific preparation, constructed upon the true principles of medicinal combination. Aloes is the base, to which are added 1, sub-carbonate of potass, 2, powdered myrrh, 3, extract of liquorice, 4, saffron, and after the decoction is made, 5, compound tincture of carnamom. By the 1st ingredient the aloes is rendered more soluble; the 2d and 3d suspend the portion not dissolved, and at the same time disguise its bitterness; the 4th imparts an aromatic flavour, and the 5th not only renders it more grateful to the stomach, but prevents any spontaneous decomposition from taking place. Its taste is improved by keeping. It is a warm, gentle cathartic. Dose, f℥ss to f℥j. Its operation is different from that of simple aloes. See *Aloes.* The following substances are incompatible with it; *strong acids, oxy-muriate of mercury; tartarized antimony; sulphate of zinc;* and *super-acetate of lead.*

DECOCTUM GUAIACI COMPOSITUM. E. Commonly called *Decoction of woods.* This decoction has fallen into disuse, and deservedly, for it can possess but little power, except as a diluent, or demulcent; the water takes up from the guaiacum only a small portion of extractive matter, and the virtues of sassafras, if any, must be dissipated by decoction.

DECOCTUM HORDEI COMPOSITUM. An elegant and useful demulcent, with an aperient tendency.

200 DIG

DECOCTUM SARSAPARILLÆ COMPOSITUM. L.D.
This decoction, which is an imitation of the once celebrated *Lisbon Diet Drink*, differs materially from the
Decoct: Guaiaci comp: from the addition of the mezereon root, which renders it diaphoretic and alterative, and useful in the treatment of secondary syphilis,
and chronic rheumatism. Dose, from f℥iv to f℥vj
three or four times a day.

DIGITALIS FOLIA. L.E.D. (Digitalis Purpurea)
Foxglove.

QUALITIES. The leaves, when properly dried,
have a slight narcotic *odour*, and a bitter nauseous
taste, and when reduced to powder, a beautiful green
colour. CHEMICAL COMPOSITION. Extractive matter,
and a green resin, in both of which its narcotic properties reside; they appear also to contain ammonia, and
some other salts. SOLUBILITY. Both water and alcohol extract their virtues, but decoction injures them.
INCOMPATIBLE SUBSTANCES. See *Infusum Digitalis.*
MED. USES. It is directly sedative, although some
maintain the contrary opinion, diminishing the fre-
quency of the pulse, and the general irritability of
the system, and encreasing the action of the absorbents, and the discharge by urine. The effects appear
to be in a great degree connected with its sensible
influence upon the body, which is indicated by feelings
of slight nausea and languor; accordingly, every attempt to prevent these unpleasant effects, or to *correct*
the operation of digitalis, by combining it with aromatic, or stimulant medicines, seems to be fatal to the
diuretic powers of the remedy. Dr. Blackall, in his
"Observations upon the cure of Dropsies," has
offered some remarks which bear upon this point, and
to which I have before referred. *See Introductory
Essay, p.* 6.

The formulæ introduced under the class of diuretics are combinations supported by high authority, but it is doubtful whether their adoption can be sanctioned upon principle; they are however well calculated to illustrate the nature of diuretic compounds, and this is the only purpose for which they were selected. Let us examine the construction of *Formula 31*, and decypher the intention of the different ingredients by their *Key letters*. The base is *Squill*, to which digitalis is added, for the purpose, we perceive, of acting in unison with it, and *Calomel*, which succeeds it, is intended to promote and direct the diuretic basis; two fœtid gums next present themselves to our notice, and these are shewn by the bracket to exert a combined action, depending, as the key letter announces, upon their medicinal similarity, but acting in the general scheme of the formula, as shewn by the exterior letter, for the purpose of fulfilling a second indication, distinct and different from that which the basis is designed to answer, i. e. to produce, not a diuretic, but an antispasmodic and stimulant effect; this question then arises for our consideration—is the latter part of the combination consistent with the former, or is the stimulant effect of the gums compatible with the sedative operation of Digitalis? The French have introduced in their new Codex an ethereal tincture, *Tinctura Ætherea Digitalis purpureæ*, in which the sedative influence of the plant must be entirely overwhelmed by the stimulant properties of the menstruum. The article *Potassæ Acetas* will furnish fresh matter, connected with this subject, and enable me to offer some more extended views respecting the popular combinations of diuretic medicines. FORMS OF EXHIBITION. In substance, tincture, or infusion, the latter form is most efficient as a diuretic. DOSE

o

of the powdered leaves gr. j, in a pill, twice a day; the augmentation of the dose should proceed at the rate of one fourth of the original quantity, every second day, until its operation becomes apparent, either on the kidnies, or on the constitution generally. If it produces such a disturbance in the primæ viæ as to occasion vomiting, or purging, its diuretic powers will be lost; in such a case the addition of a small portion of opium, or opiate confection, may be expedient. The distressing effects of an overdose are best counteracted by tincture of opium, in brandy and water, and by the application of a blister to the pit of the stomach. OFFICINAL PREP : *Infus: Digitalis.* L.E. *Tinct: Digital: L.E.D. Decoct: Digitalis.* D. It is very important that the leaves of this plant be properly collected, and accurately preserved; they should be gathered when the plant is beginning to flower, and, as it is biennial, in the second year of its growth; they should be also carefully dried, or they will lose much of their virtue; the too common method of tying them in bundles, and hanging them up to dry, should be avoided, for a fermentation is produced by such means, and the parts least exposed soon become rotten. The powdered leaves ought to be preserved in opaque bottles, and kept from the action of light, as well as of air and moisture; a damp atmosphere has, upon a principle already explained, a very injurious operation, by carrying off those faint, poisonous effluvia, with which its efficacy seems to be intimately connected.

DULCAMARÆ CAULES. L.D. (Solanum Dulcamara). The Twigs of *Woody Nightshade,* or *Bittersweet.*

The virtues of this plant are extracted by boiling water, but long coction destroys them ; the usual and best form in which it can be administered, is that of decoction or infusion. It is now rarely used, except in cutaneous affections. Officinal Prep: *Decoctum Dulcam : L.*

ELATERII POMA. L.E.D. (Momordica Elaterium). *Wild Cucumber.*

This plant appears, from the testimony of Dioscorides and other writers, to have been employed by the ancient physicians with much confidence and success. All the parts of the plants were considered as purgative, although not in an equal degree ; thus Geoffroy, " radicum vis cathartica major est quam foliorum, minor vero quam fructuum." This question has very lately been set at rest by the judicious experiments of Dr. Clutterbuck,* which prove that the active principle of this plant resides more particularly in the juice which is lodged in the centre of the fruit, and which spontaneously subsides from it ; when this substance is freed from extraneous matter, it possesses very energetic powers, and appears to me to be entitled to consideration as a distinct proximate principle, which I shall venture to call *Elatin.* See Extractum Elaterii.

ELECTUARIA. Electuaries.

This is an ancient form of prescription ; for although the term " *Electarium* " is first used by Cælius Aure-

* See London Medical Repository, Vol. xii. No. 67.

lianus, yet the ἐκλικτον, of Hippocrates, and the *Anti-dotus*, *Confectio*, *Mithridatium*, *Diascordium*, *Opiatum*, *Orvietanum*, *Philonium*, *Theriaca*, and *Requies* of other authors, were all Electuaries. They differ from *Conserves* in this, that the sugar in the latter preparations is in a greater proportion, and is intended to *preserve* the ingredients, whereas, in the former, it is merely intended to impart convenience of form. Electuaries are in general, *extemporaneous* preparations, composed of dry powders, formed into a proper consistence by the addition of syrup, honey, or mucilage; when however the latter substance is employed, the electuary very soon becomes dry and hard ; and when common syrup is used, the compound is apt to candy, and in a day or two to grow too hard for use ; this is owing to the crystallization of the sugar ; Deyeux therefore states, that the syrup should be previously exposed to the heat of a stove, as long as it forms any crystals, and that the residual liquor which, from the presence of some vegetable acid, has no tendency to crystallize, may then be advantageously applied ;— *Melasses* or Treacle may in some cases be employed, and from experiments which I have repeated with some care, I am enabled to state that the peculiar flavour of this liquid is entirely removed by a simple operation, which consists in diluting it with an equal weight of water, and then boiling it with about one eighth part of powdered charcoal for half an hour, when the liquor is to be strained, and reduced by gentle evaporation to a proper consistence, and moreover, that it appears, that active vegetable powders retain their characteristic qualities when immersed in *Treacle*, longer than in any other excipient.

In selecting and prescribing this form of exhibition, the following general rules should be observed.

I. Those substances which are nuaseous, deliquescent, which require to be given in large doses, or which are incapable of forming an intimate union with syrup, as *fixed oils, balsams,* &c. should never be prescribed in the form of an electuary.

II. The quantity of syrup directed must be regulated by the nature, and specific gravities, of the substances which enter into their composition, viz :

1. *Dry Vegetable Powders* require twice their weight of syrup, or of honey.

2. *Gummy and Resinous Powders* require an equal weight.

3. *Hard Mineral Substances* should be formed into an electuary with some conserve, as they are too ponderous to remain suspended in syrup. It deserves also to be noticed, that in consequence of the readiness with which metallic preparations undergo change, it will be generally adviseable to keep the active ingredients in the form of powder, and to add them to the syrup only just before they are required ; the Electuary of the French Pharmacopœia, which is commonly called " *Opiata Mesenterica,*" will furnish a good example, " *quantumvis molle fuerit recens, progressu temporis, ob ferrum quod ipsi inest, mirè indurescit.*"

ELEMI. L.D. (Amyris Elemifera) *Elemi.*
             Resina

This substance is what is generally termed a *gum resin,* that is, a compound consisting of gum, resin, and a volatile oil ; late researches however seem to shew that these bodies are compounds of a peculiar character, consisting of a volatile substance, something between essential oil and resin, and a constituent which possesses the properties of extractive rather than those of gum.

True Elemi has a fragrant aromatic odour, not unlike that of fennel seeds, but more potent. When powdered, it mixes with any unguent; it also combines with balsams and oils, and, by the aid of heat, with turpentine. Uses. It is only employed for forming the *mild digestive ointment*, which bears its name, viz. *Unguent: Elemi comp:* L.D.

EMPLASTRA. *Plasters.*

These are solid and tenacious compounds, adhesive in the ordinary heat of the human body; they owe their consistence to different causes, viz.

1. *To a due mixture of wax or fatty matter, and resin.* They may be said to differ only *in consistence* from liniments, ointments, and cerates, and Deyeux * accordingly proposes to distinguish them by the appellation of *Solid Ointments,* e. g. *Emplastrum Ceræ, Emp: Cumini,* &c.

2. *To the chemical combination of the semivitreous oxide of lead with oils or fat,* e. g. *Emplast: Plumbi.*

3. *To the chemical action of the component parts of the plaster on each other,* e. g. *Emplast: Ammoniaci.*

Plasters are generally kept in rolls, wrapped in paper, and when to be used they are melted and spread on leather; in performing this operation the practitioner ought not to apply a heat above that of boiling water, for if metallic oxides be present the

* Annales de Chimie, vol. 33. p. 52.

fatty matter will, at a higher temperature, reduce them, and if aromatic substances enter as ingredients they will thus suffer in their strength, besides which the fat itself will undergo a very injurious change, by a mismanaged application of heat, and the plaster will be less adhesive.

They are employed as remedies to answer two general indications; *mechanically*, to afford support to muscular parts, and to prevent the access of air; and *medicinally*, to operate as stimulants, discutients, rubefacients, or anodyne applications. That by affording an artificial support to the various parts of the body, by the application of plasters, we are capable, in certain diseases, of effecting much benefit, is a truth to be explained upon the principles of physiology, and is daily confirmed by the results of practice; thus, by giving support to the muscles of the back, how frequently the stomach is steadied and strengthened? Diseases of the kidnies, are in the same way, very frequently relieved by tight bandages around the loins; the existence of an intimate connexion between the external and internal parts is strikingly exemplified by the distressing effects which are often experienced in weak habits, such as sickness, giddiness, and other uneasy sensations, from a want of any usual compression, as that of stays, under-waistcoats, &c. where our object is simple support, we should of course select a plaster which is the most adhesive, and the least irritating. Many plasters which have gained great celebrity for their curative virtues, will be found to owe all their powers to their adhesiveness, such is the *Emplastrum Oxidi Ferri Rubri* of the Edinburgh Pharmacopœia, for it is impossible that the iron should communicate any tonic effect. The same observation applies to many of those empirical plasters which have, at different times, acquired so great a share * of popular applause.

EMPLASTRUM AMMONIACI. L. E. *Ammoniacum* reduced to a suitable consistence by distilled vinegar. It adheres to the skin without irritating it, and without being attended with any unpleasant smell.

EMPLASTRUM AMMONIACI CUM HYDRARGYRO. L. D. The Mercury in this plaster is in the state of oxidation *ad minimum*. It is discutient and resolvent, and is applicable to indurated glands, venereal nodes, and for removing indurations of the periosteum, remaining after a course of mercury; the addition of the ammoniacum encreases the stimulating and discutient powers of the mercury, which gives this plaster a superiority over the *Emplastrum Hydrargyri*. It is also powerfully adhesive.

EMPLASTRUM ASSAFŒTIDÆ. E. Emplast. Plumbi, and Assafœtida, of each *two parts*, galbanum and yellow wax, of each *one part*. I have seen it useful in flatulent cholic, when applied over, the umbilical region.

EMPLASTRUM CERÆ. L. *Emplast: Simplex.* E. This is the *Emplast: Ceræ* of P. L. 1787, the *Emplast: Attrahens* of 1745, so called because it was formerly employed to keep up a discharge from a blistered surface, and the *Emplastrum de melitoto simplex* of 1720.

EMPLASTRUM CUMINI. L. A valuable combination of warm and stimulant ingredients.

---

* A Quaker of the name of STERRY, in the Borough, prepares a plaster of this description, which is sought after with great avidity. What a blessing it would be upon the community, if every nostrum were equally innocuous !

EMPLASTRUM GALBANI COMPOSITUM. L. D. *Emplast: Gummos.* E. More powerful than the preceding plaster.

EMPLASTRUM HYDRARGYRI. L. E. The mercury in these plasters is in the state of oxidation *ad minimum ;* each drachm containing about fifteen grains of mercury, (*sixteen grains,* Edinb.) They are alterative, discutient, and sometimes sialogoque.

EMPLASTRUM LYTTÆ. L. *Emplast: Cantharidis vesicatoriæ.* E. D. A variety of substances has in different times been employed for producing vesication, but no one has been found to answer with so much certainty and mildness as the *Lyttæ.* All the others are apt to leave ill conditioned ulcers; true it is, that the emplastrum lyttæ will occasionally fail, but this is generally attributable to some inattention, or want of caution on the part of the person who prepares it; in spreading it, the spatula should never be heated beyond the degree of boiling water; the plaster also should be sufficiently secured on the part, but ought not to be bound on too tight; where the cuticle is thick, the application of a poultice for an hour, previous to that of the blister, will be useful, or the part may be washed with vinegar. In consequence of the absorption of the active principle of the *Lyttæ,* blisters are apt to occasion strangury and bloody urine; it has been a problem therefore of some importance to discover a plan, by which such an absorption may be obviated; for this purpose, camphor has been recommended to be mixed with the blistering composition, and a piece of thin gauze has been interposed between the plaster and the skin; but it has been lately found, that ebullition in water deprives the *Lyttæ* of all power of acting on the kidneys, without in the least diminishing their vesicatory properties.

In some cases the blistered parts, instead of healing kindly, become a spreading sore; whenever this occurs, poultices are the best applications; it may arise from a peculiar irritability of the constitution, although I apprehend that it not unfrequently depends upon the sophistication of the plaster with Euphorbium.

EMPLASTRUM OPII. L. E. This plaster is supposed to be anodyne, but it is very doubtful whether the opium *can*, in such a state, produce any specific effect.

EMPLASTRUM PICIS COMPOSITUM. L. *Emplast : Picis burgundiœ*, P. L. 1787. It is stimulant and rubefacient, and is often employed as an application to the chest, in pulmonary complaints; the serous exudation however which it produces, frequently occasions so much irritation that we are compelled to remove it.

EMPLASTRUM PLUMBI. L. *Emplast : Oxydi Plumbi semi-vitrei*. E. *Emplast : Lithargyri*, P. L. 1787. *Emplast : commune*, 1745. *Diachylon Simplex*, P. L. 1720. This is a very important plaster, since it forms the basis of a great many others; under the name of *Diachylon* it has been long known, and employed as a common application to excoriations, and for retaining the edges of fresh cut wounds in a state of apposition, and at the same time for defending them from the action of the air; when long kept it changes its colour, and loses its adhesive properties, and by high temperature the oxyd of lead is revived.*

* At Apothecaries Hall, this plaster, as well as others, is made in a steam apparatus, which is so well regulated, that a uniform temperature of 240° Fah: is insured during the whole process.

Emplastrum Resinæ. L. Olim, *Emplast : commune adhæsivum*, P. L. 1745. Emplast : Resinosum. E. Emplast : Lithargyri cum Resina. D. It is defensive, adhesive, and stimulant.†

Emplastrum Saponis. L.D. *Emplastrum Saponaceum.* E. The Soap Plaster is said to be a mild discutient application.

EUPHORBIÆ GUMMI-RESINA. L.

(Euphorbia Officinarum.) *Euphorbium.*

Qualities. This substance is imported from Barbary, in drops or irregular tears; its fracture is vitreous; it is inodorous, but yields a very acrid burning impression to the tongue. Chemical Composition. It is what is termed a *gum resin*, but its acrid constituent is exclusively in that portion which is soluble in alcohol. Solubility. Water by trituration is rendered milky, but dissolves only one seventh part; and alcohol one fourth of it. Uses. Internally administered, it proves very violently drastic, but is never employed except as an errhine, cautiously diluted with starch, or some inert powder.

---

† Baynton's Adhesive Plaster, differs only from this preparation in containing rather less resin, six drachms only being added to one pound of the litharge plaster. This excellent plaster is sold ready spread on calico.

Court Plaster. *Sticking Plaster.*—Black silk is strained and brushed over ten or twelve times, with the following preparation : dissolve ℥ss of gum benzoin in f℥vj of rectified spirit; in a separate vessel dissolve an ounce of isinglass in oss of water, strain each solution; mix them, and let them rest, that the grosser parts may subside ; when the clear liquor is cold, it will form a jelly, which must be warmed before it is applied. When dry, in order to prevent its cracking, it is finished off with a solution of *Tereb : Chia* 4 oz. in *tinct : benzoin* 6 oz.

Farriers use it for blistering horses, and there is good reason to believe that it is sometimes fraudulently introduced to quicken the powers of our emplastrum lyttæ. CAUTION in pulverizing this substance, the dispenser should previously moisten it with vinegar to prevent its rising and excoriating his face.

EXTRACTA. L. E. D. *Extracts.*

These preparations are obtained by evaporating the watery, or spiritous solutions of vegetables, and the native juices, obtained from fresh plants by expression, to masses of a tenacious consistence. The London college does not arrange the extracts under the titles of *watery* and *spirituous*, which is the arrangement of the Edinburgh pharmacopœia, nor under those of *simple* and *resinous*, which is the division observed in that of Dublin, but rejecting all *specific* distinctions, includes, under the *generic* appellation of extract, both the species, as well as all the *inspissated juices.* Since however the former of these arrangements will afford greater facilities for introducing the observations, which it is my intention to offer, it is retained in this work.

The chemical nature of extracts must obviously be very complicated and variable, depending in a great degree upon the powers of the *menstruum* employed for their preparation; although Fourcroy and Vauquelin considered that *one peculiar* principle was the basis of them all, which they called *Extract, Extractive,* or the *Extractive Principle.* It is distinguished by the following characters, *viz.*

It has a strong taste, varying in different plants; it is soluble in water, and in alcohol when it contains water, but is quite insoluble in *absolute* alcohol and ether; its aqueous solution soon runs into a state of putrefaction; by repeated solutions and evaporations, or by long ebullition, it acquires a deeper colour, and in consequence of its combination with oxygen, it becomes insoluble and inert, a fact which is of extreme importance, as it regards its pharmaceutical relations; it unites with alumine, and if boiled with its salts, precipitates them, hence wool, cotton, or thread, impregnated with alum, may be dyed of a fawn colour by *extractive;* its habitudes with alkalies are very striking, combining most readily and forming with them compounds of a brownish yellow colour, which are very soluble in water; if, to a colourless and extremely dilute solution of extractive, an alkali be added, a brown or yellowish tint is immediately produced, so that under certain circumstances, I have found an alkali to be a serviceable test in detecting the presence of extractive matter. The usual brown hue of the *liquor ammoniæ acetatis* is owing to the action of the ammonia, upon traces of vegetable extractive contained in the distilled vinegar.

Much confusion has arisen from the word *extract* having been employed in this double meaning, *chemically* to express a peculiar vegetable proximate principle, and *pharmaceutically* to denote any substance, however complicated in its nature, which has been obtained by the evaporation of a vegetable solution or a native vegetable juice. It is in the latter sense that it is to be understood in the present article.

The different proximate principles of vegetable matter undergo various and indefinite changes with such rapidity, when acted upon by heat, that the process of *extraction* must necessarily, more or less impair the medicinal efficacy of a plant, and not unfrequently destroy it altogether, and hence, says Dr.

Murray, "with the exception of some of the pure bitters, as gentian; or some of the saccharine vegetables, as liquorice; there is no medicine perhaps but what may be given with more advantage under some other form;" this however is not exactly true, for when care is taken in the preparation, we are thus enabled to concentrate *many* very powerful qualities in a small space, and the process lately adopted, of evaporating the solutions by the aid of steam, contributes very materially to obviate the failures which so frequently occurred from a too exalted temperature. There is, for instance, great reason to suppose that the black colour which so often characterises the extracts of commerce, is frequently owing to the decomposition and carbonization of the vegetable matter; the colour therefore of an extract becomes, in some degree, a test of its goodness.

1. WATERY OR SIMPLE EXTRACTS.

Mucilaginous Extracts of Rouelle.

These extracts must of course contain all the principles of a plant which are soluble in water, such as gum, extractive matter, tannin, cinchonin, sugar, fecula, &c. together with any soluble salts which the vegetable may contain. I have also found by experiment, that an aqueous extract may even contain, in small proportions, certain elements which although quite insoluble in water, are nevertheless partially soluble in a vegetable infusion. This law of vegetable chemistry has never been expressed, although we have repeated instances of its truth, and a knowledge of it may explain some hitherto unintelligible anomalies. It has been stated that extractive matter is perfectly insoluble in ether, but Mr. A. Thomson found re-

peatedly, that if a small proportion of resin was
present ether would in that case take up extractive
in combination with the resin which it so readily
dissolves. As Decoction or Infusion is a process,
preliminary to that of extraction, the practitioner
must refer to those articles for an enumeration of the
different sources of error which are attached to them.

EXTRACTUM ALOES PURIFICATUM. L. The resinous element of the aloes is got rid of in this preparation, on which account it is supposed in an equal
dose, to be more purgative and less irritating. *Dose*,
gr. x to xv.

EXTRACTUM ANTHEMIDIS. L. E. *Extract. Florum
Chamœmeli.* D. This extract furnishes an example
of the change effected on some plants by the process
of extraction; in this case the volatile oil is dissipated
and a simple bitter remains, possessing scarcely any
of the characteristic properties of chamomile.

EXTRACTUM CINCHONÆ. L. D. The properties
of the bark in this preparation are much invalidated,
owing to the oxidizement of its extractive matter,
which takes place to such an extent, that not more
than one half of the preparation is soluble in water;
it is not however altogether devoid of utility, and
will often sit lightly on the stomach, when the powder
is rejected. Its taste is very bitter, but less austere
than the powder. *Dose*, grs. x to ʒss. Fourteen
ounces of the bark will yield about three ounces and
a half of extract.

EXTRACTUM COLOCYNTHIDIS. L. This extract
is much milder, although less powerful than the pulp,
Dose, grs. v to ʒss. It soon becomes hard and mouldy.*

* BARCLAY's ANTIBILIOUS PILLS. Take of the *Extract of olocynth* ʒji,
Resin of Jalap (extract Jalap,) ʒj, *Almond Soap* ʒjss, *Guaiacum* ʒiij, *Tartarized Antimony*, grs. viij, essential oils of *Juniper*, *Carraway* and *Rosemary*,
of each gtt: iv, of syrup of *Buckthorn*, as much as will be sufficient to
form a mass, which is to be divided into sixty-four pills.

EXTRACTUM COLOCYNTHIDIS COMPOSITUM. L. D.
Extract. Catharticum. P.L. 1775. *Pilulæ Rudii.* P.L.
1720. This preparation has been established through
successive pharmacopœiæ, and has undergone some
modification in each; in the present edition the soap
has been omitted, and its solubility is thereby de-
creased, and its mildness as a cathartic diminished.
The omission of this ingredient was suggested by the
consideration of its being incompatible with *Calomel;*
this however is *not* the case. It presents a combination
of purgative substances which is highly judicious, and
will be found to be more powerful than an equivalent
dose of any *one* of the ingredients. *Dose*, gr. vj to ʒss.

EXTRACTUM GENTIANÆ. L. E. D. The bitter
principle suffers no deterioration in the process : it is
used principally as a vehicle for metallic preparations.

EXTRACTUM GLYCYRRHIZÆ. L. D. It is usually
imported from Spain ; in the coarser kinds, the pulps
of various plumbs and of prunes, are added; it should
dissolve in water without leaving any feculence.*

EXTRACTUM HÆMATOXYLI. L. E. D. The astringent properties of the *logwood* are preserved in the
extract, but it becomes so extremely hard, that pills
made of it very commonly pass through the body
without undergoing the least change. *Dose*, grs. x
to ʒss dissolved in cinnamon water.

EXTRACTUM HUMULI. L. The bitter taste of the
hop characterises this preparation; whether it possesses
or not any anodyne properties, seems very doubtful.
Dose, grs. v. to Əj.

* REFINED LIQUORICE. This article, which is sold in the form of
cylinders, is made by gently evaporating a solution of the pure extract
of liquorice, with half its weight of gum arabic, rolling the mass, and
cutting it into lengths, and then polishing, by rolling them together in
a box: many impurities however are fraudulently introduced into this
article, such even as *glue,* &c.

EXTRACTUM OPII. L. D. As it contains less resinous matter than crude opium, it is therefore supposed to produce its effects with less subsequent
derangement. See *Opium*. *Dose*, gr. j to v, for an
adult.

EXTRACTUM PAPAVERIS. L. D. It is a weak
opium. *Dose*, grs. ij to ℈j.

EXTRACTUM TARAXACI. L. D. The medicinal
powers of Dandelion, are asserted to exist, unimpaired
in this preparation. See *Taraxacum*. *Dose*, grs. x
to ʒj, in combination with sulphate of potass.

2. *Spiritous or Resinous Extracts.*

These may contain, with the exception of gum, all
the ingredients contained in watery extracts, besides
resin, their composition however will greatly depend
upon the strength of the spirit employed as the
solvent; but of this I shall speak more fully under
the article *Tincture*. Mr. Battley, a wholesale druggist in Fore street, London, is in the practice of preparing resinous extracts, without the intervention of
any solvent except water : his method consists in submitting the plant, after it has been well bruised and
pressed, to the operation of long continued decoction,
by which the soluble parts are extracted, and the insoluble matter is separated and procured on the surface
of the liquid, in the state of a finely divided powder;
this is removed, and when the soluble parts have by
evaporation acquired the consistence of a syrup, the
insoluble part is then intimately mixed and incorporated with it. We have certainly in this preparation
all the elements of the plant, which water and spirit
could have extracted, but have we them in the same
state, and are they calculated to produce the same
medicinal effects ? I feel some hesitation in answering

P

this question; it surely cannot be *one* and the *same* thing, whether an active resinous element be *mechanically mixed* with an extractive mass, or whether all the ingredients be at once obtained by the evaporation of a spirituous menstruum, in which they were previously *chemically combined.*

The extracts obtained by Mr. Battley's process must be less pure, as well as less soluble in the primæ viæ, and I apprehend that they will, if purgative, be more liable, on such an account, to operate with griping and uneasiness.

EXTRACTUM CINCHONÆ RESINOSUM. L.E.D. The operation of spirit in this preparation is two fold; it extracts from the bark the element which is insoluble in water, and it diminishes the tendency in the extractive matter to absorb oxygen during the process. *Dose*, grs. x to xxx.

EXTRACTUM JALAPÆ. L. E. D. It is purgative, but is liable to gripe, unless it be triturated with sugar and almonds, or mucilage, so as to form an emulsion. *Dose*, grs. x to ℈j.

EXTRACTUM RHEI. L. The powers of the Rhubarb are considerably impaired in this extract. *Dose*, gr. x to ʒss.

3. *Inspissated Juices.*

These preparations are obtained by expressing the juice of fresh plants, and evaporating them in a water bath; they are generally of a lighter colour than common extracts, and they are certainly much more active, although there is a great difference in the activity of different samples; and perhaps the *medicinal* powers of the juices themselves are very much under the control of soil and season. That they vary *in quantity* from such causes, we have ample proof, thus in moist seasons, Baumé obtained five pounds of inspissated juice from thirty pounds of *elder berries,* whereas, in dry seasons, he could rarely get more than two. From *hemlock* he procured in October, 1796, 7.5 per cent of inspissated juice, and in May of the same year only 3.7 ; on the contrary, in August 1768, 4 *per cent.* and in May, 1770, as much as 6.5 ; but in general, the product in the autumnal months was the most considerable.

The modes of preparing the inspissated juices of the same plants vary in the different pharmacopœias, and in several points that are very *essential;* some direct the expressed juices to be *immediately* inspissated, others allow them to undergo a slight degree of fermentation, and some *defecate* them, before they proceed to their inspissation.

EXTRACTUM *(Succus Spissatus* E.*)* ACONITI. L. E. The medicinal properties of this preparation are analogous to those of the recent *Wolfsbane,* viz. narcotic, and in some cases diuretic. It is however rarely used. *Dose,* at first, should not exceed gr. ¼, but it may be gradually increased.

EXTRACTUM BELLADONNÆ. L. E. See *Belladonnæ Folia. Dose,* gr. j, gradually increased to gr. v, in the form of a pill.

EXTRACTUM *(Succus Spissatus.* E. D.*)* CONII. L. Much of this extract, as it is found in commerce, has not been prepared with equal fidelity, nor with due attention to the season when the plant is in its greatest perfection ; Dr. Fothergill says, " I know from repeated experiments, that the extract which has been prepared from *hemlock,* before the plant arrives at maturity, is much inferior to that which is made when the plant has acquired its full vigour, and is rather on the verge of decline : just when the flowers fade, the rudiments of the seeds become observable, and the habit of the plant inclines to yellow, *is the proper time to collect it;*" the plants which grow in places exposed to the sun should be selected, as being more *virose* than those that grow in the shade: still however with every precaution, it will always be uncertain in strength. Orfila found that an extract prepared by boiling the dried powder in water, and evaporating the decoction, was inert; in fact, the whole of the activity of the plant resides in a resinous element *insoluble* in water, and for which I have proposed the name of *Conein*. Extract of hemlock, when judiciously prepared, is a very valuable sedative; I state this from ample experience, and when combined with Hyoscyamus, and adapted by means of mucilage and syrup, to the form of a mixture, it affords a more effectual palliative than any remedy with which I am acquainted, for coughs and pulmonary irritation. *Dose*, grs. v to ℈j or more, twice or thrice a day; in a full dose it produces giddiness, a slight nausea, and a tremor of the body; a peculiar heavy sensation is also experienced about the eyes; and the bowels become gently relaxed: unless some of these sensations are produced, we are never sure that the remedy has had a *fair trial* of its effects. Patients will generally bear a larger dose at night than at noon, and at noon than in the morning.

EXTRACTUM ELATERII. L. This substance spontaneously subsides from the juice of the wild cucumber, in consequence, I presume, of one of those series of changes, which vegetable matter is perpetually undergoing, although we are hitherto unable to express them by any known chemical law. It is therefore not an *extract*, either in the chemical, or pharmaceutical acceptation of the term, nor an *inspissated*

juice, nor is it a *fecula*,* as it has been termed; the
Dublin College has, perhaps, been most correct in
simply calling it *Elaterium*, the name given to it by
Dioscorides.

It occurs in commerce, in little thin cakes, or broken
pieces, bearing the impression of the muslin, upon
which it was dried; its *colour* is greenish, its *taste*
bitter, and somewhat acrid; and when tolerably pure,
it is light, pulverulent, and inflammable.

The early history of this medicinal substance is
involved in great perplexity, each author speaking of
a different preparation by the same name; for instance, the *elaterium* of Dioscorides must have been
a very different substance from that of Theophrastus;
and, wherever Hippocrates mentions the term, he
evidently alludes to *any* violent purgative. " *Hip-
pocrati Elaterium medicamentum est quod per alvum
expurgat.*" (*Bod: in Theophrast.*) This will, in some
degree, reconcile the discordant testimonies of different
authors, with regard to the powers of *elaterium*; for
example, Dioscorides states its dose to be from grs. ii
to ℈j—in Ætius, Paulus, and Actuarius, it is recommended to the extent of ℥ss—in Mesue from ℈ss to
℈j—in Bontius (*Med: Ind:*) from ℈j to ℥ss—Mas-
sarias exhibits it in doses of grs. vj—Fernelius and
Senneretus to ℈j—Herman from grs. v to vij—Quincy
to grs. v—and Boerhaave does not venture to give
more than grs. iv—and the practitioners of the present
day limit their dose from gr. ½ to grs. ij. Dr.
Clutterbuck, with a laudable intention to discover

---

* The juices of *iris root*, *arum root*, and *bryony root*, and those of many
other plants, allow their medicinal elements to separate and subside in
a similar manner, leaving the super-natant liquid perfectly inert; if we
must have a generic name to express such substances, it should be termed
a *feculence*, rather than a *fecula*.

some method of procuring this article at a cheaper
rate, and, at the same time, of discovering some process which might ensure a preparation of more uniform
strength, has lately performed a series of interesting
and instructive experiments,* the results of which
prove in a satisfactory manner, " that the active
principle of this plant is neither lodged in the roots,
leaves, flowers, or stalks, in *any considerable quantity ;*
nor is it to be found in the body of the fruit itself, or
in the seeds, but in *the juice around the seeds ;*" the
substance which spontaneously subsides from this
liquor, obtained without pressure, is *genuine* Elaterium, the quantity of which, contained in the fruit,
is extremely small, for Dr. Clutterbuck obtained only
six grains from *forty* cucumbers. This gentleman
communicated the detail of these experiments to the
President of the College of Physicians, who requested me, as Professor of Materia Medica, to report
upon them. I accordingly deemed it to be my duty
to enter upon a series of new experiments, which
I have lately completed, with the able assistance
of Mr. Farraday, in the laboratory of the Royal
Institution. The results of which will shew, that
although Dr. Clutterbuck found that an *eighth* part
of a grain of elaterium seldom failed to *purge vio-*
lently, yet, strange as it may appear, that *not more*
than one grain in ten of elaterium, as it occurs in
commerce, possesses any active properties, and that
this decimal part is a vegetable proximate principle,
not hitherto noticed, to which I shall give the name
of ELATIN. I shall subjoin the detail of my experi-

---

* " *Observations on the Nature and Preparation of the Elaterium*," read at
the Medical Society of London, April 24, 1819, and which were published in the Medical Repository, vol. xii. No. 67.

ments in a note, and I think it will appear, that their results will authorise me to express the chemical composition of Elaterium in the following manner.

F. Water . . . . . . ·4
⎧ B. Extractive . . . . . 2·6
I.⎨ B.DJ. Fecula . . . . . . 2·8
⎩ C. Gluten . . . . . . ·5
K. Woody matter . . . . 2·5
H. *Elatin* . . . . . ⎫
G. Bitter Principle . . ⎬ 1·2

10 grains.

Proximate Analysis of Elaterium.
Experiments. Series 1st.

A.

Ten grains of Elaterium, obtained from a respectable Chemist, and having all the sensible properties which indicated it to be genuine, were digested, for twenty-four hours, with distilled water, at a temperature far below that of boiling ; *four grains* only were dissolved.

B.

The solution was intensely bitter ; of a brownish yellow colour ; and was not in the least disturbed by alcohol, although a solution of *Iodine* produced a blue colour : the solution therefore contained no gum, and only *slight traces* of starch.

C.

The solution, after standing twenty-four hours, yielded a *pellicle* of insoluble matter, which, when burnt, appeared to resemble *Gluten*.

D.

The six grains which were insoluble in water were treated, for forty-eight hours, with alcohol of the specific gravity ·817, at 66° of *Fahrenheit* ; a green solution was obtained, but by slow evaporation *only half a grain* of solid green matter was procured. The insoluble residue obstinately adhered to, and coated the filtre, like a varnish, and completely defended the mass from the action of the alcohol, it is probable that it consisted, principally, of *Fecula.*

Experiments. Series 2nd.

E.

Ten grains of Elaterium, from the same sample, were treated with alcohol of the specific gravity ·817, at 66°. *Fah*: for twenty-four hours ;

It appears that the whole of the *Elatin* does not separate itself from its native juice, by spontaneous subsidence, and that, on this account, the supernatant liquor possesses some powers as a cathartic. We cannot be surprised therefore, that the Elaterium of commerce should be a very variable and uncertain medicine, for, independent of the great temptation

upon being filtered, and the residuum washed with successive portions of alcohol, the Elaterium was found to have lost only 1·6 of a grain. The high specific gravity of the alcohol in this experiment was important, had it been lower, different results would have been produced.

F.

The alcoholic solution, obtained in the last experiment, was of a most brilliant and beautiful green colour, resembling that of the oil of cajeput, but brighter; upon slowly evaporating it, 1·2 grains of solid green matter was obtained.

G.

The solid green matter of the last experiment was treated with boiling distilled water, when a minute portion was thus dissolved, and a solution of a most intensely bitter taste, and of brownish yellow colour, resulted.

H.

The residue, insoluble in water, was inflammable, burning with smoke, and an aromatic odour, not in the least bitter; it was soluble in alkalies, and was again precipitated from them unchanged in colour; it formed, with pure alcohol, a beautiful tincture, which yielded an odour of a very nauseous kind, but of very little flavour, and which gave a precipitate with water; it was soft, and of considerable specific gravity, sinking rapidly in water; circumstances which distinguish it from common resin; in very minute quantities it purges. It appears to be the element in which *all* the powers of the Elaterium are concentrated, and which have been denominated *Elatin*.

I.

The residuum, insoluble in alcohol, weighing 8·4 grs. (*Expt.* E) was boiled in double distilled water, when 5·9 grs. were dissolved.

J.

The above solution was copiously precipitated *blue* by a solution of *Iodine*, and was scarcely disturbed by the *Per-sulphate of Iron*.

K.

The part insoluble, both in alcohol and water, which was left after Experiment I. amounted to 2·5 grains; it burnt like wood, and was insoluble in alkalies.

which its high price holds out for adulterating it,
which is frequently done with starch, it necessarily
follows, that where the active principle of a compound bears so small a proportion to its bulk, it is
liable to be affected by the slightest variation in the
process for its preparation ; and even by the temperature of the season ; where pressure is used for obtaining the juices, a greater or less quantity of the
inactive parts of the cucumber will be mixed with the
Elatin, in proportion to the extent of such pressure,
and the *Elaterium* will of course be proportionally
weak.* There is one curious result obtained in my
experiments, which deserves notice, *viz.* that there is
a *bitter* principle in the Elaterium, very distinct from
its extractive matter, and totally unconnected with its
activity, for I diluted the solution obtained in experiment G, and swallowed it, but it produced upon me
no effect, except that which I generally experience
upon taking a powerful bitter,—an increased appetite.
The solution B was given to a person, but no effect
whatever ensued. *Dose* of good Elaterium, as it occurs in commerce, is about two grains, or it is better
to give it only to the extent of half a grain at a time,
and to repeat that dose every hour until it begins to
operate. It is probably, when thus managed, the
best hydragogue cathartic which we possess.

EXTRACTUM (*Succus Spissatus* E.D.) HYOSCYA-
MI. L. This preparation is certainly powerfully narcotic, and tends to relax rather than astringe the
bowels ; where the constitution is rebellious to opium, it furnishes a more valuable resource to the practitioner, than any other narcotic extract. *Dose* gr. v.
to Əj, in pills.

* When it has a dark green colour, approaching to black, is compact, and very heavy, and breaks with a shining resinous fracture, we
may reject it as an inferior article.

In concluding the history of Inspissated juices it deserves notice, that the London College uniformly directs, that the *feculence* should be preserved in the compound ; there can be no doubt of the propriety of such advice, but the Colleges of Edinburgh and Dublin reject it. The French Codex gives directions for two extracts from each of these substances, one containing what they please to denominate the *fecula*, the other not, thus there is " *Extractum Cicutæ absque Fecula,* " and " *Extract: Cicut: cum Fecula.* " There is one curious fact respecting these *narcotic* preparations, that most, if not all o*ᶜ* them, contain *nitre*, and *common salt.*

Manufacturing chemists, in order to give a smooth and glossy appearance to their Extracts, generally add to every lbj, about ℈ss of gum, ʒj of olive oil, and mxx of rectified spirit : there is no harm in the practice.

FERRI SUB-CARBONAS. L. Carbonas Ferri Præcipitatus. E. Carbonas Ferri. D.

Carbonate of Iron.

In the former Pharmacopœia of London, a sub-carbonate of iron was prepared, under the name of *ferri-rubigo* (rust of iron) by exposing iron filings to the action of air and water; and although the Colleges of Edinburgh and Dublin still retain this mode of preparation, yet they admit, at the same time, of another, which, like the *sub-carbonate* of the present London Pharmacopœia, is produced by precipitation. Qualities. *Form,* a chocolate brown powder. *Odour,* none. *Taste,* slightly styptic. Chemical Composition. Mr. Phillips has shewn that this precipitate is liable to vary, according to the temperature at which it is prepared, as well as from other differences of manipulation; it consists of mixtures of peroxide, protoxide, and sub-carbonate of protoxide of iron, in various proportions. SOLUBILITY. It is insoluble in water, but acids dissolve it with effervescence. FORMS OF EXHIBITION. In powder or pills, combined with aromatics. DOSE, gr. v to xxx. (*Form :* 124.)

FERRI RAMENTA ET FILA. L. FILA ET LIMATURA. E. FERRI SCOBS. D.

Iron filings and wire.

Iron seems to be a metal that proves active in its *metallic* state ; its filings may be given in the form of powder, conjoined to some aromatic, or what is perhaps more eligible, in the form of an electuary. DOSE. Grs. v to ʒss. IMPURITIES. Iron filings should be carefully purified by the application of the magnet, since those obtained from the work shops are generally mixed with copper, and other metals. For pharmaceutical purposes iron wire should be preferred, as being the most pure, since the softest iron only can be drawn, and Mr. Phillips has shewn us, in his experiments upon the " *Ferrum Tartarizatum,*" that soft iron is more easily acted upon by Tartar.

FERRI SULPHAS. L. SULPHAS FERRI. E.D. Ferrum vitriolatum. P. L. 1787. Sal Martis. P. L. 1745. Sal, seu Vitriolum Martis. P. L. 1720.
Sulphate of Iron, formerly *Green Vitriol.*

QUALITIES. *Form,* crystals, which are rhomboidal prisms transparent, and of a fine green colour ;

when exposed to the air they effloresce, and at the same time become covered with a yellow powder, owing to the attraction of oxygen; when exposed to heat, they undergo watery fusion, and at a higher temperature, the acid is driven off, and the peroxide of iron alone remains, which, in commerce, is known by the name of *Colcothar*. CHEMICAL COMPOSITION. According to Dr. Thomson it consists of 27·7 of sulphuric acid, 28·3 of protoxide of iron, and 45 of water; 8 parts, however, of this water, exists in combination with the oxide of iron. SOLUBILITY. It is soluble in two parts of water at 60°, and three-fourths at 212°. The solution reddens vegetable blues. It is insoluble in alcohol; when, however, the iron is farther oxidized, it becomes soluble in that menstruum. INCOMPATIBLE SUBSTANCES. Every salt whose base forms an insoluble compound with sulphuric acid; *the earths, the alkalies, and their carbonates; borate of soda; nitrate of potass, muriate of ammonia; tartrate of potass and soda; acetate of ammonia; nitrate of silver; acetate and super-acetate of lead; and Soaps.* Whether the medicinal virtues of a salt of iron are injured by combination with astringent vegetable matter, seems to admit of doubt. Such substances have been usually ranked amongst the *incompatibles*, but I am disposed to think without sufficient grounds, for I have frequently witnessed the salutary effects of iron, when exhibited in this questionable state of combination—may not the absorbents be more disposed to take up iron, when combined with vegetable matter, than when it is presented in a more purely mineral form? MEDICINAL USES. Tonic, astringent,*

* EATON'S STYPTIC. Calcined green vitriol ʒfs, proof spirit, tinged yellow with oak bark, oj.

AROMATIC LOZENGES OF STEEL. These consist of sulphate of iron, with a small proportion of the tincture of *Cantharides.*

emmenagogue, and anthelmintic; in large doses, it occasions griping in the bowels. Dose, gr. j to v, combined with rhubarb, or some bitter extract. (*Form:* 10, 24.) If given in solution, the water should be previously boiled, or the oxygen contained in the atmospherical air, which is diffused through it, will partially convert the salt into an *oxy*-sulphat, and render it insoluble. Officinal Prep. *Mist:* *Ferri comp: (g)* L. *Pil: Ferri comp: (g)* L.

FERRUM AMMONIATUM. L. Murias Ammoniæ et Ferri. E. D.

Ferrum Ammoniacale, P. L. 1787. *Flores Martiales. P. L.* 1745. *Ens Veneris. P. L.* 1720.

Qualities. *Form,* crystalline grains, which deliquesce; *Colour,* orange yellow; *Odour,* resembling that of saffron; *Taste,* styptic. Chemical Composition. This is a very variable composition; depending upon the degree of heat and length of time employed for its preparation. It seems to be a mixed mass, consisting of sub-muriate of ammonia, and sub-muriate of iron, the metal being in the state of red oxide; and, in the London preparation, Mr. Phillips states that a portion of sub-carbonate of ammonia is necessarily present. Solubility, f℥j of water dissolves ℨiv of it; it is also very soluble in alcohol. Med. Uses. It is tonic, emmenagogue, and aperient, but it is so uncertain in its composition and effects, that it is rarely used. Officinal Prep: *Tinct: Ferri Ammon:* L. Impurities, These are indicated by the dull and pale yellow colour of the salt; it may be purified by re-subliming it.

FERRUM TARTARIZATUM. L.
Tartras Potassæ et Ferri. E.
Tartarum Ferri. D.

Qualities. *Form*, a powder of a brownish green colour; *Odour*, none; *Taste*, slightly styptic; it attracts humidity from the atmosphere, but does not deliquesce. Chemical Composition. Mr. Phillips has devoted much attention to this subject, and he states, that as it is frequently prepared, it is a mere mixture of metallic iron, with super-tartrate of potass, coloured by oxide of iron; when however it is made with more care, a chemical compound results, which is either a triple salt, or one of those combinations which cream of tartar forms with metals, and of which I have spoken under the article *Antimonium Tartarizatum*. Solubility. It is very soluble in water, and the solution remains for a great length of time without undergoing any change, except that of depositing *tartrate of lime*, which is an incidental impurity in the supertartrate of potass. Incompatible Substances. *All strong acids; lime water; hydro-sulphuret of potass; astringent vegetables? The fixed alkalies and their carbonates* decompose the solution very slowly, unless heated; but *ammonia* and its *subcarbonate* produce upon it no effect whether it be hot or cold; this fact, observes Mr. Phillips, will enable us to exhibit iron in solution, with an alkali, without the occurrence of any precipitate. Forms of Exhibition. The perfect preparation from its tendency to deliquesce, cannot be well ordered in the form of powder; that of solution is probably the most judicious. It is supposed to add to its chalybeate virtues those of a diuretic nature. Dose, grs. x to ʒss.

FILICIS RADIX. L. E. D. (Asphidium Filix, Mas.)

Root of the *Male Fern.*

Qualities. This root is nearly inodorous; its taste slightly bitter, sweetish, sub-astringent and mucilaginous; as it contains no volatile ingredient, it may be given in decoction, but on account of its astringency, it must not be conjoined with a *chalybeate.* Dose, as an anthelmintic, ʒj to ʒiij, followed by a cathartic; its use however is superseded by more powerful and certain vermifuges. This root is sometimes boiled in ale to flavour it.

GALBANI GUMMI RESINA. L. E. D.

Galbanum.

Qualities. *Form,* variegated masses, of a yellowish brown colour; *Odour,* fœtid; *Taste,* bitter and acrid. Chemical Composition. It is one of those vegetable products to which the name of *gum-resin* has been given, see *Elemi.* Solubility. Water, wine, and vinegar, by trituration, take up one fourth of its weight, and form a milky mixture, but which is deposited by rest; a permanent suspension, however, may be effected by the intermedium of egg, or gum arabic, for which purpose the galbanum will require half its weight of gum. Alcohol takes up one fifth of its weight, and a yellow tincture results, which has the sensible qualities of the galbanum, and becomes milky on the addition of water, but no precipitate falls. By distillation, galbanum yields half its weight of volatile oil, which, at first, has a blue colour.

MEDICAL USES. It is an antispasmodic, expectorant, and deobstruent, and in a medical classification, might be placed between ammonia and assafœtida. FORMS OF EXHIBITION. No form is preferable to that of pill. *(Formula,* 71.*)* OFFICINAL PREP. *Pil. Galbani comp.* L. *Pil. Assafœtid. comp.* (a) E. *Pil. Myrrh. co.* (a) D. *Tinc. Galb.* D. *Empl. Galb.* D. *Emplast. Galb. co.* L. *Emplast. Assafœtid.* (a) E. *Emplast. Gummos.* E.

GALLÆ. L. E. D. (Cynips Quercus folii Nidus.)
Gall Nuts.

QUALITIES. *Form.* Excrescences nearly round and of different magnitudes, smooth on the surface, but studded with tuberosities; they are heavy, brittle, and break with a flinty fracture. *Odour,* none; *Taste* bitter, and very astringent. SOLUBILITY. The whole of their soluble matter is taken up by forty times their weight of boiling water. Alcohol, by digestion, dissolves .7, and æther .5 of their substance. The watery infusion possesses all the properties of the gall nut, and reddens vegetable blues. CHEMICAL COMPOSITION. Is at present involved in some obscurity; it contains tannin, gallic acid, a concrete volatile oil, and perhaps extractive and gum. M. Braconnot has also lately discovered in the gall nut a new acid, which he calls *Ellagic acid,* from the word *galle* reversed, a nomenclature, which it must be confessed, is at least free from the objections urged against that which is founded upon chemical composition. *(See Annales de Chimie, vol. ix. p.* 187, *new series; also Children's Essay on Chemical Analysis, p.* 276.*)* INCOMPATIBLE SUBSTANCES. The infusion and tincture of galls possess habitudes with which it is very important for the medical practitioner to be acquainted, not only for the purpose of directing their exhibition with success, but because the elements which impart to them their characteristic traits, viz. *Gallic acid* and *Tannin*,* are very widely diffused through the products of the vegetable kingdom, and will be found to be constantly active in their chemical, medicinal, and pharmaceutical applications. Metallic salts, especially those of iron, produce with infusion of galls, precipitates, composed of tannin, gallic acid, and the metallic oxide; of these compounds the *tanno-gallate of iron* is the most striking, being of a black colour; those of *acetate* and *super-acetate of lead* are greyish; *tartarized antimony* produces a yellowish; *sulphate of copper* a brown; *sulphate of zinc* reddish black; *nitrate of silver*, a deep olive; and *nitrate of mercury*, a bright yellow precipitate; *the oxy-muriate of mercury* produces only an opacity. *Sulphuric acid* throws down a yellowish curdy precipitate, *muriatic*, a flaky and white one, and *nitric acid* merely modifies the colour of the infusion, although it destroys its astringency; the solution of *ammonia* occasions no precipitate, but renders the colour deeper, the *carbonate* however throws down a precipitate; the carbonates of the *fixed alkalies* produce a yellowish flaky, and *lime water* a copious deep green precipitate. The *tannin* in the infusion of galls is precipitated by a solution of isinglass, or of any other animal jelly, by that of starch, and by many metallic oxides. MEDICAL USES. Galls are most powerfully astringent. FORMS

* Seguin first proved that gallic acid, and tannin or the astringent principle, are different substances; it is to the former that the property of giving a black colour to the solutions of iron is owing.

Mr. Hatchett has shewn that *tan* or *tannin*, may be artificially produced by the action of nitric acid upon various vegetable substances.

of Exhibition. In that of powder, (*Form.* 88,) in combination with other astringents, or with aromatics and bitters; as a local remedy, the gall nut enters into gargles, and injections; for *blind* piles, an ointment, composed of powdered galls, and a small proportion of opium, with simple ointment as an excipient, offers a very valuable resource. Dose, for internal exhibition, grs. x to ℈j, or more. Officinal Prep. *Tinct. Gallarum.* E. D. Observ. Those which are small, protuberant, bluish, and heavy, are the best, being those which have been collected before the *larvæ* within them had changed to the state of fly, and eaten their way out; a white, or a red hue indicates an inferior quality, and are those from which the insect has escaped. Aleppo galls are the most valuable, as being the most astringent.

GENTIANÆ RADIX. L. E. D.
(Gentiana Lutea, *Radix.*) *Gentian Root.*

Qualities. *Form,* wrinkled pieces of various lengths and thickness; *Odour,* not particular; *Taste,* intensely bitter, but not nauseous. Chemical Composition, bitter resin, extractive, and a small proportion of tannin; it contains also mucilage, in consequence of which the infusion frequently becomes ropy. Solubility. Its virtues are extracted by water and alcohol; proof spirit is perhaps its most perfect menstruum. See *Infus. Gentian. comp.* Medical Uses. It is tonic and stomachic, and its use for such purposes is of ancient date;* in dyspepsia, hysteria, and in all cases where a vegetable bitter is indicated,

---

* It takes its name from Gentius, king of Illyria, its discoverer, who was vanquished by Anicius, the Roman Prætor, A. U. 585, i. e. A. C. 167, so that it is neither to be found in Hippocrates nor Theophrastus.

it will be found a serviceable remedy. Dose, in sub-stance, from grs. x to ʒj. Officinal Prep. *Extract. Gentian.* L. E. D. *Infusum Gentiánæ comp.* L. E. D. *Tinct. Gentian comp.* L. E. D.* *Vinum Gentianæ compositum.* E.

GLYCYRRHIZÆ RADIX. L. E. D.
(Glycyrrhiza Glabra).
Liquorice Root. Stick Liquorice.

Qualities. *Taste,* sweet and mucilaginous. Che-mical Composition. Saccharine matter, mucilage, and woody fibre. Solubility. Water extracts both its principles, but by long coction it becomes bitter ; alcohol extracts only its saccharine matter. Medical Uses. It is principally employed as a demulcent in combination with other mucilaginous vegetables ; the root will yield nearly half its weight of extract. Li-quorice covers the taste of some unpalatable medicines more effectually than any other substance. Offici-nal Prep : *Decoct : Sarsaparill : comp :* L.D. *Infus : Lini,* L. *Extract : Glycyrrhizæ.* L.E.D. *Confectio Sennæ.†* L.E. Adulterations. The powdered root is generally sophisticated with flour, and some-times with powdered guaiacum ; the fraud may be de-tected by its colour being a fine pale, instead of a brownish yellow, and by its reduced, or foreign fla-vour.

* Brodum's Nervous Cordial consists of the tinctures of *Gentian, Calumba, Cardamom* and *Bark,* with the *Compound Spirit of Lavender,* and *Wine of Iron.*

Stroughton's Elixir. Is a tincture of *Gentian,* with the addition of *Serpentaria, Orange peel, Cardamoms,* and some other *aromatics.*

† Pectoral Balsam of Liquorice. The Proprietor of this nos-trum gravely affirms that f℥iss contains the virtues of a *whole pound* of Liquorice root ; but upon investigation it will be found to consist prin-cipally of *Paregoric* Elixir, very strongly impregnated with the *Oil of Linseed.*

GRANATI CORTEX. L.E.D. $\left(\begin{array}{l}\text{Punica Granatum}\\\text{Pomorum Cortex}\end{array}\right)$

Pomegranate Bark.

What has been said respecting the Gall nut, applies with equal truth to this substance.

GUAIACI RESINA ET LIGNUM. L.E.D.

(Guaiacum Officinale).

The Resin Wood of Guaiacum.

A. THE WOOD.

QUALITIES. This wood is heavier than water, and emits, when heated, an aromatic odour; *Taste*, bitterish and sub-acrid; to extract its virtues long decoction is required. It has enjoyed great reputation as a specific in the venereal disease; it was imported into Europe in 1517, and gained immediate celebrity, from curing the celebrated Van Hutten; long before this period, however, it was used by the natives of St. Domingo. Boerhaave, so late as the eighteenth century, maintained its specific powers. It seems probable that the discipline which always accompanied its exhibition, such as sweating, abstinence, and purgation, might be the means, in the warmer climates, of effecting cures which were attributed to the guaiacum. OFFICINAL PREP: *Decoct: Guaiaci comp:* E. *Decoct: Sarsaparill: comp:* L.D.

B. THE GUAIAC, or *Resin.*

QUALITIES. *Form*; it has the aspect of a gum-resin; *Colour*, greenish brown; it is easily pulverised, and the powder, which is at first grey, becomes green on exposure to air and light; which appears to depend upon the absorption of oxygen; when heated, it loses its colour; it melts by heat; and has a *sp:*

grav: of 1·2289. Solubility. *Water* dissolves out of it about 9 per cent. of extractive matter; *alcohol* 95, and *ether* 40 parts in a hundred. The *alkaline* solutions, and their *carbonates,* dissolve it readily; *Sulphuric acid* dissolves it with scarcely any effervescence, and affords a solution of a rich claret colour; *Nitric acid* dissolves it with a copious extrication of nitrous fumes; *Muriatic acid* dissolves a small portion only; but in all these cases the guaiacum is decomposed; the acids are therefore incompatible with it. Chemical Composition. The experiments of Mr. Hatchett demonstrate that it is a substance *sui generis,* and not a resin, or gum-resin. Med: Uses. Stimulant, diaphoretic,* and in large doses, purgative. Forms of Exhibition, in that of bolus, or diffused in water, by means of one half of its weight of gum arabic. Dose, gr. x to ʒss. Officinal Prep: *Mist: Guaiac:* L. *Tinct: Guaiac.* L.E.D. *Tinct: Guaiaci Ammoniat:* L.E.D. *Pulv: Aloes· comp:* (d) L.D. Adulterations. *Common resin* may be detected by the turpentine emitted when the guaiac is thrown upon hot coals; *Manchinal gum,* by adding to the tincture a few drops of sweet spirit of nitre, and diluting with water; the guaiac is thus precipitated, but the adulteration floats in white striæ.

---

* The Chelsea Pensioner. An empirical remedy for the rheumatism is well known under this name; it is said to be the prescription of a Chelsea Pensioner, by which Lord Amherst was cured; the following is its composition—*Gum Guaiac:* ʒj *Powdered Rhubarb:* ʒij— *Cream of Tartar:* ℥j—*Flowers of Sulphur:* ℥ij—*One Nutmeg,* finely powdered, made into an Electuary with one pound of *Clarified Honey.* Two large spoonfuls to be taken night and morning.

Walker & Wessel's Jesuit Drops. This is nothing more than the *Elixir Anti-venereum* of Quincey, consisting of *Guaiacum, Balsam of Copaiba,* and *Oil of Sassafras,* made into a Tincture by Spirit.

HÆMATOXYLI LIGNUM. L.E.D.
(Hæmatoxylon Campechianum). *Logwood.*

QUALITIES. The wood is hard, compact, and heavy. *Odour,* none; *Taste,* sweet and astringent; *Colour,* deep red. CHEMICAL COMPOSITION. The colouring matter of this wood has been very recently submitted to a rigid examination; the name of *Hematin* has been given to it; it affords small brilliant crystals of a reddish white colour, and slightly astringent, bitter, and acrid flavour; sulphuretted hydrogen, passed through its solution in water, gives it a yellow colour, which disappears in a few days. Gelatine throws it down in reddish flakes. The habitudes of Logwood are curious with respect to mutability of colour. The recent infusion, made with distilled water, is yellow, but that with common water has a reddish purple colour, which is deepened by the alkalies, and changed to yellow by the acids; various salts precipitate it; *super-acetate of lead; alum;* the *sulphates of copper and iron; tartarized antimony; and sulphuric, muriatic, nitric, and acetic acids,* are, on this account, incompatible with it. MED. USES. It is supposed to be astringent, and is therefore given in protracted diarrhœas, and in the latter stage of dysentery. OFFICINAL PREP. *Extract: Hæmatoxyli.* L.

HELLEBORI FŒTIDI FOLIA. L.
(Helleborus Fœtidus). HELLEBORASTER. D.
The Leaves of Fœtid Hellebore.

As this plant is merely retained in the list of materia medica, on account of its anthelmintic properties, it might be well dispensed with, since we possess many others, which are much more safe, as well as efficacious.

HELLEBORI NIGRI RADIX. L.E.D.
The Root of Black Hellebore. Melampodium.
Christmas Rose.

QUALITIES. The fibres of the root are the parts employed; they are about the thickness of a straw, corrugated, externally, of a deep dark colour, hence the epithet *black*, internally, white, or of a yellowish hue. *Odour*, unpleasant; *Taste*, bitter and acrid. CHEMICAL COMPOSITION. Its qualities appear to reside in volatile oil, gum, and resin. SOLUBILITY. Both water and alcohol extract its virtues, but the spiritous solution is the most active; long coction diminishes its powers, hence the watery extract acts more mildly than the root. MED. USES. It is a drastic cathartic, and proves therefore an emmenagogue, and hydragogue. FORMS OF EXHIBITION. It is seldom given in substance, but in the form of tincture or extract; or in that of decoction, made with two drachms of the root to a pint of water. DOSE of the powdered root, grs. x to ℈j; of the decoction, f℥j. OFFICINAL PREP. *Tinct: Hellebori Nigri.* L.E.D. *Extractum Hellebori Nigri.* E.D. ADULTERATIONS. The roots of the poisonous aconites are often fraudulently substituted; this is easily discovered, for the aconite is lighter coloured than the palest specimens of black hellebore; it is safe therefore to choose the darkest.

---

* MATTHEW's PILLS, STARKEY's PILLS. Of the Roots of *Black H.lle_bore, Liquorice*, and *Turmeric*, equal parts, *purified opium*, *Castille soap*, and *syrup of saffron*, the same quantity, made into pills, with *oil of turpentine*.

HORDEI SEMINA. L.E.D. (Hordeum Distichon. Semina, tunicis nudata.)

Hordeum Perlatum. *Pearl Barley.*

Barley is formed into *Pearl Barley*, by the removal of its husk, or cuticle, and afterwards, by being rounded, and polished in a mill. These well known granules consist chiefly of fecula, with portions of mucilage, gluten, and sugar, which water extracts by decoction, but the solution soon passes into the acetous fermentation ; the bran of barley contains an acrid resin, and it is to get rid of such an ingredient, that it is deprived of its cuticle. OFFICINAL PREP. *Decoct: Hordei.* L.E.D. *Decoct: Hord: comp:* L. D.

HUMULI STROBILI. L.E. (Humulus Lupulus Strobili Siccati.)

The Strobiles of the Hop.

CHEMICAL COMPOSITION. Resin, extractive, gum, volatile oil, tannin, an ammoniacal salt, and a bitter principle. SOLUBILITY. Boiling water, alcohol, and ether, extract their virtues ; but by decoction their aromatic flavour is lost; like most bitters, the cold is more grateful than the warm infusion ; its colour is deepened by alkalies, and rendered turbid by the mineral acids ; metallic salts also produce decomposition. MED. USES. Hops have been said to be tonic, narcotic, and diuretic; they have been recommended in the cure of rheumatism ; and, like many articles in the materia medica, which have received the sanction of respectable practitioners, they have been extolled far beyond their merit. They undoubtedly possess the advantages of a pleasant bitter, combined with a feeble narcotic ; the late Mr. Freake was very sanguine as to their powers, and at his request, I made a series of experiments at the Westminster Hospital, but I confess that their results have not established my confidence in their efficacy. OFFICINAL PREP. *Extract: Humuli.* L. *Tinct: Humuli.* L. Their use as a preservative of beer is well known ; and it is equally notorious, that various vegetable substances are daily substituted for them, such as *Quassia* and *Wormwood,* but which are inferior to the *Menyanthes Trifoliata,* or *Marsh Trefoil.* The people of Jersey are said to use the wood sage, *Teucrium Scorodonia,* it imparts however a very high colour to the beer. During the first four years that the Cape of Good Hope was in possession of the British, more than 300,000 pounds of Aloes were imported into England ; how could such a quantity be consumed ? except, as Mr. Barrow states, by the London porter brewers.

HYDRARGYRUM. L.D. HYDRARGYRUS. E.
Olim, Argentum vivum. *Mercury,* or *Quicksilver*

Mercury, in its metallic state, is never applied to any medicinal use, except in visceral obstruction, in hopes of forcing a passage by its gravity ; but under various forms of preparation, it affords a series of very active remedies. ADULTERATIONS. With the exception of Peruvian Bark, there is perhaps no active article in the materia medica more shamefully adulterated ; its impurity is at once indicated by its dull aspect ; by its tarnishing, and becoming covered with a grey film ; by its diminished mobility, in consequence

of which, its globules are unable to retain the spherical form, and therefore *tail*, as it is technically
expressed. *Lead* is discovered by dissolving it in
nitric acid, and adding to the solution, water impregnated with sulphuretted hydrogen, when, if any
be present, a dark brown precipitate will ensue.
Bismuth, by pouring the nitric solution into distilled
water, when it will appear as a white precipitate.
Zinc, by exposing the mercury to heat. *Tin* is detected by a dilute solution of nitro-muriate of gold,
which throws down a purple precipitate. The presence of lead in mercury is a most dangerous circumstance; 1 have once witnessed a case of *cholica pictonum* in consequence of it. The usual mode of purifying quicksilver, by pressing it through chamois
leather, will not separate the lead, if it be, as is generally the case, in combination with bismuth; for the
manner in which the adulteration is effected, is by
melting with a gentle heat, these two metals, and
adding the alloy to the mercury, and although this
alloy should exceed one-fourth of the whole bulk, it
will pass, together with the mercury, through chamois
leather. On standing, the bismuth will be thrown
upon the surface, in the form of a dark powder, but
the lead will remain in solution. The greatest part
of the mercury in commerce comes from Istria and
Friuli, and from the Palatinate, and as it passes
through the hands of the Dutch, we must expect to
receive it in a state of alloy. On a superficial examination, it ought not, when shaken with water, to
impart to it any colour; when agitated, or digested
with vinegar, it should not communicate a sweetish
taste; and, when exposed in an iron spoon to heat,
it ought to evaporate entirely. The French are so
well aware of the mischievous extent to which this

metal is falsified, that in their late Codex, they direct
the reduction of the *red oxyd* in order to obtain it;
the process however is far too expensive for general
adoption. The Italian Jews purify quicksilver for
their barometers, by digesting in dilute sulphuric
acid, which is by no means an improper process. The
mode directed for the purification of mercury by the
London College, (*Hydrargyrum Purificatum*) is unable to separate it *completely* from its more deleterious contaminations. It is a general opinion in
Germany, that mercury boiled in water will impart
to it an anthelmintic virtue ; this, if it happens, can
only depend upon the impurities of the mercury;
but large draughts of cold water are in themselves
anthelmintic.

HYDRARGYRUM PRÆCIPITATUM AL-
BUM. L. SUBMURIAS HYDRARGYRI AMMONI-
ATUM. D. *White Precipitate.*

QUALITIES. *Fo.m,* an impalpable powder of a
snowy whiteness ; *Odour* and *Taste,* none. CHEMI-
CAL COMP. It is a triple compound of oxide of mercury 81, muriatic acid 16, ammonia 3 parts. SOLU-
BILITY. It is insoluble in water, and in alcohol;
when triturated with lime water it does not become
black. It is only used in combination with lard as an
ointment. OFFICINAL PREP. *Unguent: Hydrarg :
præcipitati albi.* L.D.

HYDRARGYRUM CUM CRETA. L.D.
Mercury with Chalk.

This is mercury slightly oxidized by trituration,
and mixed with chalk. Grs. iij contain about one

grain of mercury. Dose, grs. v to ʒss. It is a mild and excellent mercurial, and has been known to cure syphilitic affections, when the constitution had proved rebellious to every other form of preparation. Dr. George Fordyce committed a great error, when he denied to this compound any mercurial efficacy.

HYDRARGYRI NITRICO-OXYDUM. L.

OXYDUM HYDRARGYRI RUBRUM PER ACIDUM NITRICUM. E. OXYDUM HYDRARGYRI NITRICUM. D. *Nitric Oxide of Mercury—Red Precipitate.*

QUALITIES. *Form*, small scales of a bright red colour; *Taste*, acrid and corrosive. CHEMICAL COMPOSITION. It is strictly speaking a *sub-nitrate* of mercury. SOLUBILITY. It is quite insoluble in water, but soluble in nitric acid, without any effervescence. USES. It is used only externally, as an escharotic. OFFICINAL PREP. *Unguent: Hydrargyri Nitrico-oxyd:* L. E. D. ADULTERATIONS. *Red Lead* may be detected by digesting it in acetic acid, and adding sulphuret of ammonia, which will produce a dark coloured precipitate: it should be totally volatilized by heat.

HYDRARGYRI OXYDUM CINEREUM. L. E.

PULVIS HYDRARGYRI CINEREUS. D. *Grey Oxide of Mercury.*

QUALITIES. *Form*, an impalpable grey coloured powder, which becomes paler on exposure to air and light. *Odour* and *taste*, none. CHEM. COMPOSITION. When properly prepared it is a protoxide of mercury, but as frequently found in the shops, it contains a mixture of the triple salt consisting of oxide of mercury, ammonia and nitric acid. It is rarely used. OFFICINAL PREP. *Unguent. Oxid. Hydrarg. ciner. E.*

HYDRARGYRI OXYDUM RUBRUM. L.

OXYDUM HYDRARGYRI. D.

Red Oxyd of Mercury.

The *Precipitate per se* of the older Chemists.

QUALITIES. *Form*, minute crystalline scales, of a deep red colour, inodorous, but acrid and caustic ; it is soluble in several of the acids without decomposition; it is also slightly soluble in water. USES. It is very active as a mercurial, and has been a favourite remedy with John Hunter, and other celebrated practitioners; it is however apt to affect the stomach and bowels, and is therefore now rarely employed except as an external application. DOSE, gr. j. combined with opium gss. ADULTERATIONS. It is seldom adulterated, as it would be difficult to find a substance suited to this purpose. If well prepared, it may be totally volatilized by heat.

HYDRARGYRI OXY-MURIAS. L.

MURIAS HYDRARGYRI CORROSIVUS. E. D.

Oxy-muriate of Mercury.

Corrosive Muriate of Mercury. Corrosive Sublimate.

QUALITIES. *Form*, a crystalline mass, which is easily pulverized, and undergoes a slight alteration by exposure to air, becoming on its surface opaque and pulverulent. *Odour*, none. *Taste* very acrid, with a metallic astringency. CHEMICAL COMPOSITION. According to the latest views, it is a *Bi-chloride* of mercury, consisting of one proportional of mercury, to two proportionals of chlorine. In the French Codex, it is termed "*Deuto-Chloruretum Hydrargyri*." SOLUBILITY. It is soluble in eleven parts of cold, and in three of boiling water, and in four parts of alcohol; it is also very soluble in ether, indeed this latter liquid has the curious property of abstracting it from its solution in water, when agitated with it. Its solution in water is greatly expedited by the addition of a few drops of rectified spirit, or of muriatic acid. In a solution of muriate of ammonia it is thirty times more soluble than in water, no decomposition however arises, it is therefore probable, that a triple salt is formed; it is also soluble in the sulphuric, nitric, and muriatic acids, and may be obtained again unaltered, by simply evaporating the solutions. Its watery solution is said to change to green vegetable blues, but this is an optical fallacy, *see page* 144. INCOMPATIBLE SUBSTANCES. The *carbonates of the fixed* alkalies precipitate it of a yellow hue, but the precipitates are not pure oxides; *ammonia* forms with it a white triple compound. *Lime water* decomposes it more perfectly than any alkaline body, occasioning a precipitate of a deep yellow colour, which is an oxyd of mercury containing a little muriatic acid; this result forms a useful lotion to ill conditioned ulcers, and has been long known under the title of *Aqua Phagadenica*; fℨj of lime water should be employed for the decomposition of two grains of the salt. *Tartarized antimony, nitrate of silver, super-acetate of lead, sulphur, sulphuret of potass,* and *soaps,* decompose it. *Iron, lead, copper, bismuth,* and *zinc,* in their metallic state, also decompose it, producing precipitates which consist of an amalgam of the metal employed, with calomel; hence mortars of glass or earthenware should be employed for dispensing this article; when triturated with olive oil, the oil becomes white, and when boiled with it, *calomel* is precipitated; the same happens if sugar be substituted for the oil; the volatile oils reduce it. The following vegetable infusions produce precipitates, viz. *the infusions and decoctions of chamomile, horse raddish root, calumba root, catechu, cinchona, rhubarb, senna, simarouba,* and *oak bark, tea* and *almond emulsion.* Swediaur observes, that "many authors have recommended *sublimate* combined with bark, but that a reciprocal decomposition is thus produced, by which the energies of both remedies are alike annulled;" to this ignorance, however, he thinks that many patients have been indebted for their lives, for, says he, "I see every day examples of weak and very delicate persons of both sexes, to whom ignorant practitioners prescribe, and sometimes in very large doses, the *corrosive sublimate,* with a decoction of bark, certainly without curing the syphilis, but at the same time without occasioning those grave and dangerous symptoms, which that acrid medicine would certainly produce, if given alone, or without that decoction." MEDICAL USES. It is one of the most acrid and active of all metallic preparations; in well directed doses however, it is frequently of service in secondary syphilis, and in cases of anomalous disease, when it would be improper to administer the other forms of mercury;*

---

* As this salt has been supposed to arrest the progress of syphilis more rapidly, and at the same time, to excite the salivary glands less than any other preparation of mercury, it generally forms the basis of those dangerous nostrums, which are advertised for the *cure of Syphilis, without Mercury.* The contrivers hope also to elude detection by the density and colour of the preparation.

GOWLAND'S LOTION. Is a solution of *sublimate* in an emulsion formed

its exhibition should be accompanied with mucila‑
ginous drinks; when an overdose has been taken the

of bitter almonds, in the proportion of about gr. jss to f ʒj. A solution
of this mercurial salt in Spirit of Rosemary, is also sold as an empirical
cosmetic.

NORTON'S DROPS. A disguised solution of corrosive sublimate.

WARD'S WHITE DROPS. Prepared by dissolving mercury in nitric
acid, and adding a solution of muriate of ammonia, or frequently they
consist of a solution of *sublimate* with muriate of ammonia.

SPILSBURY'S ANTISCORBUTIC DROPS.   Of *Corrosive Sublimate* Ʒij.
Prepared Sulphuret of Antimony Ʒj.   *Gentian root* and Orange *peel*, equal
parts, Ʒij.   *Shavings of Red Saunders*, Ʒj, made into a tincture with a pint
of proof spirit, digest and strain.

"THE ANTIVENEREAL DROPS," so famous at Amsterdam, were
analysed by Scheele, who found that they were composed of muriate
of iron, with a small proportion of *corrosive sublimate*.

MARSDEN'S ANTISCORBUTIC DROPS. A solution of *sublimate* in an
infusion of Gentian.

GREEN'S DROPS. The basis of these also is *sublimate*.

SOLOMON'S ANTI-IMPETIGINES. A solution of *sublimate*.

ROB ANTI-SYPHILITIQUE, *par M. Laffecteur, Medicin Chimiste*. This
popular nostrum of the French contains as a principal ingredient,
corrosive sublimate. A strong decoction of the *Arundo Phragmitis*, (the
bullrush,) is made, with the addition of *sarsaparilla* and *anniseeds* towards
the end, which is evaporated and made into a rob, or syrup, to which
the *sublimate* is added.

SIROP DE CUISINIERE. This consists of decoctions of *sarsaparilla*,
burrage flowers, white roses, senna and *anniseed*, to which *sublimate* is added,
and the whole is then made into a syrup with sugar and honey.

TERRE FEUILLETEE MERCURIELLE *of Pressavin*. This is *Tartarized
Mercury*, for it is made by boiling the oxyd of mercury (obtained by
precipitating it from a nitric solution, by potass) with *cream of tartar*.

VELNO'S VEGETABLE SYRUP. There is great obscurity with respect
to the genuine composition of this nostrum; it is supposed to consist of
sublimate, rubbed up with honey and mucilage. I have reason however
to believe that it contains *antimony*, and the syrup of marsh mallows.
Swediaur says that volatile alkali enters into it as an ingredient; this
alkali was proposed by Dr. Peyrile, as a substitute for mercury, and it
constitutes the active ingredient of the following composition, which
was proposed by Mr. Besnard, Physician to the King of Bavaria.

TINCTURA ANTISYPHILLITICA. *Sub-carb. potass*, lbj, dissolved in
Aq. Cinnam. oj. *Opii puri*, Ʒij, dissolved in *Spir cinnamom.* fʒiv. mix these
separate solutions, and put them on a water bath for three weeks,

white of egg, diluted with water, is the best antidote, for Orfila has found that albumen decomposes it, reducing it to the state of mild muriate, whilst the compound which it forms with it is inert. Dose, gr. ⅛ to ½, *see Liquor Hydrargyri Oxy-muriatis.* Caution. The salt, as it is partially decomposed by light, should be kept in opaque bottles. Adulterations. It ought to be volatilized by heat; it is frequently met with in commerce, contaminated with muriate of iron, sometimes with arsenic; the presence of calomel is at once discovered from its insolubility. Tests of its Presence. If any powder be suspected to contain this salt, expose it to heat, in a coated tube, as directed in the treatment of arsenic, but without any carbonaceous admixture, when corrosive sublimate, if present, will rise and line the interior surface with a shining white crust. This crust is then to be dissolved in distilled water, and assayed by the following tests; 1st, *lime water* will produce, if the suspected solution contain this salt, a precipitate of an orange yellow colour. 2nd, a single drop of a dilute solution of *sub-carbonate of potass* will at first produce a white precipitate, but on a still farther addition of the test, an orange coloured sediment will be formed. 3rd, *sulphuretted water* will throw down a dark coloured precipitate, which when dried, and strongly heated, may be volatilized without any alliaceous odour. A very ingenious application of galvanic electricity has been also proposed by Mr.

taking care to shake the vessel frequently; to this add *Gum arabic* ℥ij, *Carb. Ammonæ* ℥j, dissolve in *aq. Cinnamomi*, mix, filter, and keep for use. Dose, twenty-four drops three times a day, in a glass of the cold decoction of Marsh Mallow root.

The external use of these drops is also advised for local syphilitic complaints!

Silvester, for the detection of *corrosive sublimate*,
which will exhibit the mercury in a metallic state.
A piece of zinc or iron wire about three inches in
length, is to be twice bent at right angles, so as to
resemble the greek letter π, the two legs of this
figure should be distant about the diameter of a
common gold wedding ring from each other, and the
two ends of the bent wire must afterwards be tied to
a ring of this description. Let a plate of glass, not
less than three inches square, be laid as nearly hori-
zontal as possible, and on one side drop some sulphuric acid, diluted with about six times its weight
of water, till it spreads to the size of a halfpenny.
At a little distance from this, towards the other side,
next drop some of the solution supposed to contain
corrosive sublimate, till the edges of the two liquids
join together; and let the wire and ring, prepared as
above, be laid in such a way that the wire may touch
the acid, while the gold ring is in contact with the
suspected liquid. If the minutest quantity of corrosive sublimate be present, the ring in a few minutes
will be covered with mercury on the part which
touched the fluid.

HYDRARGYRI SUB-MURIAS. L.

Sub-murias Hydrargyri Mitis. E.

Sub-murias Hydrargyri sublimatum. D.

vulgo. *Calomel.*

This preparation has been known in pharmacy for
upwards of two centuries, under a variety of fanciful
names, such as *Draco mitigatus; Aquila alba; Aquila
mitigata; Manna metallorum; Panchymagogum mine-
rale; Panchymagogus quercetanus; Sublimatum dulce;*

Mercurius dulcis sublimatus ; Calomelas ; and yet there is not a name in this list that is so objectionable as the one at present adopted by our colleges : for whether we adhere to the theory of muriatic acid being the *simple* body, or accede to the new views of *chlorine*, the name is equally inappropriate ; if we regard it as a compound of muriatic acid and oxyd of mercury, it is not a *sub-*muriate, but as much a *muriate* as the corrosive sublimate ; the only difference depending upon the degree of oxidizement of the mercury, which is at a *minimum* in calomel, and at a *maximum* in sublimate. According to the new views respecting chlorine, calomel must consist of one proportional of chlorine, with one proportional of metal, and is therefore a *chloride of mercury.* (" *Proto-chloruretum Hydrargyri.*" Codex Med. Paris.)

QUALITIES. *Form.* A semi-transparent mass, consisting of short. prismatic crystals; inodorous, insipid, and of an ivory colour, which deepens by exposure to light. . SOLUBILITY. It is considered as being insoluble, since according to Rouelle, one part requires 1152 of water, at 212° for its solution. INCOMPATIBLE SUBSTANCES. *Alkalies* and *lime water* decompose it, and turn it black, in consequence of precipitating the black oxyd of the metal; it is also decomposed by *soaps, sulphurets of potass and antimony ;* and by *iron, lead* and *copper ;* hence, it is improper to employ any metallic mortar for dispensing medicines which contain it. There seems to be reason for supposing, that this preparation may undergo decomposition *in transitu,* and that therefore some substances may be *chemically,* and yet not be *medicinally* incompatible with it. If calomel be boiled for a few minutes in distilled water, to which alcoholized potass has been added, it is completely decomposed, a *mu-riate of potass*, and *black oxyd of mercury*, being the new products. MEDICAL USES. This mercurial preparation is more extensively and more usefully employed, than almost any other article in the whole range of the materia medica. It is capable of curing syphilis in every form, provided it does not run off by the bowels; and in obstructions and hepatic affections, it is, in well regulated doses, a most valuable remedy; in combination, it probably merits the appellation of *Dirigens*, more decidedly than any other remedy with which we are acquainted, for when combined with certain diuretics, it is diuretic, *(Form.* 31, 32,) and in diaphoretic arrangements, it is diaphoretic: in larger doses, it is one of the most efficient purgatives which we possess, especially in combination with other cathartics; it appears to be particularly eligible in the diseases of children; and it is singular that infants can generally bear larger doses of it than adults. DOSE, as an alterative, from gr. j to ij, night and morning; as a purgative from gr. iv to grs. x, or in some cases even to grs. xv, or Əj. FORMS OF EXHIBITION. That of pill; its insolubility and specific gravity render any other form ineligible. OFFICINAL PREP. *Pil. Hydrargyri sub-muriatis.* L.

---

* Many of the nostrums advertised for the cure of worms, contain *calomel*, as their principal ingredient, combined with *scammony, jalap, gamboge*, or some other purgative; they are uncertain and dangerous medicines; the method of exhibiting them in the form of lozenges *(worm cakes,)* is also attended with inconvenience, for the sugar and the gum generating an acid, by being kept in damp places, may considerably increase the acrimony of the mercury; besides which, the calomel is frequently diffused very unequally through the mass, one lozenge may therefore contain a poisonous dose, whilst others may scarcely possess any active matter.

CHING'S WORM LOZENGES. These consist of *yellow* and *brown*

IMPURITIES. *Corrosive sublimate* may be detected by a precipitation being produced, by the carbonate of potàss, in a solution made by boiling the suspected sample with a small portion of muriate of ammonia, in distilled water; calomel ought also, when rubbed with pure ammonia, to become intensely black, and to exhibit no traces of an orange hue.

HOWARD's *Hydro-sublimate.* Instead of subliming so as to obtain the calomel in a concrete state, as directed by the Pharmacopœia, the sublimed vapour is received in water; it is lighter than common calomel, in the proportion of three to five, and it can contain no corrosive sublimate. The French in their late *codex* have introduced a similar formula, recommended by Jewel, for obtaining calomel in a state of minute division; it consists in exposing it, in the act of sublimation, to the vapour of boiling water.

SUB-MURIAS HYDRARGYRI PRÆCIPITATUS. E.D. This is produced by precipitating a nitrate of mercury by muriate of soda; the preparation will generally contain a small portion of *sub-nitrate*, and it is on that account more liable to run off by the bowels, in small doses: in other respects it is essentially the same as that procured by sublimation.

lozenges, the former are taken in the evening, the latter the succeeding morning.

THE YELLOW LOZENGES. Saffron ℥ss, water oj, boil, and strain ; add of *White Panacea of Mercury* (Calomel washed in spirit of wine) ℔j, white sugar 28 lb, mucilage of *Tragacanth* as much as may be sufficient to make a mass, which roll out of an exact thickness, so that each lozenge may contain one grain of *panacea.* Dose, from one to six.

THE BROWN LOZENGES. Panacea℥vij, *resin of jalap* lb iijss, white sugar lb ix, *mucilage of tragacanth* q. s, each lozenge should contain gr. ½ of *panacea.*

STOREY's WORM CAKES. Calomel and jalap made into cakes and coloured by cinnabar.

HYDRAGYRI SULPHURETUM RUBRUM. L.
SULPHURATUM HYDRARGYRI RUBRUM. D. Olim,
Hydrargyrus Sulphuratus ruber. P.L. 1817—*Cinna-baris factitia,* 1745.

QUALITIES. *Form,* a red crystalline cake, inodorous, insipid, and insoluble in water, alcohol, acids, and alkalies ; although these last bodies decompose it, when melted with it; it is also decomposed by nitro-muriatic acid, which unites with the metal, and disengages the sulphur. CHEMICAL COMPOSITION. It is a *bi-sulphuret of Mercury,* i. e. it consists of two proportionals of sulphur, and one of mercury. USES. It is now only used for the purpose of mercurial fumigation, which is done by inhaling the fumes, produced by throwing ʒss of it on red hot iron ; the effect which it generally produces is violent salivation; this however does not depend upon the action of the substance, as a *sulphuret,* but upon its decomposition, and the volatilization of the metallic mercury, with sulphureous vapour. Mr. Pearson observes, that it is useful in those cases of venereal ulcers, in the mouth, throat, and nose, where it is an object to put a *sudden* stop to the progress of the disease, but that mercury must, at the same time be introduced into the constitution, by inunction, just as much as if no fumigations had been made use of. ADULTERATIONS. *Red Lead* may be discovered by digesting it in acetic acid, and by adding sulphuret of ammonia, which will produce a black precipitate; *Dragon's Blood,* by its giving a colour to alcohol when digested with it; *Chalk,* by its effervescence, on the addition of an acid. It is known in the arts under the name of *Vermilion.*

HYDRARGYRI SULPHURETUM NIGRUM.
L.E. Hydrargyrus cum Sulphure. P.L. 1787. Olim. *Ethiops Mineral.*

QUALITIES. *Form*, a very black, impalpable, insipid, and inodorous powder. CHEMICAL COMPOSITION. It is a *Sulphuret of Mercury*, i. e. it consists of one proportional of sulphur, and one proportional of mercury ; when heated in contact with the air, it is converted into a *bi-sulphuret.* SOLUBILITY. It is entirely soluble in a solution of pure potass, from which the acids precipitate it, unchanged; it is insoluble in nitric acid. MED: USES. It is supposed to be alterative, and has been given for such a purpose, in doses from gr. v. to ʒss, but its medicinal virtues are very questionable. ADULTERATIONS. It is frequently imperfect, globules of mercury being still discoverable in it by a magnifying glass, or by its communicating a whiteness to a portion of gold upon which it is rubbed ; *ivory black* may be discovered by the residue after throwing a suspected sample on a red hot iron ; it is also sometimes mixed with equal parts of crude antimony.

HYOSCYAMI FOLIA ET SEMINA. L. E. D.
(Hyoscyamus Niger)* *Henbane.*

QUALITIES. This plant, when recent, has a strong, fetid, and narcotic odour ; properties which are nearly lost by exsiccation. CHEMICAL COMPOSITION. Re-

---

* ANODYNE NECKLACES. The roots of *Hyoscyamus* are commonly strung in the form of beads, and sold under this name, to tie round the necks of children, to facilitate the growth of their teeth, and allay the irritation of teething. The application of medicated necklaces is a very ancient superstition.

sin, mucilage, extractive matter, gallic acid, and some salts. SOLUBILITY. Water feebly extracts its narcotic powers, and decoction destroys them; diluted alcohol is its best menstruum. INCOMPATIBLES. Precipitates are produced by *super-acetate of lead, ni-trate of silver*, and *sulphate of iron;* vegetable acids weaken its narcotic powers. The extract, or inspissated juice, is the best form in which it can be exhibited; see also the *Tincture;* its leaves form an anodyne cataplasm, and the smoke from its seeds, when applied by a funnel to a carious tooth, is recommended in severe fits of odontalgia. OFFICINAL PREP: *Extract: Hyoscyam: Tinct: Hyoscyam:* L.E.D.

ICHTHYOCOLLA. (Acipenser *Huso* & *Ruthenus.*)
(*The great and small Sturgeon.*)

Isinglass.   Fish Glue.

The following kinds, imported from St. Petersburg, are found in the market. *Short Staple; Long Staple; Book;* and *Leaf. Picking the Staple*, as it is called, is a peculiar art, practised by persons in this town, who gain by it a very good livelihood; they engage to return the same weight of isinglass, in shreds, as they receive in *Staple;* this, in itself, secures very fair profit, for by damping the isinglass, in order to pick it, it gains considerable weight; these persons moreover are in the habit of adulterating it with pieces of bladder, and the dried skin of soles; such frauds however are easily detected by its insolubility, for pure isinglass will dissolve entirely, and yield a clear and transparent jelly; a single grain will produce, with an ounce of water, a solution of considerable thickness; it is also soluble in acids and alkalies; and although insoluble in alcohol, yet it is not

precipitated by it from its watery solutions, unless
when added in a very considerable quantity; it is
coagulated by the infusions and decoctions of vegetable astringents; *carbonate of potass* likewise throws
down a precipitate. 100 parts of good isinglass consist of 98 of gelatine, and 2 of the phosphates of soda
and lime. Its solutions soon putrefy. Uses. It is
now rarely used except as a nutrient; its application in fining wines and turbid liquors, is well known,
and its mode of operation is equally obvious, for by
forming a skin, or fine network, which gradually
precipitates, it acts just like a filtre, with this difference, that in this case the filtre passes through the
liquor, instead of the liquor through the filtre.

INFUSA. L.E.D. *Infusions.*

These are *watery* solutions of vegetable matter, obtained by maceration, either in cold or hot water,
without the assistance of ebullition. In selecting
and conducting the operation, the following general
rules should be observed.

I. *Infusion should always be preferred to decoction,
where the medicinal virtues of the vegetable substance reside in volatile oil, or, in principles which
are easily soluble; whereas, if they depend upon
resino-mucilaginous particles, decoction is an indispensable operation.*

II. *The temperature employed must be varied according to the circumstances of each case; an infusion
made in the cold, is in general more grateful, but
less active, than one made with heat.*

III. *The duration of the process must likewise be regulated by the nature of the substances, or the*

*intention of the prescriber, for, the infusion will
differ according to the time in which the water
has been digested on the materials ; thus, the aroma
of the plant is first taken up, then, in succession, the
colouring, astringent, and gummy parts.*

Infusions are liable to undergo decompositions by
being kept, and therefore, like decoctions, they must
be regarded as *extemporaneous* preparations. Unless
the dose of them be otherwise stated, it is generally
from f℥j to f℥ij.

I. *Simple Infusions.*

INFUSUM ANTHEMIDIS. L. E. It is a good
stomachic ; and when exhibited warm, is well calculated to assist the operation of emetics. *Incompatibles.* All *soluble preparations of iron* ; *nitrate of
silver ; oxy-muriate of mercury ; acetate,* and *super-
acetate of lead* ; *solutions of isinglass ; infusion of yellow cinchona bark.*

INFUSUM CALUMBÆ. L. E. See Calumbæ Radix.

INFUSUM CARYOPHYLLORUM. L. f℥j of this infusion holds in solution the active matter of grs. vj of
cloves. *Incompatibles.* Precipitates are produced by
*sulphate of iron ; sulphate of zinc ; super-acetate of
lead ; nitrate of silver ; tartarized antimony ; lime
water,* and *yellow cinchona.*

INFUSUM CASCARILLÆ. L. It is incompatible
with the substances mentioned under *Infus: Caryophyll :*

INFUSUM CINCHONÆ. L. E. D. We obtain in this
preparation a feeble solution of the active constituents of bark, which will agree with many stomachs
that are rebellious to the stronger preparations.

INFUSUM CUSPARIÆ. L. This is a judicious form of the bark, possessing its stimulant and tonic properties.

INFUSUM DIGITALIS; L.E. This is the best form in which we can administer the *fox-glove*, where our wish is to obtain its diuretic effects as speedily as possible. *Dose*, fʒss to fʒj twice a day, *see Digitalis. Incompatibles.* We shall counteract its effects, by endeavouring to obviate its nauseating tendency by *brandy and water*, &c. Precipitates are produced by *sulphate of iron*, and the *infusion of yellow cinchona*, &c.

INFUSUM LINI. L.E. A cheap, and useful demulcent; *alcohol*, and preparations of *lead*, are of course incompatible with it; the *tinctura ferri muriatis* produces a flocculent precipitate.

INFUSUM QUASSIÆ. L. E. The proportion of Quassia directed for half a pint of water, is that of ℈j by the London, and ʒss by the Edinburgh College; the former is much too small, for in order to obtain a saturated infusion, ʒij are required for that quantity of water. *Incompatibles. The salts of iron* produce no change in it; nor is it affected by any of those substances with which it is likely to come in contact, in a medical prescription. It is highly useful in debilities of the stomach and intestinal canal; and in irregular and atonic gout. To this, as well as the other stomachic infusions, it is usual to add, at the time of prescribing them, a small quantity of aromatic tincture, or spirit.

INFUSUM RHEI. L.E. The Edinburgh infusion is stronger than that of London, and is rendered more grateful by the addition of spirit of cinnamon; these infusions, however, when given without any *adjuvants*, produce but a feeble effect. This is obvious,

since ℈j of rhubarb in substance, is at least equivalent
to ℥iss in infusion. *Incompatibles.* The *stronger acids;
the sulphates of iron and zinc ; nitrate of silver ; tartarized antimony ; super-acetate of lead ; oxy-muriate of
mercury.* and the infusions of *cusparia, cinchona, catechu, galls,* and of some other *astringent* vegetables ; the
alkalies deepen the colour, but produce no decomposition.

INFUSUM SENNÆ. L. E. D. A pint of water will
take up the active matter of ℥j of senna, but nothing
beyond that proportion; hence, there is an unnecessary waste in the London process. The quantity of
infusion directed to be made at one time, is also
injudicious, since by simple exposure to the air for
only a few hours, in consequence of the powerful
affinity of its extractive matter for oxygen, a yellow
precipitate takes place, and the infusion loses its purgative quality, and excites *tormina* in the bowels;
in preparing it therefore, we see the necessity of conducting the process in *covered* vessels, and of making
only such a portion as may be required for immediate
use; indeed, notwithstanding every precaution, the
extractive will, to a certain extent, become oxidized,
and the infusion have a tendency to gripe.   Dr.
Cullen used to say, that Senna was one of the best
purgatives, if it could only be divested of its griping
quality ; this, however, he was unable to obviate,
because he was not aware of its cause ; and therefore
conjoined it with various aromatics, instead of salts,*
which might be capable of encreasing the solubility of

---

* SELWAY'S PREPARED ESSENCE OF SENNA. This is a concentrated
infusion of Senna, in combination with an alkali. It is admirably
adapted for domestic use. It is sold at Selway's, New Cavendish-street,
Portland-place, or at Johnson's, 147, Oxford-street.

its oxidized extractive. *Soluble tartar* and *alkaline
salts* are its most useful adjuncts; it is however rarely
prescribed in practice without the addition of other
cathartics. (Form: 9, 14, 15, 27). Sydenham's favourite " *potio cathartica lenitiva,*" consisted of an
infusion of tamarinds, senna leaves, and rhubarb,
with the addition of manna, and syrup of roses. The
addition of tamarinds renders the infusion more
grateful, but less active; when made with *bohea tea,*
it is, in a great degree, deprived of its nauseous taste;
a decoction of guaiacum encreases its powers, and is
said, at the same time, to render it milder. *Incompatibles.* The infusion is disturbed by *strong acids ;
lime water ; nitrate of silver ; oxy-muriate of mercury ;
super-acetate of lead ; tartarized antimony ;* and by an
infusion of yellow cinchona.

INFUSUM SIMAROUBÆ. L. This infusion is inodorous, of a clear straw colour, with a slightly bitter
taste. It presents the best mode of exhibiting *Simarouba bark.* Dose, f3ij, beyond this it will prove
emetic. *Incompatibles. Alkaline carbonates* and *lime
water* render it ..ilky; and it is precipitated by the
following substances ; *infusions of catechu ; galls,* and
*yellow cinchona ; oxy-muriate of mercury ; nitrate of
silver ; super-acetate of lead.*

INFUSUM TABACI. L. It is never used but as an
enema, in incarcerated hernia, and in ileus.

2. *Compound Infusions.*

INFUSUM ARMORACIÆ COMPOSITUM. L. In this
preparation the stimulant property of the horse-
radish is materially aided by the mustard ; pure
alkalies, but not their carbonates, may form extemporaneous additions.

INFUSUM AURANTII COMPOSITUM. L. A grateful stomachic, having the agreeable compound taste of its several ingredients; it has the merit of sitting easily on the stomach.

INFUSUM CATECHU COMPOSITUM. L. E. This infusion is a powerful astringent, rendered grateful by the addition of cinnamon; it will keep for several months, provided the directions of the Edinburgh college be not followed in adding the syrup. In prescribing it, we must remember that it contains a large proportion of *tannin*. See *Catechu*.

INFUSUM GENTIANÆ COMPOSITUM. L. An elegant tonic and stomachic infusion. *Incompatibles*. *Super-acetate of lead* throws down a copious precipitate from the infusion, and *sulphate of iron* strikes a brown colour, but no precipitate takes place for several hours.

INFUSUM ROSÆ. L. E. D. This is an infusion of the petals of the red rose, rendered astringent and refrigerant,* by the addition of dilute sulphuric acid. *Incompatibles*. All those bodies which are decomposed by the sulphuric acid; the *sulphates of iron* and *zinc* do not immediately alter the infusion, but they *slowly* decompose it, producing precipitates of a dark colour. Dr. Clarke of Cambridge has lately detected *iron* in the petals; may not the presence of this metal enhance the tonic powers of the infusion? It affords a most elegant vehicle for the exhibition of cathartic salts. (*Form.* 8.)

* MADDEN's VEGETABLE ESSENCE. Is little else than the *Infusum Rosæ.*

IPECACUANHÆ RADIX. L. E. D.

(Callicocca Ipecacuanha.) *Ipecacuanha.*

QUALITIES. This root, when powdered, has a
faint disagreeable *odour*, and a bitter sub-acrid *taste.*
CHEMICAL COMPOSITION. The late researches of
M. Majendie, and Pelletier have detected the existence of a new vegetable proximate principle in this
root, to which ipecacuan is indebted for its emetic
properties; they have, accordingly, denominated it
Emetin.* When pure, it assumes the form of transparent brownish red scales, which are nearly inodorous, but have a slightly bitter acrid, but not nauseous
taste. *Emetin* is decomposed by a heat higher than
that of boiling water; it is soluble in water, in every
proportion, without undergoing the least change;
and, in a moist atmosphere it deliquesces; it is
also soluble in alcohol, but not in ether; *nitric acid*
dissolves it, but at the same time decomposes it;
dilute sulphuric acid has no action on it; *muriatic
acid* and *phosphoric acid* dissolve it, without altering
its nature; *acetic acid* dissolves it with great facility;
corrosive sublimate precipitates it from its solutions,

---

* A Formula for its preparation is introduced in the new CODEX of
Paris, being the one used by M. Pelletier; it is as follows. Let ℨi of the
powder of Ipecacuan be macerated in f℥ij of Ether with a gentle heat for
some hours, in a distilling apparatus; let the portion which remains,
be triturated and boiled with ℥iv of alcohol, it having been previously
macerated in it; filter, and let the remainder be treated with fresh
portions of alcohol, as long as any thing is taken up from the root;
mix these alcoholic solutions and evaporate to dryness; let this alcoholic
extract be macerated in cold distilled water, in order that every thing
soluble in that menstruum may be dissolved; filter, and evaporate to
dryness; this extract is EMETINE. In this state, however, it contains a
small quantity of *gallic acid*, but which is too inconsiderable to affect its
medicinal qualities.

but *tartarized antimony* has no effect upon them; *gallic acid*, the *infusion of galls*, and *acetate of lead*, precipitate it. Half a grain excites violent vomiting, followed by sleep, and the pat ent awakes in perfect health ! It exerts also a specific action on the lungs, and mucous membrane of the intestinal canal; when taken in an overdose, its action can be instantly paralysed by a decoction of galls. *Emetin* appears to exist in Ipecacuanha, combined in the following manner, *emettne* 16, oils 2, wax 6, gum 10, starch 40, woody fibre 20. Solubility. Alcohol takes up four parts in twenty of Ipecacuan; proof spirit, six and a half; and boiling water rather more than eight parts; one pint of good sherry wine will dissolve about 100 grains; the alcoholic is more emetic than the aqueous solution; decoction destroys the emetic property of the root. Incompatible Substances. All vegetable astringents, as *infusion of galls*, &c. *vegetable acids*, especially the *acetic*, weaken its power; Dr. Irvine found that grs. xxx, administered in f ʒij of vinegar produced only some loose stools. Forms of Exhibition: the form of powder is most energetic, although the vinous solution is both active and convenient. Dose. The medicinal operation of this substance varies with its dose, thus grs. x to ʒss, act as an emetic; grs. i to ij, as an expectorant, and in still smaller doses it proves stomachic, and diaphoretic; by combination with opium, this latter quality becomes more powerful, the primary effect of this medicine is that of stimulating the stomach, and it is equally obvious, that its secondary ones depend on the numerous sympathies of other parts, with the organs of digestion. Officinal Prep. *Pulvis Ipecacuanhæ comp.* L. E. D. *Vinum Ipecac.* L. E. D. The powder is liable to become inert, by exposure to

air and light. The root is refractory, and is reduced
to powder with difficulty, unless a few drops of oil,
or an almond or two, be previously added. It is a
curious fact that the effluvia of this root occasion in
some persons the most distressing sensations of suf-
focation I am acquainted with a lady, who is
constantly seized with a violent dyspnæa, whenever
the powder of Ipecacuan is brought into her presence.
ADULTERATIONS. There are several varieties of
Ipecacuan to be found in the market, which it is
important to distinguish; *viz.* 1, *The brown variety*,
which is the best, containing sixteen per cent of
emetin; 2, the *grey variety*, with fourteen per cent
of emetin; 3, the *white variety* with only five of
emetin. The two former varieties are those usually
met with, being imported into this country, in bales,
from Rio Janeiro; the brown is distinguished from
the grey, in being more wrinkled; the white variety
has no wrinkles whatever.

JALAPÆ RADIX. L. E. D. (Convolvulus Jalapa.)

Jalap.

QUALITIES. This root is pulverulent; *Odour*,
peculiar; *Taste*, sweetish and slightly pungent. CHE-
MICAL COMPOSITION. Resin, gum, extractive, fecula,
and some salts. The combination of the three first
principles appears requisite for the production of its
full cathartic effect. SOLUBILITY. Proof spirit is
its appropriate menstruum. FORMS OF EXHIBITION.
That of powde. is the most eligible, especially when
combined with some other powdered substance; pulverization encreases its activity, see *Pulveres*. DOSE,

gr. x to ʒss. It seems to act principally on the colon. OFFICINAL PREPARATIONS. *Pulv. Jalap. comp.* E. *Extract. Jalap* L. E. D. *Tinct. Jalap.* L. E. D. *Tinct. Sennæ comp.* (*a*) E. ADULTERATIONS. *Briony root* is sometimes mixed with that of jalap, but it may be easily distinguished by its paler colour and less compact texture; and by not easily burning at the flame of a candle. When the *teredo* has attacked it, it should be rejected.

JUNIPERI BACCÆ ET CACUMINA. L. E. D.

(Juniperus Communis.)

Juniper Berries and Tops.

The principal constituents of these berries are mucilage, sugar, and volatile oil; in the latter of which their diuretic virtues reside. FORMS OF EXHIBITION. That of an infusion, made with ʒij of the berries, to oj of hot water. Unless pains however are taken by strong contusion, to bruise and break the seeds, the preparation will contain but little of the juniper flavour. The bruised berries may be also triturated with sugar or some neutral salt, and be exhibited in substance. Dose ʒj to ʒij. OFFICINAL PREP. *Oleum. Junip.* L. E. D. *Spirit. Junip. co.* L. E. D. The taste and diuretic properties of Hollands depend upon this oil; English gin is flavoured by oil of turpentine.

KINO. L. E. D. *Kino.*

(Arboris nondum descriptæ. *Gummi Resina.* L. Eucalypti Resiniferi. *Succus Concretus.* E. Butea Frondosa. D.)

There is very considerable obscurity with regard both to the botanical history, and chemical constitution of this substance; three varieties of it are met with in the shops, viz. 1, *African Kino,* which bears the highest price, and has all the appearance of a natural production, slender twigs being often intermixed in its substance; it is of a reddish brown colour and has a bitterish astringent taste. 2. *Botany Bay Kino,* has also the aspect of a natural production, it is in more solid masses than the former species, is less brittle (for it contains a very small proportion of resin) and with its astringency, has a disagreeable sweetish taste. 3. *Jamaica Kino,* this is the one most commonly met with; it has the appearance of a dry extract, is in small fragments, of a colour more nearly approaching to black than others, and has an astringent and slightly bitter taste. There is also a fourth variety mentioned, viz. the *East India,* or *Amboyna,* but this does not appear to differ from the African variety. Chemical Composition. In all the varieties the predominant principles are tannin and extractive. Solubility. The best menstruum is diluted alcohol. Incompatible Substances, vid. *Gallæ.* Forms of Exhibition. Either in substance or in the form of watery infusion, or in that of tincture. Dose, grs. x to ℥ss. Officinal Prep. *Tinct. Kino.* L. E. D. *Elect. Catechu,* E. D. *Pulvis Sulphatis Alum. co.* E.

LIMONES. L. E. D. (Citrus Medica.) *Lemons.*
(Bacca.)

Succus—The Juice consists of *Citric acid,* mucilage, extractive matter, and small portions of sugar
and water. It may be preserved for a considerable
length of time, by covering its surface with fixed oil.
Cortex—The Rind, or Peel, is composed of
two distinct parts, the exterior, which contains glands,
filled with a fragrant volatile oil, upon which all its
properties depend, and the *interior coat,* which is
tasteless and indigestible. The flavour may be obtained by rubbing lump sugar upon it, which will
imbibe the oil, and if it be then dried, by a very
gentle heat, may be preserved unimpaired for any
length of time, and will be preferable to the volatile
oil, obtained by distillation, for the fire generally
imparts an unpleasant or empyreumatic flavour.*

LINIMENTA. L. E. D. *Liniments.*

These are external applications, having the consistence of oil or balsam. If we except the *Liniment
Æruginis,* all the officinal liniments are decomposed
by the substances which are incompatible with soaps.
Linimentum Æruginis. L. *Oxymel Æruginis.*
P. L. 1787. *Mel. Ægyptiacum.* P. L. 1745. *Unguentum Ægyptiacum.* P. L. 1720. Diluted with water,
it has been recommended as a gargle in venereal
ulcerations, but its use is hazardous; it is a detergent
escharotic preparation.

* Essential Salt of Lemons. See *Potassa Super-tartras.*

LINIMENTUM AMMONIÆ FORTIUS. L. *Oleum Ammoniatum.* E. *Linimentum Ammoniæ.* D. It consists of *liquor ammoniæ one part, olive oil two parts,* (oil eight parts, E. D.) The alkali forms with the oil a soap, which is held dissolved by the water in the *liquor ammoniæ.* It is an excellent rubefacient, and penetrating liniment.

LINIMENTUM AMMONIÆ SUB-CARBONATIS. L. *Linimentum Ammoniæ.* P. L. 1787. *Linimentum volatile,* P. L. 1745. The carbonic acid prevents the perfect formation of soap in this liniment; unlike the former one therefore, it deposits the soapy matter, on standing. It is much less stimulating than the preceding one.

LINIMENTUM CALCIS. E. D. *Oil and lime water, equal parts.* This is an *earthy* soap, formed by the combination of lime and oil; the soapy matter separates on standing, it should therefore be *extemporaneous.* In cases of burns and scalds where the cuticle has been destroyed, it is an advantageous application.

LINIMENTUM CAMPHORÆ. L. *Oleum Camphoratum.* E. D. Camphor one, olive oil four parts. It is a simple solution of camphor in fixed oil, and forms a very useful embrocation to sprains, bruises, glandular swellings, and in rheumatic affections.

LINIMENTUM CAMPHORÆ COMPOSITUM. L. *Camphor two, liquor ammoniæ six, spirit of lavender sixteen parts.* It is highly stimulating.

LINIMENTUM HYDRARGYRI. L. A pound of this liniment contains nearly ʒiv of mercury; it affects the mouth more rapidly than mercurial ointment, and hence its application requires caution.

LINIMENTUM SAPONIS COMPOSITUM. L. *Hard soap,* iij, *camphor* j, *spirit of rosemary* xvj parts. It is a stimulant and anodyne application, and in local pains, opium may be advantageously added to it. It is commonly used under the name of *Opodeldoc.**

LINIMENTUM TEREBINTHINÆ. This liniment was introduced by Mr. Kentish of Newcastle, as a dressing to recent burns, which he continued, until the eschars became loose.

LINUM CATHARTICUM. L. D. *Purging Flax.*

The qualities of this plant reside in extractive matter, hence water extracts, but long decoction injures them. MEDICAL USES. It is strongly purgative. FORMS OF EXHIBITION. ʒij of the dried herb infused in oj of boiling water. DOSE, fʒij.

LINI USITATISSIMI SEMINA. L. E. D.
Linseed, or Common Flax Seed.

These seeds contain a large proportion of mucilage, and one sixth of their weight of fixed oil; by infusion in water, a clear colourless inodorous and nearly insipid mucilage is obtained; ʒss of the unbruised seeds is sufficient for oj of water; the farina of the seed is well adapted for cataplasms. OFFICINAL PREP. *Infus. Lini.* L. *Oleum Lini.* L. E. D.

LIQUOR ALUMINIS COMPOSITUS. L.
Aqua Aluminosa Bateana. P. L 1745.

This is a compound solution of *alum* and *sulphate of zinc.* It is powerfully astringent, and is successfully used as a detergent lotion to old ulcers; as a colly-

---

* STEER's OPODELDOC. Castille soap ʒj. Rectified Spirit fʒviij. Camphor ʒiiiss. Oil of Rosemary fʒss. Oil of Origanum fʒj. Solution of Ammonia fʒvj.

rium, or as an injection in gleet, and fluor albus; it will also often answer in removing chilblains, and in curing slight excoriations.

LIQUOR AMMONIÆ. L   AQUA AMMONIÆ. E.
AQUA AMMONIÆ CAUSTICÆ. D.
Solution of Ammonia.

QUALITIES. *Form*, a limpid, colourless fluid; *specific gravity*, ·960, or, f℥j weighs about 438 grs. *Odour*, strong and pungent; *Taste*, extremely caustic. CHEMICAL COMPOSITION. A solution of ammoniacal gas in water, which varies considerably in strength in the different pharmacopœias. When prepared according to the London and Edinburgh Colleges, it contains nearly 25 per cent of ammonia, whereas the Dublin preparation does not contain more than 16. SOLVENT POWERS. It is an active solvent of many vegetable principles, e, g, *oils*, *resins*, &c. With alcohol it unites in every proportion; it assists the oxidizement of copper and zinc; and dissolves many of the metallic oxides. MED. USES. Stimulant, rubefacient, and antacid. FORMS OF EXHIBITION. In milk, or any liquid vehicle; if in decoctions, or infusions, they must be previously cooled, for at 130° the ammonia will escape in the form of gas. DOSE, mx to xxx. OFFICINAL PREP. *Linimentum Ammoniæ*, L.D. *Oleum Ammon:* E. *Spir: Ammon:* L. *Spir: Ammon: comp:* L. *Spir: Ammon: succinat:* L. *Liniment: Camphor: comp:* L. ADULTERATIONS. The presence of other salts in the solution may be discovered by saturating a portion with pure nitric acid, and applying the test for sulphuric acid *(Barytes)* and that for muriatic acid,

(*Nitrate of Silver.*) Carbonic acid is detected by its
effervescing with acids; it ought to be free from all
fetor; its strength can only be determined by taking
its specific gravity. It should be preserved in well
closed bottles, and their dimensions should be small,
for when in large vessels it often becomes carbonated
before it is half used.

LIQUOR AMMONIÆ ACETATIS. L. AQUA
ACETATIS AMMONIÆ. E.D.
Solution of Acetate of Ammonia.
olim, *Spirit of Mindererus.*

This preparation is a solution of the neutral *acetate
of ammonia*, with a proportion of carbonic acid diffused through it; it is made by saturating the sub-
carbonate of ammonia with distilled vinegar, for
which purpose it will generally be found that ℥j of
the alkali will saturate oiss of the vinegar; since,
however, the quantity of acid in distilled vinegar is
liable to a constant variation, the exact point of neutralization should be ascertained by the alternate
application of litmus and turmeric papers, for if the
proportions be not accurately adjusted, some of the
metallic salts, especially those of *antimony*, which are
often prescribed in conjunction with it, are decomposed, and thus rendered inefficacious; and on this
account an excess of alkali is to be feared more than
that of acid. It has been already stated, that a very
minute proportion of extractive matter is rendered
sensible on the addition of an alkali, hence this preparation frequently derives, from the vinegar, a brown
hue, which may be removed by filtering the solution
through a little well burnt charcoal. It also deserves

notice, that the presence of a trace of copper, derived from the copper cocks through which the vinegar has passed, will impart a *brown* tinge, whilst in larger quantities this metal yields a *blue* colour with ammonia. INCOMPATIBLE SUBSTANCES. *Acids; fixed alkalies; alum; lime water; sulphate of magnesia; corrosive sublimate; nitrate of silver;* and the *sulphates of zinc, copper, and iron.* Super-acetate *of lead* produces also a copious precipitation, but this depends upon the presence of the carbonic acid, diffused through the solution, which decomposes the salt, and forms an insoluble carbonate of lead. *Magnesia* likewise, contrary to what might be supposed, decomposes the solution, and renders it pungent, from the extrication of ammoniacal gas; this phenomenon depends upon the magnesia forming a triple acetate with one part of the ammonia, and setting the remainder at liberty. MED. USES. When assisted by warmth, and plentiful dilution, it is an excellent diaphoretic, and it produces its effects without quickening the circulation: (*Form*: 53, 62,) by keeping the surface of the body cool, its action is determined to the kidnies, and it proves diuretic, especially when combined with remedies of a similar tendency. (*Form:* 31.) DOSE, f℥iv to f℥xij.

LIQUOR AMMONIÆ SUB-CARBONATIS. L.
SOLUTIO SUB-CARBONATIS AMMONIÆ. E. AQUA CARBONATIS AMMONIÆ. D.

This is merely a solution of the *solid* sub-carbonate in distilled water, see *Ammoniæ Sub-carbonas.* DOSE, f℥ss to f℥j in any bland liquid. ADULTERATIONS.

There is frequently a deficient quantity of the sub-
carbonate in solution, its pungency being kept up by
the addition of *liquor ammoniæ*; this may be discovered by shaking it with twice its bulk of alcohol,
when a coagulum of considerable density should occur,
the absence of which will denote the sophistication of
the article. Its *specific gravity* should be 1150.

LIQUOR ANTIMONII TARTARIZATI. L.

Vinum Antimonii Tartarizati, P. L. 1787. VINUM
TARTRITIS ANTIMONII, olim, *Vinum Antimoniale.*
E. vulgo. Antimonial Wine.

During the period that I was Censor of the College,
I took considerable trouble, in conjunction with my
colleagues, to ascertain the state in which this preparation was to be generally met with in the wholesale and retail shops of the metropolis; we were satisfied, during our official visitations, that where *sound*
Sherry wine had been employed as a solvent, an
efficient and permanent solution was obtained, and
that no precipitation of the antimony took place, the
sediment which occurred being merely *tartrate of lime*,
an incidental impurity, derived from the *cream of
tartar*, of the tartarized antimony; but in a majority
of instances an inferior wine was substituted, in which
case the antimonial oxyd was found in a copious
precipitate, in combination with vegetable extractive
matter; and I have since seen this decomposition so
complete, that the super-natant liquor would not
yield any trace of the antimonial salt, when assayed
with sulphuret of potass. Under such circumstances
it might be more judicious to remove *antimonial wine*
from the list of *officinal* preparations. DOSE ɱx to

f ʒj, in any suitable vehicle, repeated every three or four hours, in which case it acts as a diaphoretic. As an emetic, it may be given to infants, in the dose of a teaspoon full every ten minutes, until the desired effect is produced. See *Antimonium Tartarizatum.*

LIQUOR ARSENICALIS. L.
SOLUTIO ARSENICALIS. E.

This is a solution of the *Arsenite of Potass*, f ʒj of which contains gr. ½ of *arsenious acid.* It was introduced into practice by Dr. Fowler, of Stafford, as a substitute for the empirical remedy known by the name of " *The Tasteless Ague Drop.*" INCOMPATIBLE SUBSTANCES. *Lime water ; nitrate of silver ; the salts of copper ; hydro-sulphuret of potass*, and *the infusions and decoctions of bark.* DOSE, m iv, gradually increased to m xxx, twice a day. See *Arsenici Oxidum.*

LIQUOR CALCIS. L. AQUA CALCIS. E.D.
Lime Water.

It is a saturated solution of lime in water; f ʒj of which contains about ¼ of a grain. INCOMPATIBLE SUBSTANCES. *All alkaline and metallic salts; borates ; tartrates ; citrates ; acids, sulphur ; spirituous preparations*, and *the infusions of all astringent vegetables.* It should be kept in close vessels, for if exposed to the air, the lime will attract carbonic acid, and become an insoluble carbonate, the addition of an *alkaline carbonate* produces the same effect instantaneously. MED. USES. It is antacid, and is there-

fore useful in dyspepsia attended with acidity; it dissolves also the slimy mucus with which disordered
bowels are so generally infested; on account of this
latter property, it has been exhibited in calculous
affections,* with a view of dissolving the cementing
ingredient of the concretion, and thereby of destroying its cohesion. Forms of Exhibition. Milk
disguises its nauseous flavour, without impairing its
virtues. Dose, f ʒj. to f ʒvj.

LIQUOR FERRI ALKALINI. L.
Solution of Alkaline Iron.

This preparation is nearly the same as Stahl's
Tinctura Martis Alkalina. Chemical Composition. It is by no means ascertained. Incompatible Substances. It is a very injudicious preparation, for it cannot be exhibited in any form without
decomposition ; *water*, especially if not distilled, and
vegetable infusions and *decoctions*, produce dense precipitates; *pure acids, alkalies*, and *spirit*, also decompose it. When we have so many valuable preparations of iron, why is this retained ?

LIQUOR HYDRARGYRI OXY-MURIATIS. L.

This solution of corrosive sublimate is intended to
facilitate the exhibition of minute doses of the salt;
f ʒj contains gr. ½; when long kept, or exposed to
light, the oxy-muriate is decomposed, and *calomel* is
precipitated ; or, what is more dangerous, it is some-

* Mrs. Stephens's Remedy for the Stone, consisted of lime, in
conjunction with an alkali.

times deposited in crystals, without decomposition;
a small portion of muriate of ammonia in the solution,
prevents this precipitation. DOSE, f℥ss to f℥ij, in an
infusion of linseed. See *Hydrarg : Oxy-murias.*

LIQUOR PLUMBI SUB-ACETATIS. L.

LIQUOR SUB-ACETATIS LITHARGYRI. D.

Aqua Lithargyri Acetati, P. L. 1767.

Solution of Sub-acetate of Lead. *olim, Extract of
Saturn.*

This preparation was introduced by M. Goulard,
of Montpellier, hence it has been commonly known
by the name of *Goulard's Extract.* QUALITIES.. It
is of a greenisn straw colour, and has an austere,
sweetish taste; when kept, it deposits a quantity of
oxide, and becomes lighter coloured. CHEMICAL
COMPOSITION. It is a saturated solution of the sub-
acetate of lead, consisting, according to Berzelius, of
one proportional of acid, and three proportionals of
oxide of lead; hence its name is correct. INCOMPA-
TIBLE SUBSTANCES. *Undistilled water; alkalies,* and
their carbonates precipitate a white subsalt; *alkaline
sulphates,* and *sulphurets; mucilage.* MEDICAL USES.
It is only used externally, in superficial and phlegmonic
inflammations of the skin, and in herpetic affections.
It has been a question, whether *Lead,* in any form,
should ever be applied to an open wound, or to an
abraded surface.*

---

* VIRGIN'S MILK. A preparation is sold under this name, which is
a *sulphate of lead,* and is prepared as follows. To a saturated solution of
Alum, add of *Goulard's extract* one third part. Shake them together;—
see *Benzoinum* for a very different cosmetic, bearing the same name.

LIQUOR POTASSÆ. L. Aqua Potassæ. E.
Aqua Kali Caustica. D.
Aqua kali puri. P. L. 1787. *Lixivium Sapo-
narium*, 1745.

Qualities. A limpid, dense, colourless solution;
a pint should weigh ℥xvj; when rubbed between the
fingers, it feels soapy, in consequence of a partial
solution of the cuticle. The solution, as usually prepared, contains small portions of muriate and sulphate
of potass, silica and lime; but these incidental impurities do not invalidate its virtues; it ought not to
effervesce with acids. Med. Uses. Antacid, diuretic, alterative, and lithontriptic; and externally,
when diluted, it acts as a stimulating lotion, and if
concentrated, as a caustic; see *Potassa Fusa.* The
operation of this, and other alkaline remedies, have
at different periods been celebrated as powerful
lithontriptics, and whilst experience has in some
cases confirmed the value of the practice, it has, in
others, proved no less decidedly its mischievous
agency; these contradictory results are, at length,
capable of explanation, for Chemistry has drawn
aside the veil that has so long obscured the history,
origin, and cure of calculous diseases, and has demonstrated, that these extraneous bodies vary in
composition, and are consequently very differently
affected by the same chemical solvents. Scheele,*
with whom the enquiry originated, conceived that
every calculus consisted of a peculiar concrete acid,
soluble in alkaline lixivia, which Morveau denomi-

* *Transactions of Stockholm.*

nated the Lithic acid; the subsequent researches
however of Fourcroy, Vauquelin, Wollaston, Pearson, Henry, Marcet, and Brande, have demonstrated
the existence of *several* distinct bodies in the composition of urinary calculi, producing varieties in
their external characters, as well as in their chemical
relations; viz. *Lithic*, or *Uric Acid*;* *Phosphate of
lime; Ammoniaco-magnesian phosphate; oxalate of
lime*, and *Cystic oxyd*;† to which may be added an
animal cementing ingredient. The varieties of calculi,
produced by the combination, or intermixture of
these ingredients, are represented in the following
tabular arrangement.‡

* The name of *uric acid* was suggested by Dr. Pearson; it is however
as Dr. Marcet observes, objectionable, on account of the close resemblance which the term bears to that of *Urea*, another and most characteristic constituent of urine, totally distinct from lithic acid.

† *Cystic oxyd*, discovered by Dr. Wollaston in the year 1805; it does
not affect vegetable colours, and has all the chemical habitudes of an
oxyd.

‡ Dr. Marcet has discovered two Calculi, which cannot be referred
to any of the species hitherto noticed, but they are not introduced
into the table, as they may never again occur. To one of these he has
given the name of *Xanthic Oxyd*, because it forms a lemon coloured
compound, when acted upon by Nitric acid. To the other nondescript
calculus, he has bestowed the name of *Fibrinous*, from its resemblance to
fibrine.

To offer more than an outline of this subject, would be altogether
imcompatible with the object of this work, the student must refer to a
paper by Mr. Brande, in the sixth volume of the Journal of the Royal
Institution; a more perspicuous and practically useful paper never
appeared. I am anxious also to recommend in the strongest terms, the
careful perusal of Dr. Marcet's work, "On the Chemical history and
Medical treatment of Calculous disorders." It merits a place in every
medical and scientific library.

A Tabular View of the Different Species of Urinary Calculi.

SPECIES OF CALCULI.	EXTERNAL CHARACTERS.	CHEMICAL COMPOSITION.	REMARKS.
1. Lithic or Uric.	Form, a flattened oval; specific gravity, generally exceeds 1·500; Colour, brownish or fawn-like; surface smooth; texture laminated.	It consists, principally, of Lithic acid: when treated with nitric acid, a beautiful pink substance results. This calculus is slightly soluble in water, abundantly, in the pure alkalies.	It is the prevailing species; but the surface sometimes occurs finely tuberculated. It frequently constitutes the Nuclei of the other species.
2. Mulberry.	Colour, dark brown; texture, harder than that of the other species; Sp. grav. from 1·428 to 1·976. Surface, studded with tubercles.	It is Oxalate of Lime, is decomposed in the flame of a spirit lamp, swelling out into a white efflorescence, which is Quick lime.	This species includes some varieties, which are remarkably smooth, and pale coloured, resembling a hempseed.
3. Bone Earth.	Colour, pale brown, or grey; surface smooth and polished; structure, regularly laminated; the laminæ easily separating into concrete crusts.	Principally Phosphate of Lime. It is soluble in muriatic acid.	
4. Triple.	Colour, generally brilliant white; surface uneven, studded with shining crystals; less compact than the preceding species; between its laminæ, small cells occur, filled with sparkling particles.	It is an Ammoniaco-magnesian phosphate, generally mixed with phosphate of lime; pure alkalies decompose it, extricating its ammonia.	This species attains a larger size than any of the others.
5. Fusible.	Colour, greyish white.	A compound of the two foregoing species.	It is very fusible, melting into a vitreous globule.
6. Cystic.	Very like the Triple Calculus, but it is unstratified and more compact, and homogeneous.	It consists of Cystic Oxide; under the blow pipe, it yields a peculiarly fetid odour. It is soluble in acids, and in alkalies, even if they are fully saturated with carbonic acid.	It is a rare species.
7. Alternating.	Its section exhibits different concentric laminæ.	Composed of several species, alternating with each other.	
8. Compound.	No characteristic form.	The ingredients are separable only by chemical analysis.	

It will appear evident from this view of the subject, that some varieties will be influenced by acids, and others by alkalies; and, that the exhibition of such remedies will be liable to aggravate, or palliate the symptoms, according to the character and composition of the offending calculus, and according to the prevailing diathesis of the patient. As a general rule, Dr. Marcet states, that *"whenever the lithic acid predominates, the alkalies are the appropriate remedies, but, that when the calcareous, or magnesian salts prevail, the acids are to be resorted to;"* but it will be asked, how are we to discover the nature of the calculous affection, so as to direct the suitable remedy? by an examination of the sediment, deposited by the recent urine, or by an analysis of the small fragments, which are frequently voided with it. The phosphates subside from the urine, as a *white*, lithic acid as a *red deposit;* and, since the phosphates are held in solution in the urine by an excess of acid, it is evident, that whenever such acidity is diminished by the hand of nature, or art, a *white* sabulous deposit will ensue;* hence, says Mr. Brande, it occurs in the urine of persons who drink soda water, or take magnesia; the remedy for such a deposit, when it takes place habitually, is a course of acidulous medicines; on the contrary, since *lithic acid* is precipitated by the acids, alkalies are naturally suggested for the prevention of that deposit. In the *compound* calculi, acids and

* The addition of ammonia will throw down an *ammoniaco-magnesian phosphate;* hence we perceive that it is liable to occur whenever the urine undergoes an incipient process of decomposition. I have in my possession a splendid specimen of this triple salt, in large and well defined octohedrons, covering a portion of a decayed beam; it was sent to me by my friend, Mr. Marshall of Half moon street, from whom I learnt that it had been taken from a privy, belonging to a Public House in the Borough.

T

alkalies may be equally injurious, or beneficial, for
since these bodies are composed of a variety of ingredients the action of any solvent will be partial, and
may convert the smooth calculus into a rough and
highly irritating body, or vice versa. In the *alter-
nating calculi*, it may be judicious to exhibit these
remedies alternately, as the symptoms of the case,
and the deposit of the urine, may indicate. After all,
however, the solvent powers of lithontriptic remedies
must be very limited, and in advanced cases we can
never expect to procure more than palliation. Independent of any chemical effect, alkaline substances
are found, by daily experience, to allay the morbid
irritability of the urinary organs, in a manner not yet
explained ; alkalies may also prove *generally* serviceable in these disorders, by acting immediately upon
the digestive organs, for the disposition of forming
calculi is always accompanied with the indications of
deranged digestion. The alkaline carbonates are found
to answer as effectually as the pure alkalies, and they
have the advantage of being less liable to disagree
with the stomach ; where an acid is indicated, the
muriatic will, in my judgment, be found as convenient
and effectual as any that can be administered. Mr.
Brande proposes *cream of tartar* for this purpose ;
upon this point I differ with him, for this salt, to say
the least, is questionable in its mode of operation ;
for although its first impression upon the stomach is
that of an acid, the subsequent processes of digestion
decompose it and eliminate its base, which is absorbed
and acts upon the urinary organs as an alkali. I have
seen a white sabulous deposite in the urine of persons
after the constant use of *Imperial* as a beverage,
which I can explain upon no other principle. Sir
Gilbert Blane has also shewn, that if a fixed alkali

be saturated with citric acid, it still acts as an alkaline remedy on the urinary organs: for some farther remarks on this subject, *see Potassæ Acetas.* During an alterative course of lithontriptic remedies, it will be beneficial to interpose occasionally, a purgative medicine, but we must not combine it with the lithontripic, for it is a law that will be hereafter expounded, *that catharsis suspends the process of absorption.* Dose of the solution of potass, m x to fʒss, in veal broth, or table beer; this latter vehicle disguises its nauseous flavour completely. Officinal Prep. *Potassa fusa,* L. E. D. *Potassa cum calce,* L. E. D. *Liquor Sulphureti Kali,* D. *Antimonii Sulphuretum præcipitatum,* L. E.

LIQUOR POTASSÆ SUB-CARBONATIS. L.

Aqua Sub-carbonatis Kali. D.

Aqua Kali præparati, P. L. 1787.

Lixivium Tartari, 1745.

Oleum Tartari per deliquium, P. L. 1720.

Qualities. It is a clear, colourless, and inodorous solution; *Spec. grav.* 1.446. Dose, m x to fʒj. See *Potassæ Sub-carbonas.*

LYTTA. L. (Lytta Vesicatoria.) Cantharis Vesicatoria. E. Cantharis. D.

Blistering or Spanish Fly. Cantharides.

The chemical history of cantharides is still involved in much obscurity; the blistering principle has been obtained by Robiquet in a separate state, when it assumes the form of small crystalline plates, with a micaceous lustre; Dr. Thomson has given to it the name of *Cantharadin*. When pure, it is insoluble in water, but it is rendered soluble by the presence of a yellow matter which exists in native combination with it; it is very soluble in oils. MEDICAL USES. Powerfully stimulant and diuretic, *(Form. 44.)*. In consulting the works of Dioscorides, Galen, and Pliny, we shall find that they entertained a notion that the *virus* was in the bodies only of the fly, and that the head, feet and wings, contained its antidote; Hippocrates prescribed them internally in dropsy, jaundice, and amenorrhæa; and yet in the end of the sixteenth century, Dr. Groenvelt was charged and sued, for giving them inwardly; he published his vindication in a small tract, entitled " *De tuto Cantharidum usu interno;*" the issue, says Quincy, (Pharm. p. 152,) ruined the unhappy doctor, but taught his envious prosecutors the safety and value of his practice. DOSE, in substance, not exceeding gr. j, with opium, or hyoscyamus. OFFICINAL PREF. *Tinct. Lyttæ.* L. *Emplast. Lyttæ.* L. *Cerat. Lytt.* L. *Unguent. infusi. Cantharid. vesicat.* E. *Unguent. Cantharid.* D. The flies do not lose their virtues by being kept.

MAGNESIA. L. MAGNESIA USTA. D.

Calcined Magnesia.

QUALITIES. *Form,* a white, very light, soft powder; *Specific gravity,* 2.3; it turns to green the more delicate vegetable blues. SOLUBILITY. Although it requires 2000 times its weight of water to hold it in solution, yet it has the property of considerably encreasing the solubility of camphor, opium and resins in the same fluid; it is soluble in solutions of the alkaline carbonates, but not in those of caustic alkalies. CHEMICAL COMPOSITION. It is an oxyd of a peculiar metal. MEDICAL USES. Antacid, and when acidity prevails, purgative; it is preferable to the carbonate whenever the bowels are distended with flatus; in other respects, its virtues are the same. See *Magnes. carb.* INCIDENTAL IMPURITIES. It ought not to effervesce with acids; lime is detected by its solution, in dilute sulphuric acid, affording a precipitate with oxalate of ammonia; the *sulphuret of lime* betrays itself, by yielding, when moistened, the smell of sulphuretted hydrogen,*

MAGNESIÆ CARBONAS. L.
CARBONAS MAGNESIÆ. E. MAGNESIA. D.
Olim, Magnesia Alba.
Carbonate of Magnesia. vulgo, *Common Magnesia.*

This preparation was formerly considered by Mr. Phillips to be a mixture of carbonate, and sub-carbonate of magnesia, an opinion which he has lately retracted; it is, says he, evidently a *carbonate*, i. e. magnesia combined with one proportion of carbonic acid, or forty-eight of carbonic acid to forty-three of magnesia. Dr. Thomson entertains a different opinion, he observes that it seems to be a mechanical mixture of carbonate of magnesia, caustic magnesia, and per-

---

* *Magnesia* was originally a *general* term, expressive of *any* substance which had the power of attracting some principle from the air, from *Magnes*, the Loadstone. The peculiar body which we now denominate *Magnesia*, was first sold as a *panacea*, by a canon at Rome, in the beginning of the seventeeth century, under the title of Magnesia alba, or Count Palma's Powder.

haps of hydrated magnesia; he found too great a diversity in its composition to permit the conclusion that it was a definite chemical compound; in a specimen purchased at Glasgow, he also found six per cent of *sulphate of lime*. I take this opportunity of stating that in some specimens which I have examined, I have also detected portions of *gypsum*. INCOM- PATIBLE SUBSTANCES. *Acids, and acidulous salts; alkalies, and neutral salts; alum; cream of tartar; nitrate of silver; acetate of mercury; oxy-muriate of mercury; super-acetate of lead; sulphates of zinc, copper and iron.* MEDICAL USES. Antacid. In cases of lithic calculi, carbonate of magnesia, in doses of $\ni$j to ζj, has been proposed by Mr. Hatchett, as a valuable substitute for alkaline remedies. Its insolubility must render its absorption equivocal; its beneficial operation must therefore principally depend upon its neutralizing any excess of acid in the primæ viæ, and in this way there can be no doubt of its lithontriptic agency; "but," says Dr. Marcet, "such is the tendency which the public has to over rate the utility of a new practice, or to take a mistaken view of its proper application, that there is every reason to believe that the use of magnesia has of late years become a frequent source of evil in calculous complaints." OFFICINAL PREP. *Hydrarg. cum Magnesia.* D. *Magnesia,* L. E. D. ADULTERATIONS. *Chalk* may be detected by adding to a suspected portion, dilute sulphuric acid, when, should any be present, the solution will be loaded with a white and insoluble precipitate; *gypsum,* by boiling a sample in distilled water, and assaying the solution by a barytic and oxalic test.*

* DALBY'S CARMINATIVE. This consists of carbonate of magnesia $\ni$ij, oils of Peppermint *m* j, of Nutmeg *m* ij, of Anniseed *m* iij, of the tinctures of Castor *m* xxx, of Assafœtida *m* xv, spirit of Pennyroyal *m* xv, of the

MAGNESIÆ SULPHAS. L. Sulphas Magnesiæ. E. D.

Magnesia Vitriolata. Sal catharticum amarum.

Bitter purging salt. Epsom salt.

QUALITIES. *Form,* small needle-like crystals. *Taste,* bitter and nauseous; when pure, it effervesces. CHEMICAL COMPOSITION. In its crystallized state, it may be considered as composed of 1 proportional of dry sulphate (Magnesia 18·5, and Sulphuric acid 37·5) and 7 proportionals of water. SOLUBILITY. f℥j of water dissolves ℥j, and the solution measures f℥xj¼; it is insoluble in alcohol. INCOMPATIBLE SUBSTANCES. *Muriates of ammonia, baryta,* and *lime; nitrate of silver ; sub-acetate,* and *super-acetate of lead. The fixed alkalies,* and *their carbonates,* precipitate from it magnesia, and its carbonate. *Phosphate of soda* occasions no immediate precipitate, unless ammonia be present, in which case the triple *ammoniaco-magnesian phosphate* will be produced. The addition of ammonia, which in the form of *Spiritus ammoniæ aromat :* is not unfrequently prescribed in conjunction with a solution of this sulphate, forms also a triple salt, and a portion of magnesia is precipitated: whenever therefore this ammoniacal stimulant is ordered with

compound tincture of Cardamoms *m* xxx; Peppermint water f℥ij. There are cheaper compositions, sold under the same name. In examining the pretensions of this combination, it must be allowed that it is constructed upon philosophical principles; this however is no reason why the physician should recommend it; the mischievous tendency of a quack medicine, does not depend upon its composition, but upon its application ; we ought to remember, says an eminent physician, that in recommending this nostrum we foster the dangerous prejudices of mothers and nurses, who are unable to ascertain the circumstances under which it should be given, or even the proper doses; if its composition is judicious, why do not physicians order the same in a regular prescription, rather than in a form, in which the most valuable remedy will be abused?

a purgative salt, the scientific physician will prefer a
solution of the sulphate of soda. FORMS OF EXHI-
BITION. Dissolved in the *Infusum Rosæ*, or in a
suitable quantity of beef tea, gruel, or any aqueous
vehicle; its cathartic powers are encreased by dilution, as well as so by the addition of a little common
salt; *magnesia* renders the taste of its solution less
nauseous; and tartarized antimony quickens its operation. DOSE, ℥ss to ℥ij, taken either at once,
or in divided doses. OFFICINAL PREP. *Enema
Catharticum. Enema Fœtid.* D. ADULTERATIONS.
Sulphate of Soda is often substituted for this salt,
which it may be made to resemble by stirring it
briskly at the moment when it is about to crystallize;
the fraud may be detected by a precipitation not
ensuing on adding carbonate of potass; if only a part
of the salt be sulphate of soda, the degree of sophistication can be learnt by the quantity of the precipitate formed; 100 parts of sulphate of magnesia,
if pure, will yield between 30 and 40 of the dry carbonate. Epsom salt, as it commonly occurs, contains
muriate of magnesia, which disposes it to deliquesce,
but lately this salt has appeared in the market in a
state of great purity and beauty; the mode of purification is founded upon the well known chemical law,
that *a saturated solution of one salt is still capable of
dissolving another*; in the present instance, therefore,
the impure crystals are washed in a saturated solution of the same sulphate, which, although unable to
act upon its kindred salt, can dissolve, with facility,
the muriate, and any other saline contamination. I
confess, however, that I am rather induced to regard
this process as chemically ingenious, than as medicinally useful, for the usual saline impurities of Epsom
salt are not only harmless, but capable of encreasing

its purgative powers, for the *double refined* sulphate is certainly less efficient as a cathartic. The presence of the *muriate* may be at once detected, by dropping upon the suspected sample some sulphuric acid, by which the disengagement of muriatic acid vapour will be produced.

MANNA. L. E. D. (Fraxinus Ornus.) *Manna.*
(*Succus Concretus.*)

QUALITIES. *Form,* flakes of a granular texture; *Colour,* whitish, or pale yellow; *Odour,* slight, but peculiar; *Taste,* nauseous sweet, with some degree of bitterness. CHEMICAL COMPOSITION. This concrete vegetable juice, besides sugar, appears to contain mucilage, and extractive, to which its taste, and other peculiar properties are owing. SOLUBILITY. It is entirely soluble in water and alcohol. MED. USES. It is now merely regarded as a laxative for children, or for weak persons. It generally requires some laxative adjunct, as castor oil, with which it may be combined, by the medium of mucilage. DOSE, for children, from ʒj to ʒiij, in warm milk. OFFICINAL PREP. *Confectio Cassiæ.* L.E.D. *Enema Cathart:* D. *Enema Fœtid:* D. *Syrup: Sennæ.* D. ADULTERATIONS. There are several varieties in the market, the best of which is flake manna, *manna cannulata,* in a stalactytic form; an article, entirely factitious, is sometimes sold for genuine manna, consisting of honey or sugar, mixed with scammony, but its colour, weight, transparency, and taste, must instantly lead to its detection.

MASTICHE. L. (Pistachia Lentiscus.) *Mastic.*
                    Resina.

The use of this resinous substance is to fill the ca-
vities of carious teeth ; a solution of it in oil of turpentine is sold as an odontalgic. The Turkish and
Armenian women use it as a masticatory for cleaning
the teeth, emulging the salivary glands, and imparting
an agreeable odour to the breath. It forms a constituent of the *Dinner Pills.* See Aloes.

MEL. L. E. D. Honey.

This well known substance appears to be merely
collected from the flowers, and not elaborated by the
internal economy of the insect, for when properly
diluted, it undergoes vinous fermentation, the product
of which is the beverage well known by the name of
Mead; such a change does not occur in any *animal*
substance. The English honey is more waxy than
those from the south of Europe. *Virgin honey* is
that wrought by young bees which have never
swarmed, and permitted to run from the comb without heat or pressure. Chemical Composition.
Sugar, mucilage, wax, and an acid, and occasionally
some essential oil. *Clarified Honey,* (*Mel Despu-
matum.* L. D.) has not the agreeable smell of crude
honey; it does not however ferment so readily, nor is
it so apt to gripe. Uses. It is principally employed
for forming several officinal preparations, i. e. *Mel-
lita.* viz. *Mel Boracis.* L. *Mel Ros :* L. D. *Oxymel.* L. D. *Oxymel Colchici.* D. *Oxymel Scillæ.*

L. D.* ADULTERATIONS. *Flour* may be detected by diffusing the honey in tepid water, by which it will be separated, and, by subsequent boiling, converted into a thick paste.

MENTHA PIPERITA. L.E. MENTHA PIPERITIS. D.

Peppermint.

All the qualities of this plant depend upon an essential oil and camphor ; it readily and strongly impregnates either water or spirit, by infusion ; its infusion, and the water distilled from the plant, are carminative and antispasmodic ; they also serve as vehicles for other medicines, to correct their operation, or to disguise their flavour. OFFICINAL PREP: *Aq: Menth: Piperit:* L.E.D. *Spir: Menth: Pip:* L.D. *Ol: Menth: Pip:* L.D. If this plant be cut in wet weather, it turns black, and is worthless.

MENTHA VIRIDIS. L. MENTHA SATIVA. D.

Spearmint.

Cold water extracts the more agreeable, and aetive parts of mint in a few hours, a longer maceration extracts the grosser and less agreeable portions, hot water more quickly extracts its virtues, but boiling water dissipates the aroma. OFFICINAL PREP: *Aqua Menth: virid:* L.D. *Infus: Menth: comp:* D. *Ol: Menth: virid:* L.D. *Spir: Menth: virid:* L.

---

* HONEY WATER. The article usually sold under this name is a mixture of essences coloured by saffron; some add a small quantity of honey, which communicates a clamminess, which retains the scent longer.

MEZEREI CORTEX. L.E.D. (Daphne Mezereum
                                (Radicis Cortex.)

Mezereon.

The inner bark of this plant, when fresh, is corrosive, and even vesicatory; the fruit is equally so;
its virulence is counteracted by camphor. It is now
seldom used except as an antivenereal remedy. From
its pungency it is one of the substances used by fraudulent brewers to communicate a strong flavour to
their beer. OFFICINAL PREP. *Decoct: Sarsaparill:
comp: L. Decoct: Daphnes: Mezerei.* E. The
Daphne Laureola is sometimes sold for Mezereon.

MISTURÆ. L.E.D. *Mixtures.*

These preparations are generally *extemporaneous,*
in which different ingredients are mingled together in
the liquid form, or, in which solid substances are
diffused through liquids, by the medium of mucilage,
or syrup : for prescribing mixtures, the following general rules may be laid down.

I. Substances, which are capable of entering into
chemical combination, or of decomposing each
other, ought not to be mixed together, unless it
be with a view of obtaining the new products as
a remedy.

II. Transparency is not a necessary condition, and
hence, insoluble powders may be advantageously
introduced into mixtures, if the following precautions be observed.

1. They must be divisible, and mechanically
miscible in the liquid.

2. They must not possess too great a specific
gravity.

3. They must not render the liquid too mucilaginous, or thick ; *thus,* f℥j *should seldom contain
more than* ʒss *of a vegetable powder,* ℈ij *of an
electuary, and conserve; or* grs xv, *or* ℈j *of an
extract.*

III. The taste, the smell, and the general aspect of
the mixture, should be rendered as pleasant as
possible, *thus, milk covers the taste of bark, of the
tinctures of guaiacum, and valerian, and of lime
water; and a light decoction of the liquorice root
disguises a bitter taste more effectually han sugar.*
But in thus accommodating our medicines to the
taste of our patient, let us be careful that we do
not invalidate their powers, which often appear
to be nearly connected with the sensible qualities which render them disgusting and objectionable.

The Physician may also produce occasional
changes in the appearance of his mixture, in
order to reconcile a delicate taste to its continuance ; he never ought however to alter the
essential part of plans which he finds advantageous.

A DRAUGHT differs merely from a mixture in quantity, it is usually taken at once, and should not exceed
f℥iss, it should be always preferred when,

1. *The remedy is to be taken in a precise dose.*

2. *Whenever it is liable to spontaneous decomposition.*

3. *Whenever the action of the atmosphere occasions*
change.

CLYSTERS. *Enemata,* may be mentioned under this
head ; they are useful resources, although they have
not escaped their due share of persecution. Paracelsus bestowed upon them the epithet, " *turpissimum
medicamentum,*" and Van Helmont, that of " *puden-*

dum medicorum subsidium." In prescribing and dispensing active substances for this form of exhibition, some care is requisite, thus, *Camphor*, unless it be carefully divided, will adhere to the rectum, and produce very unpleasant consequences; in general the dose of an active remedy given in *clysters* is allowed to be triple that taken by the mouth. A most ingenious and useful apparatus has been lately contrived by Mr. Machell, of Great Ryder Street, St. James's, for administering clysters, with which every country practitioner should become acquainted.

In apportioning the dose of mixtures, the following proportions are admissible, although not perfectly accurate. A TABLE SPOON full (*Cochleare Amplum*) f℥ss. DESERT SPOON (*Cochleare Mediocre*) more than f℥ij. TEA SPOON (*Cochleare Minimum*) f℥j. A WINE GLASS (*Cyathus*) although very variable, may be estimated as containing f℥iss. The custom of measuring the dose of a liquid by dropping it from the mouth of a phial, is very erroneous, it will therefore be proper to dilute an active medicine, that is to be so apportioned, with at least a triple quantity of water, that its real dose may not be essentially altered by any slight variation in the quantity.

MISTURA AMMONIACI. This mixture is expectorant, and may be exhibited with tincture of squills, &c. (*Form.* 50). It is slightly curdled by *vinegar*, *oxymels*, *æther*, and *oxy-muriate of mercury*.

MISTURA AMYGDALARUM. L. *Emulsio Amygdali communis.* E. *Lac Amygdalæ.* D. It is a useful demulcent, and diluent, and forms an elegant vehicle for more active medicines. *Incompatibles. Acids, Oxymel, Syrup of Squill, Spirit* and *Tinctures,* unless added in very small quantities, decompose this mixture ; *tartaric acid, super-tartrate of potass, supersulphate of potass,* and *oxy-muriate of mercury* also disturb it.

MISTURA ASSAFŒTIDÆ. L. A nauseous preparation; and where its use is indicated, it will be more
judicious to prescribe it as an extemporaneous mixture. See *Assafœtida*.

MISTURA CAMPHORÆ. L. This solution of camphor forms an elegant vehicle for more active stimulants. The camphor is separated from the water by
a solution of pure potass, by sulphate of magnesia,
and by several saline bodies.

MISTURA CRETÆ. L. D. A common and useful
remedy in diarrhœa, and may be combined with opium, catechu, or any other astringent.

MISTURA FERRI COMPOSITA. L. This is nearly
the same as the celebrated anti-hectic mixture of Dr.
Griffith; to the result of the decompositions which
take place from the mixture of its ingredients, it is
wholly indebted for its medicinal energies, thus, a
proto-carbonate of iron is formed, i. e. the iron combined with carbonic acid, is at its *minimum* of oxidation, which renders it more active than the common
carbonate, and probably less stimulant than the sulphate; this product, by means of the saponaceous
compound formed by the union of the myrrh with the
excess of alkali, is *partly* diffused and suspended in
the mixture, and *partly* dissolved, whilst, at the same
time, a *sulphate of potass* is formed, which serves to
correct the astringent influence which iron is apt to
exert upon the bowels. The iron in this preparation
is disposed to combine with an additional proportion
of oxygen, hence its ingredients should be quickly
mixed together, and it ought to be considered as an
extemporaneous preparation; it should be preserved
in a closely-stopt vessel. Its change of colour will
generally indicate its loss of efficacy.

The Dose of the above mixtures is f℥j to f℥ij twice
or thrice a day.

MOSCHUS. L.E.D. *Musk.*

QUALITIES. *Form,* grains concreted together, dry, yet slightly unctuous. *Colour,* deep brown with a shade of red; *Odour* aromatic, and peculiar, diffusive, and durable; and it has the curious property, when added in a minute quantity, to augment the odour of other perfumes, without imparting its own; this renders it a valuable article in perfumery, on which account it is a usual ingredient in lavender water. *Taste,* bitterish and heavy. CHEMICAL COMPOSITION. Resin combined with volatile oil, and a mucilaginous extractive matter, with small portions of albumen, gelatine, muriate of ammonia, and phosphate of soda. SOLUBILITY. Boiling water dissolves it perfectly; rectified spirit takes up most of its active parts, although the odour is only discovered upon dilution; sulphuric ether is its most complete menstruum. INCOMPATIBLE SUBSTANCES. The solutions are decomposed by *Oxy-muriate of Mercury ; Sulphate of Iron ; Nitrate of Silver ;* and the *Infusion of Yellow Bark.* MED: USES. Stimulant and antispasmodic. FORMS OF EXHIBITION. The best form is that of bolus, combined with ammonia, or camphor, or some other similar remedy (Form. 109), it may be also administered in a mixture, for which purpose it requires five times its weight of mucilage, consequently the London College has not directed a sufficient quantity to retain the musk in suspension : by previously triturating it with sugar, its minute division is much facilitated. DOSE, grs. x to xxx. OFFICINAL PREP *Mist: Mosch:* L. *Tinct: Mosch:* D. ADULTERATIONS. The bag containing the musk should have no appearance of having been opened : the presence of *dried blood* may be suspected, by its emitting, as it inflames, a fetid smoke; *Asphaltum* is discovered by its melting and running, before it inflames : the artificial bags are known from the deficiency of the membrane which lines the real musk bags. To increase the weight of the musk, fine particles of lead are very frequently mixed with it; this is easily detected, for by rubbing it with water the metallic particles subside.

Moschus Factitius, *Artificial Musk,* strongly resembling the real, may be formed by digesting f℥ss of *Nitric Acid,* for ten days, upon ℥j of fetid animal oil, obtained by distillation ; to this is to be next gradually added oj of *rectified spirit,* and the whole is then to be left to digest for one month : or—

2. Drop f℥iiiss of nitric acid upon f℥j of rectified oil of amber ; after standing twenty-four hours, a black, resinous pellicle, exhaling the odour of musk, will be formed.

MUCILAGO ACACIÆ. L.E. Mucilago Gummi Arabici. D.

This preparation consists of one part of gum, and two of water ; in preparing it, the dispenser is particularly recommended to pulverize the gum, and never to employ that which is purchased in the state of powder, as it is always impure, and incapable of forming a pellucid and elegant solution. Incompatible Substances. Neither the *strong acids* nor *alcohol,* when considerably diluted, occasion any disturbance in it, but *sulphuric ether,* and its *compound spirit; the tincture of muriated iron;* and *sub-acetate of lead,* produce very dense precipitates : the *super-acetate of lead* only occasions decomposition, when an alkaline salt is present in the formula: the *volatile*

U

alkali curdles the mucilage, and *hard, calcareous waters* render the mixture difficult, and often impracticable. In the pharmaceutical application of this mucilage, it should be remembered, that it contains in its composition an astringent principle, which is perhaps of but trifling consequence, except in the exhibition of some few very active metallic salts, which are certainly decomposed by it (e.g. grs. x of *nitrate of mercury* are decomposed by ʒij of gum arabic.) It contains also lime in combination with some vegetable acid. Uses ; diluted with four times its bulk of water, this mucilage forms a demulcent mixture of appropriate tenacity, which affords a convenient vehicle for several efficient remedies ; the pharmaceutical use of this mucilage depends upon the fact of its rendering expressed and essential oils, balsams, resins, gum-resins, resinous tinctures, and fatty bodies, miscible with water ; and, if a syrup be added, the union will be more perfect ; the proportions, necessary for this purpose, vary according to the nature of the substances; thus, *oils* will require about three-fourths their weight ; *Balsams* and *Spermaceti*, an equal part: *Resins*, a double quantity, and *Musk* five times its weight.

MUCILAGO ASTRAGALI TRAGACANTHÆ,
E. D. *Tragacanth Mucilage.*

Tragacanth is, strictly speaking, not soluble in water, it imbibes a large portion of it, and swells into a considerable bulk, forming a soft, but not a liquid mucilage ; on the farther addition of water, a fluid solution may be obtained by agitation, but the liquor is turbid ; and on standing, the mucilage subsides, the limpid water on the surface retaining little of the

gum; it differs from all gums in giving a thick consistence to a larger quantity of water, its power in
this respect being to that of gum arabic as twenty to
one; one part converts twenty of hot water into a
stiff mucilage. Tragacanth is not increased, but
actually diminished in solubility by the addition of
any other gum, accordingly it separates from water
with much greater facility when gum arabic is present.
This preparation, according to the Edinburgh college,
consists of one part of gum, and eight of water, the
resulting mucilage is stiff, and is principally employed
for making *troches*. The Dublin preparation contains
four times that quantity of water.

MYRISTICÆ NUCLEI. L. E.
Nux Moschata. D. *Nutmeg*.

All the properties of this well known substance
depend upon an essential oil, filling the dark coloured
veins which run through its substance, and which is
dissipated by decoction; the other components are
starch, gum, wax, and a fixed oil. The oil obtained
by expression is improperly called *oil of mace*, for it
would appear to be a triple compound of fixed oil,
volatile oil, and wax. *Mace* is the involucrum of
the nut. Medical Uses. Stimulant, and in large
doses, as from ʒij to ʒiij, narcotic, frequently producing delirium. *See Cullen Mat. Med. ii. 204.*
Frauds. Nutmegs are frequently despoiled of their
essential oil, by being punctured, and submitted to
the operation of decoction, the orifices being subsequently closed by powdered sassafras; the imposi-
tion is detected by the comparative lightness of the
nutmeg, and by its extreme fragility; the holes may
also be discovered by carefully examining the surface
of the nut, after having steeped it in hot water.

MYRRHA. L. E. D. (Arboris nondum descriptæ.
                 (Gummi-resina.   )

Myrrh.

QUALITIES. *Form,* irregularly shaped pieces, trans-
lucent, of a reddish yellow colour; *Odour,* peculiar
and fragrant; *Taste,* bitter and aromatic. CHEMICAL
COMPOSITION. Resin, gum, essential oil, and some
extractive. SOLUBILITY. When triturated with
soft, or distilled water, nearly the whole appears to
be dissolved, forming an opaque, yellowish solution,
but by rest the greater part is deposited, and not
more than one-third is actually dissolved; its solubility, however, in water, may be increased by trituration with camphor, or an alkali; rectified spirit
dissolves it, and the resulting tincture, when diluted,
becomes turbid, although no precipitate occurs. MED.
USES. Stimulant, as in *Form.* 31, 105; Expectorant,
46, 47, 52. Emmenagogue, 68. FORMS OF EXHI-
BITION. No form is so eligible as that of substance.
DOSE, grs. x to ʒj. The alkalies, in their crystalline
state, when triturated with myrrh, reduce it to the
form of a tenacious fluid. OFFICINAL PREPARATIONS.
Tinct. Myrrh. L. E. D. *Tinct. Aloes et Myrrh.* E
Tinct. Aloöes Ætherea. E. *Mist. Ferri comp.* L.
Pil. Aloes cum Myrrha. L. E. D. *Pil. Ferri cum
Myrrha.* L. *Pil. Galb. comp.* L. D. *Pil. Assafœtid.
comp.* E. *Pil. Rhei comp.* E. ADULTERATIONS.
It is subject to a variety of frauds, being frequently
mixed with adventitious gums, which are to be detected
by their foreign odour, their white or dark colour,
and by their opacity.

NUX VOMICA. $\left(\begin{array}{c}\text{Strychnus}\\\text{Nux Vomica.}\end{array}\right)$ *Nux Vomica.*

This seed has not at present a place in the British pharmacopœiæ; it presents however several points of interest to the physiologist, the physician, and the chemist. Its virulent action upon animals has been long known, and it has been administered in combination with gentian in intermittents, (*Ludovic Phar.* p. 113,) and as a narcotic in mania; it also constituted an ingredient in the famous *Electuarium de ovo,* (*Ph. Angl. p.* 263.) Dr. Fourquier has lately introduced its use in the Hospital de la Charité, in cases of partial paralysis, and, it is said, with very great success; the dose is four or five grains of the powder in pills, during the day. The French codex contains two alcoholic extracts of this substance, the one prepared with a strong spirit (22, 32, Beaumé, i, e, from sp. gr. 915 to 856,) is much more active and powerful than that made with a weak spirit, (12, 22, Beaumé, i, e, from sp. gr. 985 to 915.) M. M. Pelletier and Caventou have discovered in this substance, a peculiar proximate principle, to which its virulence is owing; it was named *Vauqueline,* in honour of the celebrated French philosopher, but in deference to the opinion of the French Academy of Sciences, the discoverers have substituted the name *Strychnine,* because "a name dearly loved, ought not to be applied to a noxious principle." (*Annales de Chimie, vol.* 8 and 10.) Strychnine is highly alkaline, and crystallizes in very small four-sided prisms, terminated by four-sided pyramids; its taste is insupportably bitter, leaving a slight metallic flavour; it has no smell; it is so extremely active and violent, that in doses of half a grain, it occasions serious effects, and

in larger ones, convulsions and death ; notwithstanding its strong taste, it is very sparingly soluble in
water, requiring 6667 parts of that fluid for its
solution at 50, and 2500 at 212°. It is very soluble
in alcohol ; with acids it forms neutral and crystal-
lizable salts ; these salts as well as their base, have
the singular property of becoming blood-red by the
action of concentrated nitric acid. Strychnine exists
in native combination in the Strychnus, with an acid,
which has some analogy with the malic, and which
Pelletier and Cavendou propose to call the *Igasuric
acid*, from the Malay name for the bean of St. Ignatius*, (Strychnus Ignatia,) in which its properties were
first examined. In conformity with such vie s, the
active principle of the tribe of Strychni is an *Igasurate
of Strychnine*. A fact which suggests the existence
of a most singular and striking analogy between the
chemical constitution of these narcotico-acrid bodies
and that of opium.

OLEA DISTILLATA. L. OL. VOLATILIA. E.
OL. ESSENTIALIA. D.
Distilled, Volatile, or Essential Oils.

The British pharmacopœiæ direct them to be
obtained by distillation only ; the French codex orders
several of them to be prepared by expression. QUA-

---

* *Strychnine* was obtained from the beans of St. Ignatius by the following process ; a portion of the beans being grated was heated in a close
vessel, under pressure, with sulphuric ether, by which an oily matter
was dissolved ; the residuum then yielded by the action of alcohol, a
yellowish brown, very bitter substance, which being boiled with pure
magnesia and filtered, the colouring matter was washed out, and the
Strychnine and magnesia, in a state of mixture, remained on the filtre.
The strychine was then separated by alcohol, and thus obtained in a
state of great purity.

LITIES. *Form*, liquid, sometimes viscid; *specific grav.* various, oil of turpentine, which is the lightest, being only 0.792, whilst the oils of cloves, cinnamon, and allspice exceed 1030, and that of sassafras, which is the heaviest, amounts to 1.094; these latter oils hold resin in solution, they of course sink in water. *Odour*, penetrating and fragrant; *Taste*, acrid; they are volatilized at a temperature somewhat below that of boiling water; they are very inflammable. SOLUBILITY. Very soluble in alcohol, forming what are termed, in perfumery, *Essences ;* in water they are very sparingly soluble; the solutions are known in pharmacy under the title of *distilled waters :* they are also dissolved by ether, and the *fixed* oils ; when digested with ammonia, some of the less odorous acquire a considerable degree of fragrance, whilst, on the contrary, fixed alkalies universally impair their odour; they are rapidly decomposed by nitric and sulphuric acids, and their action is sometimes attended with instant inflammation. Volatile oils, from continued exposure to the air, absorb oxygen, and become resinous, by which they lose their volatility, fragrance and pungency, hence they should be preserved in small opaque phials, completely full and well stopped. MEDICAL USES. They act as powerful stimulants and aromatics; they remove nausea and flatulence, correct the griping of certain purgatives, and cover the offensive taste of various remedies. See *Aquæ distillatæ*. The following is a list of the species admitted into our British pharmacopœiæ; those designated in *italics* are principally for internal use. OLEA *Anisi, Anthemidis, Carui, Juniperi*, Lavandulæ, *Menthæ Piperitæ, Menthæ viridis*, Origani, *Pimentæ, Pulegii, Rosmarini, L.* OLEA VOLATILIA, *Juniperi communis*, Juniperi Sabinæ, Lavandulæ Spicæ, Lauri

Sassafras, *Menthæ Piperitæ, Myrtæ Pimentæ, Pim-pinellæ Anisi,* Rorismarini Officinalis, E. Olea *Juniperi, Pimento,* Corticis et Ligni Sassafras, *e Se-minibus Anisi, Carui,* et *Fœniculi dulcis,* Florum Lavandulæ, Foliorum Sabinæ, *Herbæ florescentis Menthæ Piperitidis, Herbæ florescentis Menthæ Sativæ,* Origani, *Pulegii, Rorismarini, Rutæ,* D. Adulterations. *Fixed Oils* may be detected by moistening writing paper with the suspected article and holding it before a fire; if the oil be entirely essential, no stain of grease will remain; as castor oil is more soluble in spirit than the others, it is the one generally selected for this fraudulent purpose, and the addition of alcohol restores the sophisticated oil to its proper degree of consistency. *Alcohol* is dis-covered by adding water, which, if it be present, occasions a milkiness, and at the same time, an in-crease of temperature. *Cheaper oils,* as that of tur-pentine, are recognised by their peculiar odour, which may be developed by rubbing a drop upon the hand and holding it to the fire, or, by the dense black smoke with which they burn. The oil of aniseed, as it crys-tallizes at 50°, is frequently sophisticated with wax, spermaceti or camphor; the fraud is detected by warming the oil, when the crystals, if genuine, will dissolve.

OLEA EXPRESSA. L. D.
Olea Fixa, sive Expressa. E.
Expressed or Fixed Oils.

These are obtained from animal matter, by fusion,

* Huiles Antiques. The basis of the best of these oils, is the oil of Ben, from the nuts of the *Guilangia Moringa;* or oil of hazel, which is a very good substitute, since it is inodorous, colourless, and may be kept for a considerable period without becoming rancid: it is therefore well adapted to receive and retain the odour of those vegetables that yield but a small proportion of essential oil.

and from vegetables, by expression, or decoction with water. Qualities. *Odour*, none; *Taste*, mild; they boil at 600, but undergo decomposition, becoming acrid and empyreumatic; the oil, in this state, was formerly used in medicine under the name of *philosophers oil.** By exposure to air they absorb oxygen and become rancid; they congeal at a temperature of 32°, and some even above that. When the oil is expressed by heating the plates of the press, or by previously roasting the seeds, it is more disposed to become rancid; *cold drawn* oils are on this account to be preferred for the purposes of pharmacy. Solubility. They are insoluble in water, and, except castor oil, nearly so in alcohol and ether; with caustic alkalies they combine and form soaps; when aided by heat they readily unite with oxide of lead, forming the solid compound well known by the term *plaister*. They unite also very readily with each other, and with volatile oils. Solvent Powers. They dissolve sulphur, and form a kind of balsam with it; they also possess the power of extracting and dissolving the narcotic and acrid principles of several vegetable and animal substances, in consequence of which, the French pharmacopœia directs a series of preparations under the term " *Olea Medicata;*" thus, there are olea Cicutæ, Hyoscyami, Solani, Stramonii, Nicotianæ;+ which are made by digesting with a gentle heat, one part of the subject in two parts of olive oil.‡

* Oil of Bricks. So called because this empyreumatic oil was sometimes obtained by steeping a brick in oil, and submitting it to distillation.

+ Roche's Embrocation for the Hooping Cough. Olive oil mixed with about half its quantity of the oils of cloves and amber.

‡ The editors have also unaccountably retained the *Oleum de Lumbricis!*

OLEUM AMYGDALARUM. L. E. D.

Oil of Almonds.

This oil, whether procured from the *sweet* or *bitter* almond, has the same properties, for the bitter principle resides exclusively in combination with the mucilage; that from the latter keeps longer without raucidity. It is sometimes made from old Jordan almonds, *by heat*, in which case it very soon grows fotid. Nut oil, *Oleum nucum Coryli*, has been proposed as a substitute for that of almonds; in China it is drank with tea, instead of cream. MEDICAL USES. For forming emulsions, in coughs, and other pulmonary complaints. FORMS OF EXHIBITION. It may be formed into an *emulsion* by the intermedium of *mucilage*, the *yolk of an egg*, or by that of an *alkali*.

1. BY MUCILAGE. This is in general a more convenient medium than the yolk of an egg; one part of gum, made into mucilage, will be sufficient for the diffusion of four parts of oil, (see *Mucilago Acaciæ*,) the oil and mucilage must be carefully triturated together, and the water then gradually added; the emulsion thus formed, is permanent, and the addition of a moderate quantity of acid, spirit, or tincture, will not produce decomposition. *See Form. 73.*

2. BY ALKALIES. This oil, by uniting with alkalies and water, forms an elegant and grateful mixture, for which purpose the following proportions are to be observed, every f3j of oil requires *m* viij of liquor potassæ, and f℥iss of distilled water. INCOMPATIBLE SUBSTANCES. *Acids; oxymel; syrups of poppies and squills; tartrate and super-tartrate of potass; super-sulphate of potass; oxy-muriate of mercury; resins; hard water. See Form. 74.*

OPIUM. L. E. D. (Papaver Somniferum. *Capsularum immaturarum Succus concretus.*) (Turcicus.)

Turkey Opium.

Two kinds are found in commerce, distinguished by the names of *Turkey* and *East India* Opium. Qualities. *Form.* Turkey opium occurs in flat pieces, of a solid compact texture, and possessing considerable tenacity; by long exposure to the air it becomes hard, breaks with a shining fracture, and affords a yellowish powder. *Colour,* reddish-brown or fawn-like. *Odour,* peculiar, heavy, and narcotic. *Taste,* at first, a nauseous bitter, which soon becomes acrid with some degree of warmth. It is inflammable. Solubility. It is partially soluble in water, alcohol, ether, wine, vinegar, and lemon juice; when triturated with hot water, five parts in twelve are dissolved, six suspended, and one part remains perfectly insoluble and resembles *gluten.* By long boiling, its soporific powers are impaired, and ultimately destroyed : the alcoholic is more highly charged with its narcotic principle than the aqueous solution, but spirit, rather below proof, is its best menstruum. The watery solution, when filtered, is transparent, and reddens the colour of litmus; it undergoes no change on the addition of alcohol, but precipitates occur from *pure ammonia,* and from the *carbonates of fixed alkalies ;* from the solutions of *oxy-muriate of mercury, nitrate of silver, acetate and super-acetate of lead,* the *sulphates of copper, zinc and iron,* and from an *infusion of galls.* Chemical Composition. Resin, gum, bitter extractive, sulphate of lime, gluten, and a peculiar alkaline body, to which the narcotic virtues of opium are owing, and to which the appropriate name of *Morphia* has been assigned; and it appears,

moreover, that this new alkaline body exists in combination with an unknown acid, which has therefore
been denominated the *Meconic acid;* so that the
narcotic principle of opium is *Morphia* in the state of
a *meconiate*, or perhaps of a *super-meconiate*.

For these important facts we are indebted to the
successive labours of Derosne,* Sertuerner, and Robiquet. And the French codex contains, in its appendix,
formulæ for the preparation of morphia according to
the directions of these two latter chemists.†

* *Annales de Chimie, vol. 45.* The Salt of Derosne, however, as the
experiments of Robiquet seem to shew, is not, as Sertuerner supposed,
a *meconiate of morphia*, but another acid, characterized by a different train
of properties, and which may be separated from opium by a somewhat
circuitous process. Farther experiments are required upon this subject.

† Robiquet's Process. Three hundred parts of pure opium are to
be macerated, during five days, in one thousand parts of common water;
to the filtered solution, fifteen parts of perfectly pure magnesia, (carefully avoiding the *carbonate*,) are to be added, boil this mixture for ten
minutes, and separate the sediment, by a filter, washing it with cold
water until the water passes off clear; after which, treat it alternately
with hot and cold alcohol; (12, 22 Bé.) as long as the menstruum takes
up any colouring matter; the residue is then to be treated with boiling
alcohol (22, 32, Bé.) for a few minutes. The solution, on cooling, will
deposit crystals of *Morphia*.

Rationale of the Process. A soluble *meconiate of magnesia* is thus formed,
whilst the sediment consists of *Morphia*, in the state of mixture, with
the excess of magnesia; the boiling alcohol, with which this residuum
is treated, exerts no action upon the magnesia, but dissolves the *Morphia*,
and on cooling surrenders it in a crystalline form. A repetition of the
treatment with boiling alcohol will procure a fresh crop of crystals,
and the process should be continued until they cease to appear.

Sertuerner's Method. It differs from the preceding in substituting
ammonia for magnesia, and in adding to the sediment, separated as
before mentioned, as much sulphuric acid as is sufficient to convert the
Morphia into a sulphate, which is subsequently decomposed by a farther
addition of ammonia; the precipitate thus produced, is then dissolved
in boiling alcohol, which on cooling, surrenders the *Morphia*, in a state
of crystalline purity. It appears however that the *Morphia* produced
by this latter method, is less abundant and more impure and coloured,
than that which is furnished by the process of Robiquet.

Characters of Morphia. When pure, it crystallizes
in very fine, transparent, truncated pyramids, the bases
of which are either squares or rectangles, occasionally
united base to base, and, thereby forming octohedra.
It is sparingly soluble in boiling water, but dissolves
abundantly in heated alcohol and ether, and the solutions are intensely bitter. It has all the characters
of an alkali ; affecting test papers, uniting with acids,
and forming neutral salts, and decomposing the compounds of acids with metallic oxides. It unites with
sulphur by means of heat, but the combination is
decomposed at the same instant; it is incapable of
forming soap with an oxidized oil. It fuses at a
moderate temperature, when it resembles melted sulphur, and like that substance, crystallizes on cooling ;
it is decomposed by distillation, yielding carbonate
of ammonia, oil, and a black resinous residue, with a
peculiar smell; when heated in contact with air, it
inflames rapidly; the voltaic pile exerts but little
action upon it, yet, when mixed with a globule of
mercury, the latter appears to become encreased in
bulk, and to change consistence. Its habitudes with
different bodies have not hitherto been sufficiently
investigated, but they are highly important, in as
much as they will explain the operation of those
various medicinal compounds, into which opium
enters as a principal ingredient. Morphia acts on the
animal body as a most powerful agent, three half
grains taken in succession, with intervals of half an
hour, by the same person, produced violent vomiting,
and alarming faintings, and yet its comparative insolubility must materially diminish its potency; hence,
under certain circumstances, vegetable acids render
narcotic extracts more efficient. The following history of its saline compounds may be useful.

The *Carbonate* crystallizes in short prisms.

The *Acetate* in soft prisms, very soluble, and extremely active.

The *Sulphate*, in arborescent crystals, very soluble.

The *Muriate*, in plumose crystals, much less soluble; when evaporated, it concretes into a shining white plumose mass on cooling.

The *Nitrates*, in prisms grouped together.

The *Meconiate*, in oblique prisms, sparingly soluble.

The *Tartrate* in prisms.

Morphia is separated from the above combinations by ammonia.

Morphia is very soluble in olive oil, and according to the experiments of M. Majendie, the compound acts with great intensity; with extractive matter morphia forms a compound, which is almost insoluble in water, but very soluble in acids.

The *Meconic acid*, when separated from the residuum of the magnesian salt, as described above, does not appear to possess any medicinal activity. Its distinguishing *chemical* character is, that it produces an intensely red colour in solutions of iron oxidized *ad maximum*.

East India Opium, is an inferior species; it differs from *Turkey Opium*, in its *texture* being less compact, and much softer; its *colour* darker; its narcotic *odour* fainter, but combined with a strong empyreuma, and in its *taste* being more bitter, but less acrimonious. According to the experiments of Mr. A. T. Thomson, *Turkey Opium* contains three times more morphia than the *East India* variety. This latter, when triturated with water, is taken up without any residuum, hence it contains no gluten, but the sulphate of lime is more abundant, as appears from the relative proportion of precipitate produced by oxalic

acid. The solution of the acetate of barytes, whilst
it occasions no disturbance in the solutions of the
Turkey variety, produces a copious precipitate with
the East Indian. MED. USES. Are so well known
that a few practical remarks will suffice.

Chemistry, it appears, has developed the principle
of its activity, and accumulated experience has established the value and importance of its medicinal
applications, but Physiology is still unable to demonstrate the manner in which it produces its effects.
It must be admitted, that its primary operation is
that of a powerful and diffusible stimulant, but it is
immediately followed by narcotic and sedative effects,
which are far greater than could have been inferred
from the degree of previous excitement, and hence,
much keen controversy has arisen in the schools concerning its *modus operandi.* In very large doses, the
primary excitement is scarcely apparent, but the
powers of life are instantly depressed, drowsiness
and stupor succeed, and when the dose is excessive,
these are followed by delirium, stertorous breathing,
cold sweats, convulsions, and apoplectic death. Its
stimulant effects are apparent only in small doses, by
which the energy of the mind, the strength of the pulse,
and the heat of the body, are considerably increased,
but all the secretions and excretions, except the
cuticular discharge, are diminished ; for example, the
fæces of persons, after the use of opium, are not unfrequently clay coloured, from the suspension of the
biliary secretion ; this circumstance suggests some
important precautions with respect to its exhibition.
Opium, when properly directed, is capable of fulfilling two great indications ; 1st, of supporting the
powers of life, and 2nd, of allaying spasm, pain, and
irritation, and of blunting that morbid susceptibility

of impression, which so frequently attends fever. It
must be differently administered, as it is designed to
fulfil one or other of these indications ; where its
primary or stimulant operation is required, as in diseases of debility, as, for instance, in fevers of the
typhoid type, it should be given in small doses, at
short intervals, so as to sustain a uniform and regular
state of excitement. But, where the object is to
mitigate pain, allay irritation, and produce sleep, it
ought to be exhibited in full doses, at distant intervals. Its use is contra-indicated in all cases where
inflammatory action prevails, as in pulmonary affections, attended with an accelerated circulation, and a
dry hard cough.* In combination, the powers of
opium are wonderfully extended ; by diminishing
the sensibility of the stomach and bowels, it becomes
a valuable and efficacious *corrigent* to many important
medicines, and thus frequently favours their absorption and introduction into the system, as for instance,
in the exhibition of mercurial alteratives, (*Form :*
34), and in certain diuretic combinations, (*Form : 28,*
35, 38), in combination with antimonials, and with
ipecacuan, its narcotic powers are obviated, and
sudorific results are obtained. See *Pulv. Ipecac. co.*

* Opium is the Quack's sheet anchor. The various nostrums advertised as " *Cough Drops,* for the cure of colds, asthmas, catarrhs, &c·"
are preparations of Opium very similar to paregoric elixir. PECTORAL
BALSAM OF LIQUORICE, and ESSENCE OF COLTSFOOT, are combinations
of this kind. GRINDLE's COUGH DROPS, are a preparation of this kind,
made with Rectified, instead of Proof Spirit, and consequently more
highly charged with stimulant materials. " The mischief," observes
Dr. Fothergill, " that has proceeded from the *healing* anodynes of
quacks, can be scarcely imagined, for in coughs, arising from sup-
pressed perspiration, or an inflammatory diathesis, Opiates generally do
harm.
SQUIRE's ELIXIR. Opium, camphor, anise and fennel seeds, made
into a tincture, and coloured with cochineal.

and Form. 53, 55, 60, 61, 66. Forms of Exhibition.
In substance, or under the form of tincture: when we
wish to continue the operation of opium, and not to
obtain its full effects at once, it may be advantageously combined with some substance capable of
retarding its solution in the stomach, as *gum resins*.
See *Pilulæ*. A watery infusion, made by infusing
powdered opium in boiling water, will often operate,
without producing that distressing nausea, and head-
ache, which so frequently follow the use of this substance. When the stomach rejects altogether its
internal exhibition, it may be successfully applied in
the form of frictions, along the spine, with the camphor liniment, or what is more efficacious, in combination with olive oil; a piece of solid opium introduced into the rectum, or dissolved in some appropriate solvent, and injected as an enema, affords also
considerable relief, in spasmodic affections of the
bowels, and in painful diseases of the prostrate gland,
or bladder. Incompatible Substances. *Oxy-
muriate of mercury; acetate of lead; alkalies; infusions of galls*, and *of yellow cinchona*. Orfila states that
the decoction of *Coffee* is less energetic, as an antidote, than the infusion. When we intend the opium
to act as a sedative, we should not combine it with
stimulants. The Edinburgh College certainly erred
in this respect, when they made pepper an ingredient
in their *Pilulæ Opiatæ*. In combination with vegetable acids its narcotic powers are encreased, in consequence of the formation of soluble salts, with *morphia*.* When the opium however has passed out of

* The Black Drop, or *The Lancaster*, or *Quaker's Black Drop*. This
preparation, which has been long known and esteemed, as being more
powerful in its operation, and less distressing in its effects, than any
tincture of opium, has, until lately, been involved in much obscurity;

the primæ viæ, vinegar and acids are then the best
remedies for counteracting its effects; (see *Introductory
Essay*, page 25.) Dose, must be varied according
to the intention of the prescriber, the constitution of
the patient, and the nature of the disease. A quarter
of a grain, frequently repeated, will keep up its ex-
hilarating influence; from gr. j to ij act as a narcotic;
its power on the system soon becomes weaker; and
from habitual use is so much impaired that very large

the papers however of the late Edward Walton, of Sunderland, one of
the near relations of the original proprietor, having fallen into the
hands of Dr. Armstrong, that gentleman has obliged the profession by
publishing the manner in which it is prepared, and is as follows:—
" Take half a pound of Opium sliced; three pints of good Verjuice,
(juice of the wild crab,) and one and a half ounce of nutmegs, and half an
ounce of Saffron. Boil them to a proper thickness, then add a quarter
of a pound of sugar, and two spoonsful of yeast. Set the whole in a
warm place, near the fire, for six or eight weeks, then place it in the
open air until it becomes a syrup; lastly, decant, filter, and bottle it
up, adding a little sugar to each bottle." One drop of this preparation
is considered equal to about three of the Tincture of Opium. P. L.
It would appear that an *Acetate of Morphia* is formed, which is more
active, and less distressing in its effects, than any other narcotic combination.

The *French Codex* contains directions for preparing a compound, very
similar to the *Black Drop*; viz.

VINUM OPIATUM FERMENTATIONE PARATUM, or, *Gutta, seu Laudanum Abbatis Rousseau*. Take of white honey twelve ounces; warm
water, three pounds; dissolve the honey in the water, pour it into a
matrass, and set it aside in a warm place: as soon as fermentation has
commenced, add four ounces of good opium, having previously dissolved, or rather diffused it in twelve ounces of water; allow them to
ferment together for a month, then evaporate, until ten ounces only
remain, filter, and add four ounces and a half of alcohol.

LIQUOR OPII SEDATIVUS. Under this name, Mr. Battley, of Fore-
street, London, has introduced a narcotic preparation, which it is
generally supposed owes its efficacy to the *acetate of morphia*; on being
kept, however, I found that it underwent some important change,
during which so much air was disengaged as to blow out the cork from
the bottle with violence. This is a great objection to its admission
into practice.

doses are required to produce its usual effects. Russel observes that the effects of opium, on those addicted to its use, are at first obstinate costiveness, succeeded by diarrhea and flatulence, with loss of appetite and a sottish appearance ; the teeth decay, the memory fails, and the unhappy sufferer prematurely sinks into the grave. OFFICINAL PREP. Gr. j of opium is contained in *Confect. Opii.* L. grs. 36. *Elect. Opii.* E. grs. 43. *Elect. Catechu.* E. grs. 193. *Elect. Catechu comp.* D. grs. 199. *Pil Saponis cum opio.* L. grs. 5. *Pil. Opiat.* E. grs. 10. *Pil. e Styrace.* D. grs. 5. *Pulv. Corn. ust. cum Opio.* L. grs. 10. *Pulv. Cret comp. cum Opio.* L. grs. 40. *Pulv. Ipecac. comp.* L. E. grs. 10. *Pulv. Kino comp.* L. grs. 20. *Tinct. Opii.* L. m 19. *Tinct. Camphor. comp.* L. f℥ss. *Tinct. Opii ammon.* E. f℥j. *Troch. Glycyrr. cum. Opio.* E. ℥j. *Vinum Opii.* L. m 17. ADULTERATIONS. The *Turkey Opium*, when good, is covered with leaves, and the reddish capsules of some species of *rumex;* the inferior kinds have none of these capsules adhering to them. It is frequently adulterated with the extract of liquorice ; it should be regarded as bad, when it is very soft, or friable, of an intensely black colour, or mixed with many impurities, or when it has a sweetish taste, or marks paper with a brown, continuous streak, when drawn across it. It frequently happens that in cutting a mass of opium, bullets and stones have been found imbedded in it, a fraud which is committed by the Turks, from which the retailer alone suffers.

OVUM. L. (Phasianus Gallus.) *The Egg of the*
        (*Ovum.*   ) *domestic Fowl.*

VITELLUS, The *Yolk,* or *Yelk,* is principally employed in pharmaceutical operations, for rendering
oils and balsams miscible with water. It is gently laxative.

Oleum e vitellis, Oil of eggs. Obtained by boiling
the yolks, and then submitting them to pressure; 50
eggs yield about 5 oz. of oil. It is introduced into
the Paris Pharmacopœia, being much employed on
the Continent for *killing* mercury.

ALBUMEN. Used principally for clarifying turbid
liquors.

TESTA. Similar to other absorbents.

PILULÆ. L.E.D. *Pills.*

These are masses of a consistence sufficient to preserve the globular form, and yet not so hard as to be
of too difficult solution in the stomach. The subject
offers some interesting points of inquiry. The following general rules will enable the practitioner to
select those substances to which the form of pill is
adapted, and to reject those to which it is not suitable,
as well as to direct, *extemporaneously,* the mode of
preparation.

I. THE SELECTION OF SUBSTANCES.

1. *Suitable Substances* are 1. All remedies which
operate in small doses, as *Metallic Salts,* and 2. Those
which are designed to act slowly, and gradually, as
certain *Alterative* medicines, or, 3, which are too
easily soluble, when exhibited in other forms, as

Gamboge, &c. 4, Substances which are not intended to act until they reach the larger intestines, as in pills for habitual costiveness ; *see Aloes.* 5, Bodies whose specific gravities are too considerable to allow their suspension in aqueous vehicles. *Efflorescent* salts may also be exhibited in this form, but they ought to be first deprived of their water of crystallization, or the pills composed of them will crumble into powder as they dry.

2. *Unsuitable Substances* are, 1. Those which operate only in large doses. 2. Which deliquesce. 3. Whose consistence is such as to require a very large proportion of dry powders, to afford them a suitable tenacity, as *oils, balsams,* &c. 4, Substances that are so extremely insoluble, that when exhibited in a solid form they pass through the canal unaltered, as certain *extracts.*

Many remedies which are incompatible with each other in solution, may be combined in pills, unless indeed their medicinal powers are adverse or inconsistent, or their divellent affinities sufficiently powerful to overcome their state of aggregation.

II. Their Formation into Masses.

This is a subject of far greater importance than what is usually assigned to it, as will be more fully explained in the sequel.

1. Many substances, as *vegetable extracts*, may be formed into pills without any addition ; others, as *gum resins,* become sufficiently soft by being beaten, or by the addition of a drop or two of spirit, or *liquor potassæ.* Some dry substances react upon each other, and produce, without the addition of any foreign matter, soft and appropriate masses. The *Pilulæ Ferri Compositæ* of our Pharmacopœia, afford a very

striking example of this peculiar change of consistence,
which the mut·al ·eaction of the ingredients produces
by simple triture. The *Pilulæ Aloes Compositæ* offer
another instance, for the extract of gentian, upon
being triturated with aloes, produces a very soft mass,
so that the addition of syrup, as directed by the Pharmacopœia, is quite unnecessary.

2. Many substances are, in themselves, so untracta-
ble, that the addition of some matter foreign to the
active ingredients, is absolutely essential for imparting convenience of form. It. is generally considered
that very little skill or judgment is required in the
selection of such a substance, provided it can fulfil
the *mechanical* intention just alluded to—the fact
however is, that *the medicinal power of the pill may
be materially controlled, modified, or even subverted,
by the mode in which it is formed into a mass.* Where
the active element of a pill is likely to be improved
by minute division, a gummy or resinous constituent
may be usefully selected ; under the history of Aloes,
I have alluded to a popular pill, known by the name
of the *dinner pill,* in which case, the *mastiche* divides
the particles of the aloes, and modifies the solubility
of the mass. The *Pilulæ Opii* of the former Pharmacopœia of London, consisted of equal proportions of
opium and extract of liquorice, and the mass was so
insoluble that its effects were extremely uncertain
and precarious ; in the present edition, soap has been
very judiciously substituted ; but in certain cases
where we wish to protract the influence of opium, or
that of any other active body, so as not to obtain its
full effects at once, we may, very advantageously,
modify its solubility, by combining it with a gum resin, or some substance which will have the effect of
retarding its solution in the stomach. The *Pilula*

c Styrace of the Dublin college, presents itself as an efficient example of this species of pharmacentical address. I am well acquainted with many extemporaneous formulæ, whose utility has been fully sanctioned by experience, and I have no hesitation in believing that their salutary mode of operation, would receive a plausible explanation from this simple law of combination. Dr. Young has very justly stated, in his Medical Literature, that the *balsam of copaiba* envelopes metallic salts, so as to lessen their activity; he says, that the sub-carbonate of iron, made into pills with copaiba, was given for some weeks without any apparent effect; and, that a few hours after the same quantity had been given, with gum only, the fœces were perfectly black. I do not know a more striking and instructive proof of the influence of a glutinous or viscid constituent, in wrapping up a metallic salt, and defending the stomach from its action, than is presented in the case published by the medical attendant Mr Marshall, in consequence of the attempt of Eliza. Fenning to poison the family of Mr Turner of Chancery-lane, by arsenic, which she providentially administered in a heavy yeast dumpling. *Soap* is very frequently used for the formation of pill masses, and it is an excellent constituent for substances likely to be injured by meeting with an acid in the *primæ viæ;* many resinous bodies may also be reduced to a proper consistence by soap, although in prescribing it, its levity should be attended to, or, otherwise, the pills will be too bulky; in general, it will combine with an equal portion of any resinous powder, as *Rhubarb, Jalap; &c.;* it is of course ineligible where the substances are decomposed by alkalies, as *Tartarized Antimony;* this last precaution will also apply to *aromatic confection* as a vehicle, on account of the carbonate of lime contained in it. The *Conserve of Roses* has the advantage of retaining its consistency much longer than mucilage, but, as it contains an uncombined acid, it is frequently inadmissible; it could not, for instance, be with propriety employed with the precipitated sulphuret of antimony. Pills, made with mucilage, are apt to crumble when they are rolled out; this is the case with the *Pilula Hydrargyri submuriatis;* some extract therefore would be a more convenient constituent; in this particular case, however, the addition of a few drops of spirit would supersede the necessity of any constituent.

Crumb of bread furnishes a convenient vehicle for those salts which are ponderous, active in very small doses, or which are liable to be decomposed by other vehicles, but an objection is attached even to this, for it is liable to become so dry and hard when kept, that pills made with it, will frequently pass undissolved. Swediaur mentions this fact with reference to Plenck's mercurial pill, as well as to one of corrosive sublimate, and he proposes, for this reason, to substitute *starch;* the addition however of a small portion of sugar will prevent the bread from becoming thus indurated, and with such a precaution it may be very safely employed. For the purpose of forming active vegetable powders into pills, such as Digitalis, Conium, &c., I am informed by Mr. Hume of Long Acre, that, in his experience, *melasses* or *treacle*, is the best constituent that can be selected; for it undergoes no decomposition by time, but maintains a proper consistency, and preserves the sensible qualities of the plant quite unimpaired for many years. I have deposited in the cabinet of the college, specimens of such pills, of *hemlock* and *foxglove*, which retain the characteristic odour of these vegetables, notwith-

standing they have been now made for several years.
Honey has likewise the property of preserving vegetable substances ; *seeds* may be kept in it for any length
of time, some of which, on being taken out, washed,
and planted, will even vegetate. It has also been
used for the preservation of animal matter; the bodies
of the Spartan kings, who fell at a distance in battle,
were thus preserved, in order that they might be
carried home.

3. In the formation of pills, the ingredients should
be hastily rubbed together, whenever they are liable
to be injured by long exposure to the air; thus, in
the formation of *Pilula Hydrargyri sub-muriatis*,
the compound is rendered less active by long continued triture. *See Pulveres.*

4. In dividing pill masses, it is usual to add to,
and envelope them in magnesia; where calomel is
present I have satisfied myself, by experiment, that a
muriate of magnesia is formed, and it is owing to this
partial decomposition, that the surface of the pill
exhibits a greenish hue ; starch, powder of liquorice, or
orrice root, might perhaps, under such circumstances,
be more judiciously preferred. In Germany, the
powder of *Lycopodium* is generally used. Formerly,
the pill was covered with gold leaf, which protected
it from the influence of the stomach, and frequently
rendered it unavailing.

It has been observed, that many of the pill masses,
directed in our pharmacopœias, are liable to become
so hard and dry, by being kept, that they are unfit
for that division for which they were originally intended ; indeed, Dr. Powell considers it doubtful
whether the greater number of articles had not better
be kept in powder, and their application to the
formation of pills left to extemporaneous direction ;

the necessity of this is farther apparent, when we learn, that it is a common practice for the dispenser to soften these masses by the application of a hot spatula, or pestle, which sometimes carbonizes, and frequently decomposes them.*

III. Their Form of Prescription.

In our extemporaneous directions, it is necessary to apportion with accuracy the quantity of active materials, which we may wish each pill to contain, and since the proportion of the *constituent*, can rarely be exactly defined, the equable division of the whole mass, into a given number of pills, will be safer than defining the weight of each pill.

A pill, the bulk of whose ingredient is vegetable matter, ought not to exceed five grains in weight, but where the substances which compose it are metallic and ponderous, it may without inconvenience weigh six or even eight grains.

Pilulæ Aloes Compositæ. L. Extract of aloes *two parts*, extract of gentian, (*d.*) *one part*, with oil of carraway; (*c.*) to which syrup is unnecessarily added. It is a useful pill in habitual costiveness. *Dose*, grs. x to ℈j.

---

* Some extracts become so hard, that in the state of pill, they pass unchanged; this has occurred to me with the *extract of logwood.* Astringent vegetable matter, in combination with iron, is frequently characterised by a hardness that is not exceeded by ebony, and which is perfectly insoluble; the action of iron upon the petals of the red rose furnishes a very striking instance of this fact; if the petals be beaten in an iron mortar, for some hours, they ultimately become converted into a paste of an intensely black hue; which, when rolled into beads and dried, is susceptible of a most beautiful polish, still retaining the fragrance of the rose. I have seen a necklace of this description; indeed these beads form an article of extensive commerce with the Turks, and are imported into Europe, through Austria, under the name of *Rose Beads*, or *Rose Pearls.*

PILULÆ ALOES ET ASSAFŒTIDÆ. E. Powdered aloes, assafœtida (d.) and soap, (h.) *equal parts.* Anodyne and cathartic, a very useful combination in dyspepsia attended with flatulence. *Dose,* grs. x.

PILULÆ ALOES CUM MYRRHA. L. *Pilulæ Rufi,* P. L. 1745. Extract of aloë, *two parts,* saffron and myrrh, (d.) *one part,* syrup, q.s. This is a very ancient form of preparation, and is described by Rhazes. It is stimulant and cathartic. *Dose,* grs. x to ℈j.

PILULÆ ALOES CUM COLOCYNTHIDE. E. This pill is known by the popular name of *Pil. Coccia.* κοκκίον, signifies a seed, and the term was first applied to this preparation by Rnazes. It consists of *eight parts* of aloes, and scammony; *four* of colocynth; and *one part* of oil of cloves, (c.) and of sulphate of potass with sulphur, olim, *Sal Polychrest.* It is more powerful in its operation than the simple aloetic pills.

PILULÆ CAMBOGIÆ COMPOSITÆ. L. Gamboge, extract of aloe, and compound powder of cinnamon *one part;* soap *two parts;* see *Introductory Essay,* p. 21.

PILULÆ FERRI COMPOSITÆ. L. This combination is analogous to that of Griffith's mixture. *Dose,* gr. x to ℈j.

PILULÆ GALBANI COMPOSITÆ. L. *Pil. Gummosæ,* P. L. 1745. We are here presented with a combination of fœtid gums, in which Assafœtida is the most potent article. Antispasmodic, and Emmenagogue. *Dose,* grs. x to ℈j.

PILULÆ HYDRARGYRI. L. E. D. *Pil. Mercuriales.* P. L. 1745. vulgo, The *Blue Pill.* The mercury in this preparation, is not, as it was formerly considered, in a state of mere mechanical division, but in that of a black oxide, upon which its activity as a remedy undoubtedly depends; for mercury in its metallic state is entirely inert with regard to

the living system. Various substances have at different times been triturated with the mercury, for the
purpose of *extinguishing* or *killing* it, by effecting the
mechanical division, and subsequent oxidation of its
particles; *Conserve of Roses* is now generally preferred
for this purpose, although Swediaur suspects that the
astringent principle of this conserve invalidates the
effects of the mercury, " I have," says he, "given
these pills to several patients for a long time, without
any symptom of salivation." The practice of this
country has established a very different opinion. What
says Mr. Abernethy to this ? When any of the gums
are employed for *killing* the metal, the pills soon
become hard and brittle, and after some time, the
mercury is liable to run into its metallic state. The
pill mass, when rendered thinner by the addition of a
little water, and extended on a piece of paper, ought
not to exhibit any metallic globules ; in this examination however we must be careful not to be betrayed,
by the fallacious appearance which is frequently presented, by small crystals of saccharine matter. The
relative proportion of mercury contained in the mass
can be ascertained only by its weight. The *blue pill*
is made at Apothecaries Hall, by a very ingenious
machine, actuated by steam, and which rubs as well
as rolls the materials, and it is said, that the pill thus
made is more active than that produced in the ordinary
way. MEDICAL USES. It is by far the best form
for the internal exhibition of mercury; where it is
intended to act upon the system, as an alterative,
it should be administered in doses of from grs. iv to vj ;
if it occasion any action on the bowels, it may be
conjoined with opium ; sometimes a few grains of
rhubarb, exhibited every morning, will impart such a
tone to the intestines, as to enable them to resist the

mercurial irritation : when exhibited in doses of grs.
x to Əj, it acts as a mild, but efficient purgative.
One grain of mercury is contained in *four* grains of
the mass, made according to the London and Dublin
formulæ, and in three grains according to that of
Edinburgh. For the specific effects of mercury, see
Ung. Hydrarg.

PILULÆ HYDRARGYRI SUB-MURIATIS COMPO-
SITÆ. L. E. Olim, *Plummer's Pills.* They consist
of *one part* of calomel, and precipitated sulphuret of
antimony (*e.*) and *two parts* of guaiac (*d.*) made into form
with mucilage. It is a very useful alterative, especially in cutaneous eruptions, and in secondary syphilitic symptoms, particularly when affecting the skin.
Dose, grs. v to x.

PILULÆ OPIATÆ. E. Opium *one part;* extract of
liquorice *seven parts;* Jamaica pepper *two parts.* It
is a compound of questionable propriety.

PILULÆ RHEI COMPOSITÆ. E. Rhubarb, aloes,
and myrrh, with oil of peppermint. When such a
combination is indicated, it is better to prescribe it
extemporaneously, for the mass, by being kept, will
become less efficacious.

PILULÆ SAPONIS CUM OPIO. L. *Pil. Opii.* P. L.
1787. By substituting soap, for extract of liquorice,
these pills are now rendered more soluble in the
stomach, and are consequently more efficient. Five
grains contain one of opium.

PILULÆ SCILLÆ COMPOSITÆ. L. A stimulating
expectorant ; but as squill is always impaired by keeping, it ought to be an extemporaneous combination.
It is surely injudicious thus to multiply our officinal
formulæ.

PIMENTÆ BACCÆ. L. E. (Myrtus Pimenta.
Pimento. D (*Baccæ.*)

Pimenta Berries. Jamaica Pepper. All-spice.

QUALITIES. *Odour,* aromatic and agreeable, combining that of cinnamon, cloves and nutmegs; hence the term *all*-spice. *Taste,* warm and pungent, resembling that of cloves. These qualities reside principally in the cortical part of the berry. CHEMICAL COMPOSITION. It contains a volatile oil, very like that of cloves, resin, extractive, tannin, and gallic acid. SOLUBILITY. Water, alcohol, and ether, extract its virtues. MEDICAL USES. Principally to cover the disagreeable taste of other remedies; it is also a very useful adjunct to dyspeptic medicines.* OFFICINAL PREPARATIONS. *Aq. Piment.* L. E. D. *Ol. Piment.* L. E. D. *Pil. Opiat.* E. *Syrup. Rhamni.* L.

PIPERIS LONGI BACCÆ. L. E. D.

Long Pepper.

The chemical and medicinal properties of this substance, are similar to those of black pepper, *which see.* The varieties in the market are distinguished by the names *short* long pepper, and *long* long pepper.

PIPERIS NIGRI BACCÆ. L. E. D.

Black Pepper.

CHEMICAL COMPOSITION. An oily matter, which appears to be the source of its odour and taste; fecula,

* RYMER'S CARDIAC TINCTURE. Little else than a disguised tincture of *all-spice.*

and extractive. SOLUBILITY. Its virtues are entirely extracted by æther, and alcohol; and partially
by water, 550 pints being required to extract all the
sapidity of lbj of pepper. MEDICAL USES. It appears
to be a more general and permanent stimulus than
other species of equal pungency on the palate; it
may be combined with bitters, and exhibited in nausea,
dyspepsia, retrocedent gout, or as a stimulant in
paralysis; it is also a valuable coajutor to bark, in
obstinate intermittents. DOSE, grs. v to Ɔj, or more.
OFFICINAL PREPARATIONS. *Emplast. Meloes vesicat.
comp.* E. *Unguent. piper. nig.* D. *White* pepper is
made by separating the first skin of the berry, by
soaking it in salt and water. ADULTERATIONS. The
powdered husk of the mustard seed is universally
mixed with powdered pepper, and is regularly sold
for this purpose by the mustard manufacturer, under
the technical title of P. D. *(Pepper Dust;)* there are
besides other admixtures less innocent. *Whole Pepper*
is also frequently factitious; artificial pepper-corns,
composed of peas-meal, both white and black, are
mixed with real pepper-corns, and sold as genuine
pepper; the method of detecting the fraud is very
simple; throw a suspected sample into water; those
that are artificial will fall to powder, or be partially
dissolved, while the true pepper-corns will remain
whole.

† WARD'S PASTE, for fistula, piles, &c. The following is the receipt
for preparing this celebrated composition. Take of Black Pepper and
Elecampane, powdered, equal parts lbss, of the seeds of Fennel lbiss,
of Honey and Sugar, equal parts, lbj; beat, and well mix together all
the ingredients, in a mortar. *Dose,* the size of a nutmeg three times a
day.

PIX ARIDA. L. (Pinus Abies. *Resina Concreta.*)
PIX BURGUNDICA. E. D. *Burgundy Pitch.*

This substance is procured by making incisions
through the bark of the Norway Spruce fir, whereas
frankincence (Abietis resina) is a spontaneous exudation from it. It is now entirely confined to external use, as a rubefacient spread on leather; it is very
adhesive. OFFICINAL PREP: *Emplast: Picis Bur-
gund:* D. ADULTERATIONS. A factitious sort, man-
nufactured in England, is often met with; it is to be
distinguished by its friability, and its want of viscidity and unctuosity, and the absence of that peculiar
odour which characterises the genuine specimens.

PLUMBI SUB-CARBONAS. L.   CARBONAS
PLUMBI, vulgo *Cerussa*, E. CERUSSA, *Sub-acetas
Plumbi.* D.

Cerusse, or *White Lead.*

CHEMICAL COMPOSITION. The composition of
this substance has not until lately been well understood, and hence the different appellations bestowed
upon it by the different colleges. SOLUBILITY. It
is insoluble in water, but soluble in pure potass.
USES. It is only employed externally, being sprinkled
on excoriated parts; the safety of such a practice
however is questionable. OFFICINAL PREP: *Unguent: Ceruss:* D. *Plumbi Super-acetas* (f) L.E.D.
ADULTERATIONS. *Chalk* may be detected by assaying its solution in cold acetic acid, with oxalate of
ammonia; *Carbonate of barytes,* by adding to a portion
of the same solution, sulphate of soda, very largely
diluted with distilled water; and *Sulphate of barytes,*
or *Sulphate of lead,* by the insolubility of the white
lead in boiling distilled vinegar.

PLUMBI OXYDUM SEMI-VITREUM. L.E.
LITHARGYRUM. D.
Litharge.

It is a yellow protoxide of lead, which has been melted, and left to crystallize by cooling. It is only employed in pharmacy, for forming other preparations of lead, and the following officinal plasters, *Emplast : Plumbi:* L.E.D. *Ceratum Saponis.* L. It is added to wines, to remove their acidity; evaporate the suspected liquor to a thick fluid, add charcoal, and calcine in a crucible; in the space of an hour metallic points will be obtained, consisting of lead, surrounded by a quantity of yellow protoxide. *See Orfila.*

PLUMBI SUPER-ACETAS. L. *Cerussa Acetata.*
P.L. 1787. *Saccharum Saturni,* 1745.
ACETAS PLUMBI. E. Acetas Plumbi. D.
vulgo, Sugar of Lead.

QUALITIES. *Form,* irregular masses, resembling lumps of sugar, being an aggregation of acicular, four-sided prisms, terminated by dihedral summits, which are slightly efflorescent; by careful crystallization it may be obtained in quadrangular prisms. *Taste,* sweet and astringent. CHEMICAL COMPOSITION. Although termed a *Super-*acetate, it appears to be a neutral salt, and, that its power of reddening vegetable blues is attributable to a partial decomposition, for, when dissolved in water containing the least portion of carbonic acid, a white carbonate of lead is precipitated, and a corresponding portion of acetic acid is necessarily disengaged. According to the experiments of Berzelius, this salt, in its anhydrous state, consists of one proportional of acetic

acid, and one proportional of oxide of lead; so that
the proportion of the metallic base is one third of
that in the *sub*-acetate. SOLUBILITY. It is dissolved
in 25 parts of water, hot or cold; it is also soluble
in alcohol. When common water is employed the
solution is quite turbid, unless a small proportion of
acetic acid be previously added. INCOMPATIBLE
SUBSTANCES. *The alkalies, alkaline earths, and their
carbonates; most of the acids; alum; borax; the sulphates, and muriates; soaps; all sulphurets; ammoniated, and tartarized iron; tartarized antimony.; undistilled water.* The solution of *acetate of ammonia*
decomposes this salt, in consequence of the carbonic
acid which is generally diffused through it. Certain
bodies appear likewise to be incompatible with the
compounds of lead, not from the *chemical* changes
they induce, but from the contrary effects they produce upon the body; thus Mercury appears to invalidate their powers, and to counteract their effects; as
we may have observed in treating saturnine cholic.
I suspect also that antimony operates in the same
manner; M. Merat relates a case of an apothecary
who was cured of a desperate saturnine cholic, after
having taken, in the course of eight days, eighty
grains of tartarized antimony. MED : USES. I feel
no hesitation in pronouncing this salt of lead to be
one of the most valuable resources of physic; from
the results of numerous cases, I state with confidence,
that it is more efficient in stopping pulmonary, and
uterine hemorrhage, than any other known remedy,
and, that its application is equally safe and manageable,
but it must not be combined with substances capable
of decomposing it, nor must it be simultaneously administered with the medicines which are frequently
prescribed in conjunction with it, as an *Infusion of*

Roses, with *Sulphate of Magnesia*. Alum has also been in some cases added to it, with the intention of increasing its astringency. It is evident that under such circumstances an insoluble and inert *Sulphate of lead* will be produced. The experiments of Orfila confirm the truth of these facts, and shew, that such substances act as counter-poisons for the salts of lead. According to my experience, those vegetable acids which decompose the acetate of lead, and form insoluble salts with its base, are not *medically* incompatible, when administered simultaneously with it, although no scientific physician would prescribe such a mixture; this fact is shewn by the circumstance of potations, containing malic and tartaric acids, not having been found to invalidate the efficacy of this salt; whether the stomach, in the first instance, prevents the decomposition, and its necessary results, or allows the operation of the usual affinities, and then, subsequently, decomposes the insoluble compound which results from them, by the abstraction and *digestion* of its vegetable constituent, are questions for future enquiry, when the laws of gastric chemistry shall be better understood, and more justly appreciated. FORMS OF EXHIBITION. In that of pill, guarded by opium; it will be prudent to recommend an abstinence from all potation, except that of cold water, or draughts composed of diluted acetic acid, for at least an hour after the ingestion of the pill. DOSE gr. $\frac{1}{2}$ to gr. j. OFFICINAL PREP: *Cerat: Plumb: superacetat:* L.*

---

* ROYAL PREVENTIVE. This pretended prophylactic against venerea virus is a solution of *Super-acetate of lead*.

POTASSA CUM CALCE. L.E. KALI CAUSTI CUM CUM CALCE. D.

The addition of lime to potass renders it less deli quescent, and more manageable, as an escharotic.

POTASSA FUSA. L. POTASSA. E. KALI CAUS TICUM. D.
Lapis infernalis. P.L. 1720.

QUALITIES. *Form*, a white brittle substance, extremely caustic and deliquescent, and possessing, in an eminent degree, all the properties denominated *alkaline.* SOLUBILITY, f$\mathfrak{z}$j of water dissolves $\mathfrak{z}$vij; it is also soluble in alcohol. CHEMICAL COMPOSITION. This preparation, independent of its impurities, is the *hydrated protoxide of potassium.* MED. USES. It is a most powerful caustic (*causticum commune acerrimum*), and is frequently employed to establish an ulcer, or, instead of incision, to open a tumour; as an internal remedy it is only employed in solution. See *Liquor Potassæ.*

POTASSÆ ACETAS. L. ACETAS POTASSÆ. E.

ACETAS KALI. D. *Kali Acetatum.* P.L. 1787.— *Sal diureticus.* P.L. 1745.—*Terra foliata Tartari— Sal Sennerti.—Magisterium Purgans Tartari—Sal essentiale vini, Oleum Tartari Sennerti—Sal digestivus Sylvii, &c.*

QUALITIES. *Form*, masses of a foliated, laminar texture, extremely deliquescent; *Odour*, slight and peculiar; *Taste*, sharp and pungent. SOLUBILITY, f℥j of distilled water at 60° dissolves 404 grains, or 100 parts of it are soluble in 105 parts of water; the solution soon undergoes spontaneous decomposition; it is soluble in four times its weight of alcohol. CHE-MICAL COMPOSITION. It consists of one proportional of each of its components, or 45 potass, and 48 acetic acid. INCOMPATIBLE SUBSTANCES. It is decomposed by *tamarinds*, and *most sub-acid fruits;* by almost every acid, as well as every variety of neutral salt, whether *alkaline, acid,* or *metallic.* MED. USES. In small doses, diuretic; in larger ones, mildly cathartic. DOSE. ℈j to ℨj to produce the former, ℨij to ℨiij to excite the latter of these effects. FORMS OF EXHIBITION. It is not admissible in powders or pills, but should be always exhibited in solution. (*Form :* 36, 38, 39.) In the course of the present work, references have been frequently made to this article, for an explanation of certain views regarding the chemical powers of the digestive organs, as well as the operation of several remedies, dependent upon them : I beg therefore to observe, that the results of experiments, carefully conducted, and of observations faithfully recorded, during the exercise of my profession, have fully satisfied me that the digestive organs possess the power of readily decomposing all saline compounds, into which *vegetable* acids enter as ingredients, and of eliminating their alkaline base, which, being in the course of circulation carried to the kidnies, excites them into action, and promotes the excretion of urine; and that it is in this way, the *acetate, citrate, super-tartrate,* and other combinations of potass, or soda, prove diuretic : on the other hand, it is equally evident, that salts containing the *mineral* acids are not under the control of the decomposing powers of the *chylo-poietic* organs, and consequently do not undergo any changes *in transitu ;* although some of these salts, especially the more soluble ones, are absorbed, and stimulate the urinary organs by their contact; this happens with *nitrate of potass,* which may be chemically detected in the urine of those persons who have taken it. *Sulphate* of potass however, from its insolubility, is not readily absorbed, and its composition will not allow the development of its base; it has not therefore any tendency to produce an influence upon the urinary secretion. But it must be observed, that the diuretic operation of any saline body that acts by absorption, is at once suspended* if a catharsis is induced, either by the largeness of the dose, its encreased solubility, or by the effect of its combination with any other remedy ; for it is a law, that *the processes of assimilation and absorption are arrested, or very imperfectly performed during any alvine excitement :* the different effects of the saline compounds of the alkalies, with tartaric acid, elucidate in a very striking manner the truth of this law—thus super-tartrate of potass, or *cream of tartar,* in well regulated doses, acts, as we all know, upon the kidnies ; the tartaric acid being in this case abstracted, and assimilated by the digestive process, and the alkaline base at the same time, eliminated, and subsequently absorbed ; but if we increase the solubility of the compound, by reducing it to the state of a neutral tartrate (*soluble tartar*), or by combining it with boric acid, or some body that has a similar effect ; or what is equivalent to it, if we so encrease the dose of the cream of tartar,

* The *secondary* diuresis, which sometimes succeeds catharsis, offers an apparent exception to this law ; but this must not be confounded with that, which is the result of a *primary* action upon the urinary organs by the absorption of a specific stimulant.

that catharsis follows its administration, then diuresis will not ensue, since no decomposition can, under such circumstances, take place. *(See Introductory Essay, p.* 21.) *Nitre,* and those salts which are carried to the kidnies, without previous decomposition, are subject to the same law, for if we combine them with purgatives, their presence can no longer be recognised in the urine; (see *Scillæ Radix, and Terebinthinæ Oleum.)* By a parity of reasoning we might infer, that by associating saline diuretics with substances capable of rendering the powers of digestion more acute, we should be more likely to ensure their successful operation; that such is actually the fact is satisfactorily proved by the unequivocal results of daily experience, for alkalies, and their compound salts, are never more active than when exhibited in combination with vegetable bitters; and the invigorating influence of *bitter extractive* upon the digestive organs, has been already explained. *(See Historical Introduction, page* xl. *Note.)* For the same reason, although purgatives, when *simultaneously* exhibited with this class of diuretics, will invalidate their powers, they may, nevertheless, when previously exhibited, be the means of assisting their operation; for it is probable that the absorbents are more ready to take up medicinal bodies, after a full evacuation of the bowels. *(See Introductory Essay, p.* 9*).* This view of the operation of saline diuretics, appears to me to offer much matter of practical importance, shewing the circumstances which are most likely to assist, or invalidate the operation of this class of medicinal substances, it admonishes us, for instance, not to combine them with those bodies, whose *primary* operation is upon the bowels, nor with substances capable of so affecting them, *chemically,* as to render them unsusceptible of the necessary changes *in transitu*, as would happen were we, for example, to exhibit the acetate of potass, in the acidulated infusion of roses. At the same time, it seems to suggest some hints that might lead to a more just and practical arrangement of diuretic remedies in general.

ADULTERATIONS. *Tartrate of potass* is discovered by adding a solution of tartaric acid, which will occasion with it a copious precipitate ; the *sulphates*, by their forming with acetate of lead, or muriate of baryta, precipitates insoluble in acetic or muriatic acid. The brown tinge which it frequently exhibits depends upon the same cause as that which usually imparts colour to the *Liquor: Ammon: Acet:* This salt is also sometimes contaminated with *lead;* which arises from its having been prepared by decomposing the *super-acetate of lead* by *carbonate of potass.*

POTASSÆ CARBONAS. L. E.
Carbonate of Potass.

QUALITIES. *Form,* crystals which are four-sided prisms, with dihedral summits, permanent in the air : *Taste,* slightly alkaline, without acrimony. CHEMICAL COMPOSITION. It is a *bi-carbonate,* consisting of two proportionals of carbonic acid, and one proportional of potass ; and in its crystalline form, it also contains water equal to one proportional. SOLUBILITY It is soluble in 4 parts of cold, and in 5 6ths of its weight of boiling water, in which it is partially decomposed, carbonic acid being emitted during the solution; it is quite insoluble in alcohol. MED. USES. In cases where an alkali is indicated, this preparation offers an agreeable and efficient remedy ; and experience has shewn that its additional propor

tion of carbonic acid, does not in the least invalidate
its alkaline agency. In disordered states of the
digestive functions, alkalies frequently act with surprising effect; in calculous affections their value has
been already noticed (see *Liquor Potassæ*), and the
stomach appears to bear the protracted exhibition of
the carbonate of potass, or soda, with more temper
than it does that of any other alkaline combination;
and, on account of the increased quantity of carbonic
acid which this salt contains, it is preferable for
effervescing draughts. (See *Acid: Citric:* and *Form:*
59, 75.) INCOMPATIBLE SUBSTANCES. *Acids* and
acidulous salts ; borax ; *muriate of ammonia; acetate
of ammonia ; alum ; sulphate of magnesia ; lime water;
nitrate of silver ; ammoniated copper ; muriate of iron ;
sub-muriate, and oxy-muriate of mercury ; super-
acetate of lead ; tartarized antimony ; tartarized iron ;
the sulphates of zinc, copper, iron, &c.* DOSE, grs.
x to ʒss.

POTASSÆ NITRAS. L.E.   NITRUM. D.
Nitre or *Salt Petre.*

QUALITIES. *Form,* crystals, which are six-sided
prisms, usually terminated by dihedral summits :
Taste, bitter and sharp, with a sensation of cold.
CHEMICAL COMPOSITION. It consists of one proportional of nitric acid, and one proportional of
potass. SOLUBILITY. It dissolves in seven parts of
water at 60°, and in its own weight at 212°. Its solubility is considerably increased by adding muriate of
soda to the water; its solution is attended with a
great reduction of temperature ; it is quite insoluble
in alcohol. INCOMPATIBLE SUBSTANCES. *Alum ;
sulphate of magnesia ; sulphuric acid, the sulphates*

of zinc, copper, and iron ; according to the usual laws
of affinity, it should be also decomposed by *sulphate
of soda*; this however only takes place at the temperature of 32°, and then but partially. Med. Uses
Refrigerant, in which case, the draught should be
swallowed immediately after the solution of the salt
is complete, for if it be allowed to stand for some
time, its effect with regard to cooling is not nearly so
evident (see *Form :* 84), as a diuretic, its powers are
too inconsiderable to be employed, except in combination (*Form :* 30, 37, 43) ; a solution of ʒj to fʒvj
of rose water forms a good detergent gargle, and a
small portion allowed to dissolve slowly in the mouth,
will frequently remove an incipient inflammation of
the tonsils : for it *modus operandi* as a diuretic, see
Potassæ Acetas. Dose, grs. x to xv, as a diuretic, or
refrigerant. Grs. xxv to xl are aperient, and in large
doses it excites vomiting, bloody stools, convulsions,
and even death. The best antidotes are opium and
aromatics Impurities As it occurs from the hand
of nature it is far from pure and even by art it is freed
with difficulty from sea salt ; the presence, and quantity of which, in any specimen, may be learnt by
adding nitrate of silver to its solution as long as any
precipitate is produced

POTASSÆ SUB-CARBONAS. L. F.
Sub-Carbonas Kali. E.
Kali Præparatum, P. L. 1787   *Sal Absinthii*
Sal Tartari. 1745.

Before the nature of this salt was well understood, it
received various appellations, according to the different
methods by which it was procured, and it was supposed
to possess as many different virtues, as *Salt of Wormwood, Salt of Tartar, &c.*

Qualities. *Form*, coarse white grains, so deliquescent, that by exposure to air, they form a dense solution, (*Oleum Tartari per deliquium*, P. L. 1720.) Chemical Composition. This salt, although far from being pure, is sufficiently so for every phar maceutical purpose. It consists of one proportional of acid, and one proportional of potass, with variable quantities of *sulphate of potass, muriate of potass, siliceous earth*, and *alumina.* Solubility. It is dissolved by twice its weight of water ; the residue, if any, may be considered as impurity ; it is insoluble in alcohol ; with oils it combines, and forms soaps. Incompatible Substances. They are enumerated under *Potassæ carbonas.* Medical Uses. Antacid, and diuretic, (*Form.* 29,) but it is far less pleasant than the carbonate ; it is principally used for making saline draughts, see *Acid. Citric.* and *Form.* 35. Dose, grs. x to ʒss. Officinal Prep. *Potassæ Acetas, (f)* L. E. D. *Liquor Potassæ,* (g) L. E. D. *Potassæ Sulphuretum, (f)* L. E. D. *Potassæ Tart. (f)* L. E. D. *Liquor Arsenicalis, (f.h).* Adulterations. Its degree of purity may be estimated by the quantity of nitric acid, of a given density, requisite for the saturation of a given weight. The purest *sub-carbonate* is that obtained by incinerating *cream of tartar*, since most of the impurities are decomposed by the heat during the process. *Sub-carbonas Potassæ Purissimus.* E.

POTASSÆ SULPHAS. L. E. Sulphas Kali. D.
Kali Vitriolatum, P. L. 1787.
Tartarum Vitriolatum, 1745, and 1720.
Sal de duobus, &c.

Qualities. *Form*, crystals which are short, six-sided prisms, terminated by six-sided pyramids ; some-

times the body of the prism is wanting, when a dode-
cahedron results; they are slightly efflorescent, and
when heated, they decrepitate. SOLUBILITY. f3j
of water dissolves only grs. 24 : the salt is insoluble
in alcohol. INCOMPATIBLE SUBSTANCES. It is
partially decomposed by the nitric and muriatic acids,
in which case, a portion of the base being saturated,
a corresponding portion of *bi-sulphate* results; this
fact illustrates a chemical law of some importance,
viz. *that a substance less weakly attracted by another
than a third, will sometimes precipitate this third from
its combination with the second, in cases wherein a* super,
or sub-*salt is readily formed*. The history of tartrate
of potass will furnish farther illustrations. Sulphate
of potass, when in solution, is entirely decomposed
by *lime* and *its compounds;* by *oxymuriate of mercury ;
nitrate of silver ;* and by *sub-acetate* and *super-acetate
of lead.* MEDICAL USES On account of its insolubility, it does not possess much activity as a purgative, but is said to be powerfully deobstruent ; it
should be exhibited in the form of powder, and in
conjunction with rhubarb, or some other purgative
medicine. DOSE, grs. x to 3ss. From its hardnes
and insolubility, it is a most eligible substance for
triturating and dividing powders. OFFICINAL PREP
Pulvis. Ipecac. co. L. E. D. Under the name *Sulphas
Potassæ cum Sulphure*, the Edinburgh college retains
the preparation formerly known by the name of *Sal
Polychrest;* and as it is produced by deflagrating
nitre with sulphur, the product, besides sulphate of
potass, contains *bi-sulphate* and *sulphuret of potass*
It possesses no superiority over the common sulphate

POTASSÆ SUPER-SULPHAS. L.

Sal Enixum of Commerce

QUALITIES. *Crystals*, long hexangular prisms; *Taste*, sour, and slightly bitter. CHEMICAL COMPOSITION. It is a bi-sulphate, consisting of two proportionals of acid, and one proportional of base. SOLUBILITY. It is soluble in twice its weight of water, as well as in alcohol. MEDICAL USES. It affords a convenient mode of exhibiting sulphuric acid, combined with a saline purgative, in a solid form; as it is more soluble, so it is more active than the sulphate. DOSE, grs. x to ʒij. It forms a grateful adjunct to rhubarb. See *Form. 22.*

POTASSÆ SULPHURETUM. L. E.

SULPHURETUM KALI. D.

Kali Sulphuratum, P. L. 1787. *Hepar Sulphuris*

QUALITIES. *Form*, a hard brittle mass; *Colour*, liver brown, hence the old name of *hepar; Taste,* acrid and bitter; *Odour*, none, when dry, but if moistened, it yields the stench of sulphuretted hydrogen. CHEMICAL COMPOSITION. It is not a perfect chemical sulphuret, as the alkali employed for its preparation is in the state of *sub-carbonate;* it consists of sulphur, potass, and a proportion of carbonic acid. SOLUBILITY. Although soluble in water, it is changed during its solution, the greatest portion being converted into an *hydroguretted sulphuret*, and a part into *sulphate of potass.* INCOMPATIBLE SUBSTANCES. *Acids; acidulous salts; earthy and metallic salts.* MED. USES. It presents us with a form in which sulphur is soluble in water; it is diaphoretic, and has been found advantageous in cutaneous affections, (*Form* 54,) and in arthritic and rheumatic complaints; from its known chemical action on metallic salts, it has been proposed as an antidote to such poisons.

POTASSÆ SUPER-TARTRAS. L. E.

TARTARUM, CRYSTALLI. E.

Super-Tartrate of Potass, Crystals of Tartar.

QUALITIES. *Form,* small irregular crystals, brittle, and which when reduced to powder are termed *cream of tartar; Taste,* harsh and acid. CHEMICAL COMPOSITION. It is a *bi-tartrate* consisting of two proportionals of acid, and one proportional of potass. SOLUBILITY. It requires 120 parts of water at 60°, and 30 parts at 212°, for its solution; it is slightly soluble in alcohol. The watery solution of this salt was first observed by Berthollet to undergo a spontaneous decomposition, by keeping, during which a mucous matter is deposited, and there remains a solution of carbonate of potass coloured with a little oil. It has long been regarded a pharmaceutical desideratum, to encrease the solubility of *cream of tartar;* Vogel discovered that it might be accomplished by combining it with boracic acid, and, accordingly, a formula has been introduced into the Codex Medicamentarius of Paris, for preparing a " *Tartras Acidulus Potassæ Solubilis, admixto Acido Boracico.*" The following is the process. Let thirty parts of boracic acid, and twenty parts of distilled water be heated together in a silver dish; as soon as this has been effected, add, in divided portions, 120 parts of super-tartrate of potass, taking care to shake the mixture continually; the whole will soon liquefy ("*mire liquescent*,") and by continuing the heat, a pulverulent mass will result. As it is extremely deliquescent it must be carefully preserved from the contact of the air; it dissolves in its own weight of water at 55°, and in half its weight at 212. It is probable, that the result is a new salt, in which the boracic and tartaric acids are in combination, but grant even, that the chemical identity of the super-tartrate is preserved inviolate in the compound, I would ask, what medical advantage can possibly attend the discovery? the peculiar value of cream of tartar depends, doubtless, upon its comparative inso-lubility, as I have already stated in the *Introductory Essay*, p. 21, and farther, under the head of *Potassæ Acetas;* modify this, and you will instantly change the medicinal effects of the salt; for, like the neutral tartrate, it will act upon the bowels, and therefore cease to undergo those changes, *in transitu*, which are essential to its characteristic operation. Alum also has been observed by Berthollet to have, in some measure, the same effect in increasing the solubility of cream of tartar. INCOMPATIBLE SUBSTANCES. *Alkalies* and *alkaline earths;* the *mineral acids*, &c. MEDICAL USES. In doses of ʒiv to ʒvj, it acts as a hydragogue cathartic, occasioning a considerable dis-charge of serous fluid into the intestines; when however it is often repeated, it is liable to occasion debility of the digestive organs, and consequent ema-ciation : in smaller doses it acts as a diuretic, (*Form.* 40,) ʒj in oj of boiling water, flavoured with lemon peel and sugar, forms, when cold, an agreeable cooling beverage, well known by the name of *Imperial.* As it decomposes the carbonate of potass, the union of these two salts will afford a very pleasant purgative draught. (*Form.* 19.) OFFICINAL PREP. *Pulv.*

Jalap. comp. (a, i,) E. *Pulv. Scammon.* E. *Pulv. Sennæ comp.* L. *Ferrum Tartarizatum, (f)* L. *Antimonium Tartarizatum, (f)* L.E.D. *Soda Tartarizata, (f)* L. E. D. ADULTERATIONS. Super-sulphate of potass, *Sal Enixum,* is the substance with which tartar is usually adulterated; it may be detected by its superior solubility, and by the solution affording, with muriate of baryta, a precipitate insoluble in muriatic acid.

POTASSÆ TARTRAS. L.   TARTRAS POTASSÆ.
Olim Tartarum Solubile. E.   TARTRAS KALI. D.

Kali Tartarizatum, P. L. 1787.

Tartarum Solubile, P. L. 1745.

QUALITIES. *Form* This salt, although ordered to be crystallized, is generally kept in its granular form. *Taste,* bitter and cool. CHEMICAL COMPOSITION. It consists of one proportional of acid, and one proportional of base. SOLUBILITY. When in its crystalline form, it is soluble in its own weight of water, but in its ordinary granular form, 4 parts are required for its solution; hence, compared with the insoluble super-tartrate, it has justly acquired the name of *soluble* tartar; when long kept in solution, its acid is decomposed, and its alkali remains in the state of a *sub-carbonate.* It is also readily soluble in alcohol. INCOMPATIBLE SUBSTANCES. *Magnesia; baryta,* and *lime; sub-acetate* and *super-acetate of lead,* and *nitrate of silver* decompose it. All acids, and *acidulous*

---

* ESSENTIAL SALT OF LEMONS. The preparation sold under this name, for the purpose of removing iron moulds from linen, consists of cream of tartar, and super-oxalate of potass, or *salt of sorrel,* in equal proportions.

salts, tamarinds, and other *sub-acid vegetables,* by neutralizing a proportion of the base, convert it into the state of super-tartrate; this fact offers another illustration of the chemical law of affinity, explained under the head of *super-sulphate of potass.* The practitioner should bear this in his recollection, for I have frequently seen a dose of *soluble tartar* directed in the acidulated *infusion of roses;* the result was of course very different from that which the author of the prescription intended to produce. Medical Uses. It is a mild and efficient purgative, and forms a very valuable adjunct to resinous purgatives, or to senna, the griping properties of which it corrects, by accelerating their operation. Dose, ʒj to ℥j, in solution.

PULVERES. *Powders.*

The form of powder is, in many cases, the most efficient and eligible mode in which a medicinal substance can be exhibited, more especially under the following circumstances.

1. *Simple Powders.*

1. Whenever a remedy requires the combination of all, or most of its principles, to ensure its full effects, as *Bark, Ipecacuan, Jalap, &c.*

2. Where medicinal bodies are insoluble, and indisposed to undergo those essential changes, *in transitu,* which render them operative; for it must be remembered, that by minute division, every particle is presented to the stomach, in a state of activity, being more immediately exposed to the solvent, or decomposing, powers of that organ.

z

3. Where the mechanical condition of the substance is such, as to occasion irritation to the stomach, as the *Sulphuretum Antimonii,* or in external applications, to produce an improper effect upon the skin, as *Hydrargyri nitrico-oxydum.*

The degree of fineness to which substances should be reduced by pulverization, in order to obtain their utmost efficacy, is an important question. The impalpable form appears to be extremely injurious to some bodies, as *cinchona, rhubarb, guaiacum,* and certain aromatics, in consequence of an essential part of their substance being dissipated, or chemically changed by the operation; Fabbroni, for instance, found by experiment that cinchona yielded a much larger proportion of soluble extractive, when only coarsely powdered. I think it may be laid down as a general rule, that *extreme pulverization assists the operation of all substances, whose active principles are not easily soluble, and, that of compound powders, whose ingredients require, for their activity, an intimate intermixture; whilst, it certainly injures, if not destroys, the virtues of those which contain, as their active constituents, a volatile principle, easily dissipated, or extractive matter, which is readily oxidized.*

2. *Compound Powders.*

The disintegration of a substance is much accelerated and extended by the addition of other materials, hence the pharmaceutical aphorism of Gaubius; "*Celerior atque facilior succedat composita, quam simplex pulverisatio.*" Thus, several refractory vegetable bodies, as *myrrh, gamboge, &c.* are easily reduced by triturating them with sugar, or a hard gum; and some gum resins, as *assafœtida,* or *scammony,* by the addition of a few drops of almond oil : upon the same

principle the Pharmacopœia directs the trituration of
aloes with clean white sand, in the process for preparing *Vinum Aloes*, to facilitate pulverization, and
to prevent the particles of aloes, when moistened by
the liquid, from running together into masses; some
dispensers very judiciously adopt the same mechanical
expedient in making a tincture of myrrh; so again,
in ordering a watery infusion of opium, it will be
judicious to advise the previous trituration of the
opium with some hard, and insoluble substance, as
directed in the *Pulvis Cornu Usti cum Opio*, otherwise its particles will adhere with tenacity, and the
water, accordingly, be unable to exert a solvent operation upon its substance. It is equally evident that
in the construction of compound medicinal powders,
the addition of an inert ingredient, which the mere
chemist might condemn and discard, as useless, not
unfrequently acts a very important part in the combination, owing to its effects in dividing and commi-
nuting the more active constituents: the *sulphate of
potass*, in Dover's powder, acts merely in dividing,
and mixing more intimately the particles of opium
and ipecacuan : the *phosphate of lime* appears to act
in the same mechanical manner, in the Antimonial
Powder ; so again, in the *Pulvis Contrajervæ compositus*, the prepared oyster shells may be a necessary
ingredient : in the *Pulvis Jalapæ compositus*, of the
Edinburgh college, the cream of tartar greatly increases the activity of the jalap, by breaking down its
substance, and dividing its particles. The old combination of *Pulvis Helvetii*, consisted of alum, and
dragon's blood, and there can be no doubt, but that
the effect of this latter ingredient, which has been
often ridiculed, was to retard the solution of alum in
the stomach, in consequence of which, the preparation

was likely to produce less inconvenience, and could
therefore be administered in larger doses; the
Edinburgh college has substituted, in the *Pulvis
Aluminis compositus*, gum Kino, which may have the
same effect in modifying the solubility of the alum.

In rubbing together different substances, it is necessary to remember, that there are many saline bodies,
which in the dry state, become moist, and even liquid,
by triture with each other, and that they are consequently susceptible of mutual decomposition. This
change is effected by the action of water, derived
from the following sources.

1. *From the water of crystallization.* This always
operates when the proportion contained in the original
ingredients is greater than that which the products
can dispose of, that is to say, whenever the capacity
of the new compound for water is less than that of
the original ingredients. By previously driving off
this water by heat, we shall of course avoid such a
source of solution, and no liquefaction can ensue.
Thus, if recently burnt quicklime be triturated with
calomel, the resulting mixture will be white, shewing
that no decomposition can have arisen, but add a few
drops of water, and it instantly assumes a dark aspect
If *crystallized* sulphate of copper be triturated with
super-acetate of lead, the resulting mixture will
assume a fine green colour, but if the sulphate of
copper be previously heated, and its water of crystallization driven off, no change of colour will be produced: if for super-acetate of lead, we substitute
muriate of lime, and the sulphate of copper be *crystallized*, we shall obtain a result of a yellow colour,
but if the sulphate of copper, be *anhydrous*, the
product will be colourless, becoming, however, instantly yellow, like the former, on the addition of a

drop of water; and, on a farther addition of this
fluid, the yellow product, in both instances, will be
rendered blue, which proves that a chemical decomposition has taken place, and that a muriate of copper
has resulted, for this salt is rendered *yellow* by a
small, and *blue* by a larger proportion of water. The
Cuprum Ammoniatum presents another illustration,
for the ingredients, when rubbed together, become
extremely moist, and undergo a chemical decomposition. Certain resinous bodies also, as *myrrh*,
become liquid by triture with alkaline salts, in which
case the resin and alkali form a soluble compound,
which the water of crystallization, thus set at liberty,
instantly dissolves.

2. *From aqueous vapour in the atmosphere.* The
water of the atmosphere does not act upon these
occasions, unless it be first attracted and absorbed by
one of the triturated bodies, e. g. if super-acetate of
lead, and recently burnt alum, be triturated together,
no change will be produced; but, if the burnt alum
be previously exposed for a short time to the atmosphere, these bodies will in that case become liquid.

The physician, without this chemical knowledge,
will be often betrayed into the most ridiculous blun-
ders; an instance of which very lately came to my
knowledge, in a prescription, for the relief of cardialgia
and constipation, in a case of dyspepsia; it directed
sulphate of soda and *carbonate of potass*, in the form of
a powder; but the *fiat* of the physician, upon this
occasion, only served to excite the ridicule of the
dispenser, who soon discovered that the ingredients
in his mortar dissolved into a liquid.

During the exhibition of powders, containing insoluble matter, it is always important to maintain a
regularity in the alvine excretions, or an accumulation

may take place, attended with very distressing symptoms. Dr. Fothergill relates a case of this kind which succeeded the use of powdered bark ; and Mr. Brande has communicated a similar instance of mechanical obstruction, produced by the habitual use of magnesia. I could also add, if it were necessary, some striking facts, of a similar tendency, which occurred from eating bread, that had been adulterated with pulverized *felspar*. This precaution seems more particularly necessary in the case of children, whose bowels are very impatient of extraneous and insoluble contents.* The dose of a powder ought not to exceed ʒj; and, when taken, should be diffused in water, wine, or any other convenient vehicle; resinous and metallic powders require a thick and consistent one, as syrup, since they subside from those which are more fluid.

Powders should be preserved in opaque, or green bottles, as they are materially affected by the action of light and air. Many of the compound ones should be considered as extemporaneous, and ought to be prepared only when they are required.

The practitioner is particularly cautioned against purchasing any medicine, in its powdered form, for so universal is the system of adulteration, that regular formulæ are observed for sophisticating powders, and

---

* It is perhaps not generally known, that the *sugared plumbs*, sold to children, consist very frequently of *Paister of Paris;* the introduction of such a substance into the intestines, may often prove a source of mischief. I also understand, that it is no uncommon fraud to adulterate biscuits with the same substance. I confess I felt a great inclination to oppose the practice, lately suggested, of improving bad flour by the addition of *Magnesia*; I object to the introduction of any foreign, and insoluble substance, into our daily bread, and I am satisfied, that the result of medical experience will sanction such an objection.

Mr. Gray, in his " *Supplement to the Pharmacopœias*,"
has given us several specimens, under the title of
Pulveres reducti, p. 320.

PULVIS ALOES COMPOSITUS. L. Pulvis Aloes
cum Guaiaco. D. It consists of Aloes *3 parts*,
Guaiacum 2 *(d.)*, and compound powder of cinnamon
1 *part (k)*. It combines sudorific and purgative
effects. *Dose*, grs. x to ℈j. See *Form.* 17.

PULVIS ALOES CUM CANELLA. D. and P. L.
1807. Aloes 4 *parts*, white canella *(c)* 1 *part*. It is
known in the shops by the name of *Hiera Picra*.
The compound is more adapted to the form of pills
than that of powder. It is very generally used by
the lower classes, infused in gin. *Dose*, grs. x to ℈j.

PULVIS ANTIMONIALIS. L.D. Oxidum Antimonii cum Phosphate Calcis. E. This preparation
was introduced into the Pharmacopœia, as the succedaneum of the celebrated *fever powder of Dr. James*,*
the composition of which was ascertained by Dr.
George Pearson. *(Phil. Trans.* lxxxi. 317.) It
consists of 43 parts of the phosphate of lime, mixed,
or perhaps chemically combined, with 57 parts of oxide
of antimony, of which a portion is vitrified ; and it is
probable, that the difference of the two remedies
depends, principally, upon the quantity of oxide
which is vitrified : the specification of the original
medicine is worded with all the ambiguity of an
ancient oracle, and cannot be prepared by the process
as it is described. Experience has established the
fact, that *James's powder* is less active than its imitation; it affects the bowels and stomach very slightly,

* JAMES'S ANALEPTIC PILLS.—These consist of James's Powder,
gum ammoniacum, and the pill of Aloes with Myrrh, *(Pil. Rufi)* equal
parts, with a sufficient quantity of the tincture of Castor, to make a
mass.

and passes off more readily by perspiration ; in general however the difference is so inconsiderable, that we need not regret the want of the original receipt. As it is quite insoluble in water, it should be given in powder, or made into pills. It is diaphoretic, alterative, emetic, or purgative, according to the extent of the dose, and the state of the patient ; in combination it offers several valuable resources to the intelligent practitioner. (See *Form.* 17. 48, 55, 57, 61.)

PULVIS CINNAMOMI COMPOSITUS. L. Cinnamon bark *four*, Cardamom seeds (*a*) *three*, ginger root (*a*) *two*, long pepper (*e*) *one part*. It is principally used to give warmth to other preparations, e. g. *Pulv. Aloes comp.* L.D.

PULVIS CONTRAYERVÆ COMPOSITUS. L. Contrayerva *five*, prepared shells, *eighteen parts*. Dose, grs. x to xl. It is said to be stimulant and diaphoretic.

PULVIS CORNU USTI CUM OPIO. L. Opium *one part*, burnt hartshorn *eight*, powdered cochineal *one part*. Ten grains contain one of opium.

PULVIS CRETÆ COMPOSITUS. Prepared chalk *twelve parts*, tormentil root (*d*), acacia gum (*i*), of each, *six*, cinnamon bark *eight* (*d*), long pepper (*d*) *one part*. It is antacid, astringent, and carminative. *Dose*, grs. v to ℈j.

PULVIS CRETÆ COMPOSITUS CUM OPIO. L. Compound powder of chalk *thirty-nine parts*, Opium *one part*.

PULVIS IPECACUANHÆ COMPOSITUS. L. E. D. Ipecacuan *one part*, Opium (*e.*) *one part*, sulphate of potass (*k.i.*) *eight parts.* This combination has been long established in practice, as a valuable sudorific, under the name of *Dover's Powder*. It affords one of the best examples of the power which one medicine possesses of so changing the action of another, as to produce a remedy of new properties ; in this combination, the opium is so modified, that it may be given with perfect safety ànd advantage, in inflammatory affections, accompanied with increased vascular action : it would seem, that whilst the Opium increases the force of the circulation, the Ipecacuan relaxes the exhalent vessels, and causes a copious diaphorhesis : the sulphate of potass is also an important ingredient, for experience has fully proved, that ipecacuan and opium, in the same proportions, have not so powerful an effect without it ; its action must be purely mechanical, dividing and mixing the active particles more intimately, and it appears that the success of the remedy depends very much upon its being finely powdered. *Dose,* grs. v to ℈j, diffused in gruel, or in the form of a bolus. (See *Formulæ* 56, 57, 58.) The saline constituent in the original *Dover's Powder,* was the result of the deflagration of nitre, and was therefore deliquescent ; its dose was as much as from 40 to 70 grains. In the *Codex* of Paris, this compound is directed to be prepared by melting together *four parts* of sulphate of potass, with an equal proportion of nitrate of potass ; to which, when nearly cold, is to be added, and well mixed by triture, *one part* of pulverized extract of opium ; the powders of ipecacuan and liquorice root, of each *one part,* are to be added last. It is evident that the proportions of opium and ipecacuan in this combination, are less than those in ours, and yet it is said to be more powerfully diaphoretic, on account of the nitre. An arrangement, which is indebted for its medicinal virtue to a similar mode of operation, is presented in *Formula* 66.

Pulvis Scammoniæ Compositus. L. Scammony, and hard extract of jalap, of each *four parts*, ginger root, (*c.*) *one part*. The Edinburgh preparation, of the same name, differs very materially in composition, its ingredients being scammony and cream of tartar, in *equal parts*.

Pulvis Tragacanthæ Compositus. L. Powdered Tragacanth, acacia gum, and starch, of each *one part;* refined sugar, *two parts*. From what has been already stated under the head of mucilage of tragacanth, it appears to be a superfluous, if not an injudicious demulcent; and since starch is insoluble in cold water, the object for introducing it is not very obvious.

QUASSIA, L.E.D. (Quassia Excelsa.)   *Quassia.*
                  (*Lignum.*   )

This wood owes all its properties to a peculiar bitter principle, which has been examined by Thomson, and named *Quassin;* it is solid, slightly transparent, and of a yellowish-brown colour. (See *Infusum Quassiæ.*)

RHEI RADIX. L.E.D. *Rhubarb.*

Two varieties of this root are known in the shops, viz. *Turkey,* or *Russian,* and *East Indian,* or *Chinese.*

1. Turkey, or Russian. (*Rheum Palmatum.*)

Qualities. *Form,* small round pieces, rather compact, and heavy, perforated in the middle; *Colour,* lively yellow, with streaks of white; it is easily pulverized, affording a powder of a bright buff - yellow colour. CHEMICAL COMPOSITION. Gum, resin, extractive, tannin, gallic acid, and a peculiar colouring matter, with traces of alumen and silex ; the white, or flesh-coloured streaks, pervading its substance, consist of sulphate and oxalate of lime : according to the experiments of Mr. John Henderson, there is, besides, a peculiar vegetable acid, to which he has given the name of *Rheumic* acid, but M. De Lassaignes has satisfactorily proved that this is no other than the oxalic acid : the purgative powers of the root appear to be intimately connected with its extractive and resinous elements, but the subject is still involved in considerable obscurity. SOLUBILITY. Water at 212° takes up 24 parts in 60, see *Infusum Rhei :* by decoction, its purgative qualities are lost, and it becomes more bitter and astringent ; alcohol extracts 2·7 from 10 parts, (see *Tinct. Rhei.*) MED. USES. In this substance, Nature presents us with a singular, and most important combination of medicinal powers, that of an astringent, with a cathartic property, the former of which never opposes, or interferes with, the energy of the latter, since it only takes effect when the substance is administered in small doses, or, if given in larger ones, not until it has ceased to operate as a cathartic ; this latter circumstance renders it particularly eligible in cases of diarrhœa, as it evacuates the offending matter, before it operates as an astringent upon the bowels. It seems to act more immediately upon the stomach and small intestines, and therefore in relaxed and debiliated states of these organs, it will prove an easy and valuable resource ; it may, for such an object, be exhibited in conjunction with alkalies, bitters, and other tonics. *(Form. 93.)* Its cathartic property is most efficient when given in substance. It was formerly supposed, that by toasting rhubarb, we increased its astringency, but this process merely diminishes its purgative force, so that a larger dose may be taken. The colouring matter of rhubarb may be detected in the urine of persons to whom it has been exhibited; it does not however appear to possess any specific powers as a diuretic. Dose, grs. vj to x as a tonic; ℈j to ʒss as a purgative, the operation of which is considerably quickened by the addition of neutral salts; the super-sulphate of potass forms also a very useful adjunct, and its acidulous taste completely covers that of the rhubarb. Its powder, when sprinkled upon ulcers, is found to promote their healthy granulation. OFFICINAL PREP. *Infus: Rhei.* L.E. *Vinum Rhei Palmati.* E. *Tinct: Rhei.* L.E.D. *Tinct: Rhei comp:* L. *Tinct: Rhei cum Alöe.* E. *Tinct: Rhei cum Gentian:* E. *Pil: Rhei comp:* E.

2. EAST INDIAN, or CHINESE. (*Rheum* * *Undulatum ?*)

QUALITIES. *Form,* long pieces, sometimes flat, as if they had been compressed; they are heavier, harder, and more compact than those of the preceding species, and are seldom perforated with holes; *Odour,* stronger; *Taste,* more nauseous; white streaks less numerous, and it affords a powder of a redder shade than *Turkey* rhubarb. CHEMICAL COMPOSITION. It differs from the *Turkey* in containing less tannin and resin, and according to the experiments of Mr.

* Dr. Rehman asserts that it is the root of the same species as that which produces the Turkey variety, but that it is prepared with less care.

A. T. Thomson, less oxalate of lime, in the ratio of 18 to 26. It contains, however, more extractive and gallic acid. SOLUBILITY. Water takes up one half of its weight, but the infusion, although more turbid, is not so deep coloured as that of Russian hubarb; alcohol extracts 4 parts in 10. Its habitudes with acids, alkalies, and neutral salts, differ likewise from those of the Russian variety, as Mr. A. T. Thomson has exhibited in a very satisfactory manner. (*London Dispensatory*, *Edit.* 2, *p.* 339.) ADULTERATIONS. The inferior kinds of *Russian, East Indian,* and even *English* rhubarb, are artfully dressed up, and sold under the name of Turkey rhubarb. I am well informed that a number of persons in this town, known in the trade by the name of *Russifiers*, gain a regular livelihood by the art of dressing this article, by boring, rasping, and then colouring the inferior kinds; for which they charge at the rate of eighteen-pence per pound. The general indications of good rhubarb are, its whitish or clear yellow colour, and its possessing the other characteristic properties as above mentioned; it ought also to possess in an eminent degree the peculiar odour, for when this is dissipated, the powers of the medicine are nearly destroyed. In the form of powder, rhubarb is always, more or less, mixed with foreign matter; the detection of which can be alone effected by a trial of its efficacy

RICINI OLEUM. L.E.D. (*Ricinus Communis.*)
Castor Oil.

QUALITIES. *Form,* a viscid and colourless, or pale straw-coloured oil; it is nearly inodorous, but excites, on being swallowed, a slight sensation of

acrimony in the throat. It has all the chemical habitudes of the other expressed oils, except those which
relate to its solubility in alcoholic and ethereal menstrua. MED. USES. It is mildly cathartic, and is
particularly eligible in cases where stimulating purgatives would prove hurtful. FORMS OF EXHIBI-
TION. The most efficacious mode of administering it
is by floating it upon tincture of senna, or peppermint
water, or some other similar vehicle; it is also sometimes given, with success, in coffee, or mutton broth,
or suspended in water, by the intervention of mucilage, yolk of egg, (*Form*. 13), or by honey, which
at the same time contributes to its laxative operation;
alkalies, although they form an emulsion with it,
convert it into a saponaceous compound, and impair
its cathartic force. DOSE, f$\mathfrak{z}$ss to f$\mathfrak{z}$iss. ADULTE-
RATIONS. It is usually adulterated with olive oil,
or poppy oil, and, when to a considerable extent,
scammony is added to quicken its operation. There
is, however, a peculiarity in castor oil, which serves
to distinguish it from every other fixed oil, viz. its
great solubility in highly rectified spirit; for instance,
f$\mathfrak{z}$iv of alcohol of 820 will mix uniformly with any
proportion of castor oil, whereas it will not dissolve
more than f$\mathfrak{z}$j of *Linseed Oil;* when the spirit is
diluted, its action on both these oils, is equally diminished, so that common *spirit of wine* has but little
power even over castor oil; but here chemistry again
interposes its aid, for by the addition of camphor,
spirit of 840 is enabled to dissolve castor oil, whilst
it has no influence upon the other fixed oils; castor
oil is also very soluble in sulphuric æther.

SACCHARUM. L.E.D. *Sugar.*

Sugar, as a pharmaceutical agent, is employed for accelerating the pulverization of various resinous substances, and when exhibited with the most acrid of them, it prevents their adhesion to the coats of the intestines, by which they might irritate and inflame them; it is also extensively used on account of its power in preserving animal and vegetable substances. (See *Conservæ.*) Milk, boiled with fine sugar, will keep for a great length of time, and might be very conveniently employed during a long voyage. Dr. Darwin also observes, that fresh meat cut into thin slices, either raw or boiled, might be preserved in coarse sugar or treacle, and would furnish a very salutary and nourishing diet to our sailors. Sugar exerts also some chemical affinities, which are highly interesting to the pharmaceutic chemist. Vogel has published a paper to shew, that when sugar is boiled with various metallic oxides, and with different metalline salts, it has the property of decomposing them ; sometimes reducing the oxide to the state of metal, and at others, depriving the oxide only of one of the proportionals of oxygen, thus, *sulphate of copper,* and *nitrate of mercury,* are precipitated in a metallic form, whilst *peroxide of mercury,* and *acetate of copper,* are converted into protoxides ; *corrosive* sublimate is changed into *calomel,* but *calomel* is not susceptible of any further decomposition. All those metallic salts, which have the power of decomposing water, are not affected by sugar, as those of *iron, zinc, tin,* and *manganese.*

SAPO. L.E.D. *Soap.*

1. Durus. *(Hispanicus.)* *Hard,* or *Spanish Soap*

Chemical Composition. Oil 60·94, soda 8·56, water 30·50, the water is partially dissipated by being kept, and the soap therefore becomes lighter. Solubility. Water dissolves about one-third of its weight of genuine soap, and forms a milky solution; alcohol also dissolves it, and affords a solution nearly transparent, although somewhat gelatinous.* Incompatible Substances. 1. All acids and acidulous salts; which combine with the alkali, and develope the oil. 2. Earthy salts, e. g. *Alum ; muriate,* and *sulphate of lime ; sulphate of magnesia.* 3. Metallic salts. *Nitrate of silver; ammoniated copper; tincture of muriated iron ; ammoniated iron acetite, sub-muriate,* and *oxy-muriate of mercury ; super-acetate of lead ; tartarized iron ; tartarized antimony* ; *sulphates of zinc, copper, and iron.* 4. All astringent vegetables. 5. Hard water. Medical Uses. In large doses it is purgative, in smaller ones, it is decomposed *in transitu,* and its alkali is carried to the kidnies; in this way it may act as a lithontriptic; or it may produce its effects by correcting any acidity which may prevail in the *primæ viæ,* for the weakest acid is capable of decomposing soap, and of uniting with its alkaline base; a solution of soap in lime water was long regarded as one of the strongest solvents of urinary calculi, that could be administered with safety, but the result of such a mixture is an insoluble soap of lime, and a solution of soda; in habitual constipation, and in biliary obstructions, it

* Transparent Soap is made by carefully evaporating the alcoholic solution.

is frequently prescribed in conjunction with rhubarb, or some, bitter; in which cases it can only act as a laxative, or as a chemical agent, in increasing the solubility of the substance with which it is united It has been also given in solution as an antidote to metallic poisons ; as an external application, it is used in the form of liniment, (see *Linimenta.*) Or-FICINAL PREP. *Pil : Saponis cum Opio. (h.)* L. *Pil: Scillæ comp: (i.)* L. *Pil: Aloet: (h.)* E. *Pil: Aloes et Assafœtia. (h.)* E. *Pil: Aloes cum Zinzib: (h.)* D. *Pil: Colocynth: comp: (h.)* D. *Emplast: Saponis.* L. E. *Ceratum .Saponis.* L. *Liniment: Saponis comp:* L. *Liniment: Saponis cum Opio.* L.

II. SAPO MOLLIS. *Soft Soap.*

This differs from *hard soap*, chiefly in its consist-ence, which is never greater than that of hog's lard ; it is transparent, yellowish, with small seed-like lumps of tallow diffused through it: the alkali employed for its formation is a ley of potass, instead of that of soda.

SARSAPARILLA. L. E. D. (Smilax Sarsaparilla.)
                                   (*Radix.*   )
Sarsaparilla.

QUALITIES. *Form,* long and slender twigs, cover-ed with a wrinkled brown bark ; *Odour,* none ; *Taste,* mucilaginous, and slightly bitter. CHEMICAL COMPOSITION. Its virtues appear to reside in fecula. SOLUBILITY. It communicates its active principle, most completely, to boiling water. (See *Decoct: Sarsaparillæ.)* MED. USES. According to Mo-nardes, it was imported by the Spaniards into Europe in 1549, as a specific remedy for the venereal disease; but it soon fell into disrepute, and so it continued until about the middle of the last century, when it was again brought into esteem by Hunter and Fordyce, as a medicine calculated to assist the operation of mercury, as well as to cure those symptoms, which may be called the *sequelæ* of a mercurial course. DOSE, of the powdered root, ℈j to ʒj, three times a day. In selecting the roots, it will be right to choose such as are plump, not carious, nor too dusty on breaking; but rough, and which easily split longitudinally. OFFICINAL PREP. *Decoctum Sarsaparillæ.* L.E D. *Decoct: Sarsaparillæ comp:* L.D. *Extractum Sarsaparillæ.* L.

SASSAFRAS. L.E.D. (Laurus Sassafras.)
(*Lignum, Radix et Cortex.*)
The Wood, Root, and Bark of Sassafras.

QUALITIES. *Odour,* fragrant; *Taste,* sweet and aromatic. CHEMICAL COMPOSITION. The qualities of this plant depend upon an essential oil and resin. SOLUBILITY. Its active parts are soluble in water and alcohol. MED. USES. It is said to be diaphoretic, and diuretic; and has been employed in cases of scurvy, rheumatism, and in various cutaneous affections; it also formerly enjoyed the reputation of being an antisyphilitic remedy. Its powers are very questionable. OFFICINAL PREP. *Oleum Sassafras.* L.E.D. *Decoct: Sarsaparillæ comp:* L.D. *Decoct: Guaiac:* L.E.D. *Aqua Calcis comp:* D.*

---

* GODFREY'S CORDIAL.—The following receipt for this nostrum was obtained from a wholesale druggist, who makes and sells many hundred dozen bottles, in the course of the year. „There are however several other formulæ for its preparation, but they are not essentially different.

SCAMMONIA. L.E.D. ⎧Convolvulus Scammonia⎫
                  ⎩   Gummi-resina.   ⎭
SCAMMONIUM. D. *Scammony.*

QUALITIES. *Form,* blackish-grey cakes; *Taste,*
bitter and subacrid: *Odour,* heavy, and peculiar;
when rubbed with water, the surface lathers, or *lacti-
fies. Specific gravity* 1·235. CHEMICAL COMPOSI-
TION. Resin is the principal constituent; 16 parts of
good *Aleppo* Scammony yield 11 parts of resin, and
$3\frac{1}{2}$ of watery extract. That from *Smyrna* contains
not more than half the quantity of resin, but more
extractive, and gum. SOLUBILITY. Water, by trituration, takes up one-fourth; alcohol two-thirds, and
proof spirit dissolves all, except the impurities. IN-
COMPATIBLE SUBSTANCES. Neither acids, metallic
salts, nor ammonia, produce any change in its solutions, but the fixed alkalies occasion yellow precipitates; and yet they do not appear to be *medicinally*
incompatible with it; thus Gaubius, " *Scammoneum
acidi commixtio reddit inertius; alcali fixum, contra,
adjuvat.*" The mineral acids appear to destroy a part
of the substance, without in the least altering the rest.
The discrepancy which exists in authors, respecting
the power of this drug, seems to have arisen from its
operation being liable to uncertainty, in consequence
of peculiar states of the alimentary canal; for instance,
where the intestines are lined with an excess of
mucus, it passes through without producing any
action, but where the natural mucus is deficient, a
small dose of scammony may irritate, and even inflame

Infuse ℥ix of Sassafras, and of the seeds of Carraway, Coriander, and
Anise, of each ℥j, in six pints of water, simmer the mixture, until it is
reduced to four pints; then add lbvj of Treacle, and boil the whole for
a few minutes; when it is cold, add f℥iij of the tincture of Opium.

the bowels. MED. USES. It is an efficacious and powerful cathartic, very eligible in worm cases, and in the disordered state of bowels, which so commonly occurs in children. DOSE, grs. iij to xv, in the form of powders triturated with sulphate of potass, sugar, or almonds; when given alone, it is apt to irritate the fauces; it may be also administered in a solution, effected by triturating it in a strong decoction of liquorice, and straining. (*Form.* 16, 20) OFFICI-NAL PREP. *Confect: Scommon:* L.D. *Pulv: Scammon: co.* L.E. *Extract: Colocynth: co.* L. *Pulv: Sennæ co.* L. ADULTERATIONS. Two kinds of Scammony are imported into this country, that from *Aleppo,* which is the best; and that from *Smyrna,* which is more compact and ponderous, but less pure : it is commonly mixed with the expressed juice of the *cynanchum monspeliacum;* it is also sophisticated with *flour, sand,* or *ashes;* their presence may be detected by dissolving the sample in proof spirit, when the impurities will sink, and remain undissolved; there is however a compound, bearing the name of Scammony, to be met with in the market, which is altogether factitious, consisting of jalap, senna, manna, gamboge, and ivory black. Good Scammony ought to be friable, and when wetted with the finger, it should *lactify,* or become milky : the powder should manifest its characteristic odour, which has been compared to that of old ewe milk cheese.

SCILLÆ RADIX. L.E.D.   (Scilla Maritima.)
Squill Root.   (Bulb.)

QUALITIES. *Odour,* none: *Taste,* bitter, nauseous, and acrid; when much handled, it inflames, and ulcerates the skin. By drying, the bulb loses about

four-fifths of its weight, and with very little diminution of its powers, provided that too great a heat has
not been applied. CHEMICAL COMPOSITION. According to Vogel, gum 6—tannin 24—sugar 6—bitter
principle (*Scillitin*, which is white, transparent, and
breaks with a resinous fracture) 35—woody fibre 30.
SOLUBILITY. Squill gives out its virtues so perfectly to any of the ordinary menstrua, as to render the
form of its exhibition, in that respect, a matter of in-
difference. INCOMPATIBLE SUBSTANCES. *Alkalies*
diminish their acrimony and bitterness, and are probably *medically* inconsistent with their diuretic qualities, but farther experiments are required to decide
this question : *vegetable acids* produce no effect upon
their sensible qualities, but are said to increase their
expectorant power. MED. USES. According to the
dose, and circumstances, under which it is administered, it proves expectorant, diuretic, emetic, or
purgative; as an expectorant, it can never be employed where pulmonary inflammation exists, for in
such cases, instead of promoting, it will check any
excretion from the lungs; its combination with a
diaphoretic will frequently increase its powers,
and, generally, be a measure of judicious caution.
(See *Form:* 48.) As a diuretic, it seems to act by
absorption, and we accordingly find, on the authority
of Dr. Cullen, that, *when the squill operates strongly
on the stomach and intestines, its diuretic effects are less
likely to happen ;* he therefore found, that by accompanying it with an opiate, (*Form:* 28) the emetic and
purgative operation may be avoided, and the squill be
thereby carried more entirely to the kidneys. Experience, moreover, has taught us the value of combining this medicine with some mercurial preparation,
by which its diuretic powers are very considerably

augmented, (*Form: 31, 32, 34,*) but we must take care that it does not occasion purging. In the exhibition of squill, it has been often delivered as a rule, to give it to the extent necessary to induce nausea, as a test of the medicine being in a state of activity: after what has been observed it is unnecessary to dwell upon the mischievous tendency of such a practice. As an emetic, it has been advised in solution, in cases of hooping cough, but its extreme uncertainty renders it unfit for exhibition, unless as an adjunct to emetic combinations, as in *Form: 3.* Dose. Of the dried root gr. j to iv. Officinal Prep. *Acetum Scillæ,* * L.E.D. *Pil: Scill: somp:* L.E.D. *Pulv: Scill:* E. D. *Syrup: Scill: maritim:* E. *Tinct: Scill:* L.D.

SENNÆ FOLIA. L.E.D. (Cassia Senna.)
Senna Leaves.

Qualities. *Odour,* faint and sickly; *Taste,* slightly bitter, sweetish, and nauseous. Chemical Composition. Extractive, resin, mucilage, and saline matter. Med. Uses. See *Infus: Sennæ.* Officinal Prep. *Confectio Sennæ.* L.E.D. *Extract: Cassiæ Sennæ.* E. *Infus: Sennæ.* L. D. *Infus: Tamarind: cum Senna.* E.D. *Pulv: Sennæ comp:* L. *Tinct: Sennæ.* L.D. *Tinct: Sennæ comp:* E. *Syrup: Sennæ.* L.D. Adulterations. The leaves of senna are imported from Alexandria in a state of adulteration, being mixed by the merchants of Cairo, with the leaves of *Cynanchum Oleafolium,*

---

* This is a very ancient preparation, thus *Ausonius,*
　　" Scillato decies si cor purgeris aceto,
　　Anticipitesque tuum Samii Lucomonis acumen."

[Arguel) and with those of *Colutea Arborescens* ; the former are distinguished by their greater length, as well as by their structure, which differs from the leaves of Senna in having a straight side, and being regular at their base, and in not displaying any lateral nerves on the under disk ; the latter are so different from Senna leaves, that there is no difficulty in at once recognising them. The *Tripoli Senna* contains a much larger proportion of *Cynanchum*, and of the other adulterations; as a general rule, those leaves which appear bright, fresh, free from stalks and spots, that are well and strongly scented, smooth and soft to the touch, thoroughly dry, sharp pointed, bitterish, and somewhat nauseous, are to be preferred.

SINAPIS SEMINA. $\left(\begin{array}{cc} Sinapis\ Nigra. & \text{L.} \\ Alba. & \text{E.D.} \end{array}\right)$

Mustard Seeds.

CHEMICAL COMPOSITION. Fecula, mucilage, a bland fixed oil, an acrid volatile oil, on which their virtues depend, and an ammoniacal salt. SOLUBI-LITY. Unbruised mustard seeds, when macerated in boiling water, yields only an insipid mucilage, which, like that of linseed, resides in the skin; but, when bruised, water takes up all their active matter, although it is scarcely imparted to alcohol. MED. USES. It is a beneficial stimulant in dyspepsia, chlorosis, and paralysis ; for which purpose, a tea spoonful of the bruised seeds may be administered ; or, a *whey* may be made, by boiling a table spoonful of the bruised seeds in oj of milk, and straining ; of which a fourth part may be taken three times a day, (see also *Form:* 106). The farina made into a paste, with crumbs of bread and vinegar, affords one of the most powerful external stimulants which we can apply, and is technically termed a *Sinapism*. If a table spoonful of powdered mustard be added to oj of tepid water, it operates briskly as an emetic. OFFICINAL PREP. *Cataplasm: Sinap*, L.D. *Emplast: Meloes comp :* E.* ADULTERATIONS. Fine powder, or flour of mustard, as it occurs in commerce, contains only one-sixth part of genuine mustard, the remainder consists of flour, coloured by turmeric, and made pungent by the addition of powdered capsicum.

SODA TARTARIZATA. L. TARTRAS SODÆ ET POTASSÆ. E. TARTARUS SODÆ ET KALI. D. olim. *Sal de Seignette. Sal Rupellensis,* or *Rochelle Salt.*

QUALITIES. *Form,* irregular prismatic crystals, very slightly efflorescent. CHEMICAL COMPOSITION. It is a triple salt, formed by neutralizing the excess of acid in super-tartrate of potass with soda. SOLUBILITY. It is soluble in five parts of water at 50°. MED. USES. Similar to those of *Potassæ Tartras*.

SODÆ CARBONAS. L.E. *Carbonate of Soda.*

This salt, when properly prepared, is a *bi-carbonate* of soda ; its taste is very slightly alkaline, and it is

* WHITEHEAD'S ESSENCE OF MUSTARD.—This consists of *oil of turpentine, camphor,* and a portion of *spirit of rosemary;* to which is added a small quantity of *flour of mustard.*
WHITEHEAD'S ESSENCE OF MUSTARD PILLS.—Balsam of Tolu, with resin !

much less soluble in water than the sub-carbonate;
its chemical habitudes, as connected with its medicinal applications, are similar to those of the *carbonate of potass*, which see. MED. USES. As it is
less nauseous, so is it more eligible than the *sub-
carbonate*; in other respects, its effects are the same,
vid. Sodæ Sub-carbonas. DOSE, grs. x to ʒss.*

SODÆ MURIAS. L.E.

SAL COMMUNE, Murias Sodæ. D.

Muriate of Soda. Common Salt.

QUALITIES. *Form*, that of regular cubes, which
do not deliquesce, unless contaminated with muriate
of magnesia. CHEMICAL COMPOSITION. It consists,
according to Berzelius, of 46·55 of muriatic acid, and
53·44 of soda; according to the new theory, however,
this salt must be considered as a true *muriate of soda*,
only while it remains in an aqueous solution; for
when it is reduced to dryness, the muriatic acid, and

---

* SODAIC POWDERS.—Contained in two distinct papers, one of which
is blue, the other white; that in the former consists of ʒss of the *carbonate of soda*, that in the latter, of grs. xxv of *tartaric acid*. These powders
require half a pint of water. It is very evident that a solution of these
powders is by no means similar to " *Soda Water*," which it is intended
to emulate; for in this latter preparation, the soda is in combination
only with carbonic acid; whereas, the solution of the " *Sodaic Powders*"
is that of a neutral salt, with a portion of fixed air diffused through it.

PATENT SEIDLITZ POWDERS.— These consist of two different powders; the one, contained in a white paper, consists of ʒij of *Tartarized
Soda*, and ɘij of *Carbonate of Soda*; that, in the blue paper, of grs. xxxv
of tartaric acid. The contents of the white paper are to be dissolved in
half a pint of spring water, to which those of the blue paper are to be
added; the draught is to be taken in a state of effervescence. The acid
being in excess renders it more grateful, and no less efficacious, as a
purgative.

the soda become both decomposed, and the hydrogen, of the former, uniting with the oxygen of the latter, they both pass off in the form of water, while the chlorine of the muriatic acid unites with the metallic base of the soda, to form *chloride of sodium*, in the proportion of 22 sodium, to 33·5 chlorine. SOLUBILITY. It is equally soluble in cold and in hot water, one part of the salt requiring rather more than 2½ parts. MED. USES. The effects of salt upon the animal and vegetable kingdoms, are striking and important, and have furnished objects of the most interesting enquiry, to the physiologist, the chemist, the physician, and the agriculturist; it appears to be a natural stimulant to the digestive organs ; and that carnivorous animals are instinctively led to immense distances in pursuit of it; the reader is referred to " *Parkes on the Repeal of the Salt Laws;*" and to an interesting work by Sir Thomas Bernard, entitled, " *Case of the Salt Duties, with Proofs and Illustrations.*" Salt, when taken in moderate quantities, promotes, while in excessive ones, it prevents digestion : it is therefore tonic and anthelmintic, correcting that disordered state of the bowels which favours the propagation of worms. In Ireland, where, from the bad quality of the food, the lower classes are greatly infested with worms, a draught of salt and water is a popular and efficacious anthelmintic. *Form:* 123, is a prescription by Rush, who says, that in this manner he has administered many pounds of common salt, with great success, in worm cases. In the first volume of the Medical Transactions, we shall find an interesting account of a cure of this disease by salt, after the failure of other remedies ; I beg also to refer the practitioner to another case illustrative of its anthelmintic powers, published by Mr. Marshall,

(London Medical and Physical Journal, vol. xxxix, No. 231,) which is that of a lady who had a natural antipathy to salt, and was, in consequence, most dreadfully infested with worms, during the whole of her life. In very large doses, *salt* proves purgative; it is also absorbed, and carried to the kidneys, but it undergoes no decomposition *in transitu,* nor does it appear to possess any considerable powers as a diuretic; its solution in tepid water, in the proportion of ℥ss—℥j in oj of water, forms the common domestic enema. Dose, when intended to act as a cathartic, from ℥ss to ℥j very largely diluted, when to answer the other intentions, from grs. x to ʒj.

SODÆ SUB-BORAS. L.D. Boras Sodæ. E.

Borax.

Qualities. *Form,* irregular hexaedral prisms; slightly efflorescent. *Taste,* alkaline and styptic; when heated it loses its water of crystallization, and becomes a porous friable mass *(calcined borax).* Chemical Composition. Boracic acid, 34—soda, 17—water, 49. Solubility. It is soluble in 20 parts of water at 60°, and in 6 parts at 212°. Incompatible Substances. It is decomposed by *acids ; potass ;* and the *sulphates,* and *muriates* of the *earths,* and by those of *ammonia.* Med. Uses. It is only employed in the form of powder, mixed with 8 or 10 parts of honey, as a detergent linctus in aphthæ, &c. Officinal Prep. *Mel Boracis.* L. Adulterations. *Alum,* and *fused muriate of soda,* are the substances with which it is sometimes sophisticated, to discover which, dissolve it in distilled water, and after saturating the excess of base with nitric acid, assay the solution with nitrate of barytes and nitrate of silver.

SODÆ SUB-CARBONAS. L.E.D.

Sub-carbqnate of Soda.

QUALITIES. *Form*, octohedrons, truncated at the summits of the pyramids ; it effloresces when exposed to the air, and at 150° Fah. undergoes watery fusion, its crystals containing as much as seven proportionals of water; *Taste*, mild, but alkalescent. CHEMICAL COMPOSITION. Soda 29·5—carbonic acid 20·7. SOLUBILITY. It is soluble in two parts of water at 60°, and in considerably less than its weight of boiling water; it is insoluble in alcohol. INCOMPATIBLE SUBSTANCES are enumerated under *Potassæ Carbonas.* MED. USES, are similar to those of the sub-carbonate of potass, but it is preferable to it for internal use, as being more mild, and less nauseous; and, moreover, Fourcroy states it as his opinion, that soda is more eligible for medicinal purposes than potass, on account of its analogy with animal substances, which always contain it, while, on the contrary, no portion of potass is found in them. Are the absorbents more disposed to take up soda than potass? The results of experience do not appear to sanction such a conclusion. FORMS OF EXHIBITION. It may be administered in solution, in an electuary, or in pills ; when exhibited in the latter form, it must be previously deprived of its water of crystallization, (*Sodæ Sub-carbonas exsiccata.* L.) or the pills will fall into powder as they dry. DOSE, gr. x to ʒj, twice or thrice a day.

SODÆ SULPHAS. L.E.D.

Natron Vitriolatum, P.L. 1787. *Sal Catharticus
Glauberi.* P.L. 1745.

QUALITIES. *Form*, transparent, prismatic crystals,
which effloresce; when exposed to heat, it undergoes
watery fusion, that is, it melts in its own water of
crystallization. *Taste*, saline and bitter. CHEMICAL
COMPOSITION. Sulphuric acid 24·64,—soda 19·36—
water 56. SOLUBILITY. f℥j of water at 60° dissolves ℥iiiss; in boiling water it is considerably more
soluble; it is quite insoluble in alcohol. INCOM-
PATIBLE SUBSTANCES. The same *as those which
decompose *sulphate of magnesia.* MED. USES. A
common and useful purgative; its nauseous taste may
be, in a great degree, disguised by the addition of a
small quantity of lemon juice, or *cream of tartar.*
DOSE, ℥ss to ℥ij. In an effloresced state it is just
equal in efficacy to double the weight of that which
is in a crystalline form. It is rendered more active
by being combined with other purgative salts, especially with sulphate of soda, and the compound is
more soluble and less nauseous; (*Form* 8, 10.) A
portion of triple salt, a *magnesio-sulphate of soda,*
probably results from the combination, a salt, which
may be frequently detected in parcels of sulphate of
magnesia, and may be known by its crystals, which
are regular rhomboids; it is also contained, according
to Dr. Murray, in the brine, or *mother liquor* of sea
water; and it constitutes the whole of that salt which
was formerly sold under the name of " *Lymington
Glauber's Salts.*"

* CHELTENHAM SALTS.—A factitious compound has been long
vended, as a popular purgative, under this name; it is formed by tri-

SPARTIUM. L.E. ⎛Spartii *Cucumina.* L.⎞
　　　　　　　　⎝　　　*Summitates.* E.⎠
　　　　GENISTA. D.

　　　The tops of Broom.

QUALITIES. When bruised, they yield an unpleasant *odour*, and a nauseous bitter taste. SOLU-
BILITY. Water and alcohol, alike extract their

turating together the following salts. *Sulphate of Soda,* grs. 120. *Sulphate of Magnesia,* grs. 66. *Muriate of Soda,* grs. 10. *Sulphate of Iron,*
grs. ½. As a purgative it is very efficacious, and superior, probably, to
that which is actually obtained by the evaporation of the Cheltenham
water itself, for, notwithstanding the high pretensions with which it
has been publicly announced, it will be found to be little else than
common *Glauber's salt.* This fact has been confirmed by the experiments
of Mr. Richard Phillips, *(Annals of Philosophy,* No. lxi) who observes,
that the "REAL CHELTENHAM SALTS contain no *chalybeate property,*"
but are merely sulphate of soda, mixed with a minute quantity of soda,
and a very small portion of common salt." It could not be imagined
that the salt should contain oxide of iron, even in a state of mixture,
much less in combination, for carbonate of iron is readily decomposed
by ebullition, and the oxide of iron is precipitated before the salt can be
crystallized. A preparation, under the name of *Thomson's* Cheltenham
Salts, is accordingly manufactured in London, by evaporating a solution, consisting of sulphate of soda, and sub-carbonate of soda.

　　"EFFLORESCENCE OF REAL CHELTENHAM SALTS." The preceding
salt deprived of its water of crystallization.

　　"EFFLORESCENCE OF REAL MAGNESIAN CHELTENHAM SALTS,'
MADE FROM THE WATERS OF THE CHALYBEATE MAGNESIAN SPA.
This is asserted to be a *sub-sulphate* from nature, which combines both a
pure and a *sub-sulphated* magnesia in its composition; "but," says Mr.
Phillips, "neither nature, nor art, has ever produced such a combination; in truth, it consists of *Epsom salt,* with small portions of magnesia,
and muriate of magnesia, or muriate of soda.

　　MURIO-SULPHATE OF MAGNESIA AND IRON. The preparation thus
named by Mr. Thomson, was found by Mr. Phillips to consist of
Epsom salt, deprived of part of its water of crystallization, and dis-
coloured by a little rust of iron, and containing a small portion of
muriate of magnesia.

　　Thus it appears, that not one of these preparations is similar to the
water which is drank at the Spa; in order to remedy this difficulty, Mr-

active matter. MED. USES. They certainly act as a powerful diuretic, and even prove so to animals that browse upon them. I have frequently exhibited them in the Westminster Hospital, with very great success, in the form of decoction. (See *Form.* 41.)

SPIRITUS. L. SPIRITUS STILLATITII.
Distilled Spirits.

These are the solutions of the essential oils of vegetables in diluted alcohol, or proof spirit; they are obtained by distilling spirit with the recent vegetables; sometimes, however, they are extemporaneously made by at once dissolving the oils in the spirit. (See *Spiritus Tenuior.*) MED. USES. Like the *distilled waters*, they serve as vehicles for the exhibition of more active medicines; they are also occasionally employed as grateful stimulants. It is unnecessary to dwell on each of these simple spirits, as their virtues are the same as those of the substances from which they are extracted, united to the stimulus of the alcohol. The following are officinal:—*Spirit: Anisi.* L. *Spir: Anisi comp:* L. D. *Armoraciæ comp:* L. *Carui.* L. E. D. *Cinnamomi.* L. E. D. *Juniperi comp:* L.D. *Lavandulæ.* L.E.D. *Lavandulæ comp:* L.E.D. *Menth: Pip.* L.D. *Menth. Virid:* L. *Myristic:* L. E. D. *Pimentæ.* L. D. *Pulegii.* L. *Raphani comp:* D. *Rosmarini.* L.E.D.

Thomson prepared the "ORIGINAL COMBINED CHELTENHAM SALTS" by evaporating the waters to dryness: but a very small share of chemical penetration is required to satisfy us that no process of this description can remedy the defect described, for as Mr. Phillips has observed, the chalybeate properties of the water *must* be essentially altered by such an operation.

SPIRITUS AMMONIÆ. L.D.

ALCOHOL AMMONIATUM. E.

Spiritus Salis Ammoniaci dulcis. P.L. 1745. *Spiritus Salis Ammoniaci.* P.L. 1720.

This is a solution of ammoniacal gas in spirit; in which a small portion of the sub-carbonate is also generally present. It is a powerful stimulant, but it is principally employed in the basis of the following compounds; viz. *Spirit: Ammoniæ comp:* L.E.D. *Spirit: Ammoniæ fœtid:* L.E.D. *Tinctura Castorei comp:* E. *Tinct: Guaiaci comp:* E. *Tinct: Opii Ammoniat:* E.

SPIRITUS AMMONIÆ AROMATICUS. L.D.

ALCOHOL AMMONIATUM AROMATICUM. E.

Spiritus Ammoniæ Compositus. P.L. 1787. *Spiritus Volatilis Aromaticus.* P.L. 1745. *Spiritus salis volatilis oleosus.* P.L. 1720.

This is a solution of several essential oils, *Cinnamon, Cloves,* and *Lemon.* L.—*Rosemary* and *Lemon.* E.—*Lemon* and *Nutmeg.* D. in the spirit of ammonia. It is a valuable stimulant, and an agreeable adjunct, and efficacious corrective to other remedies, see *Form:* 97, 106. Dose, f3ss to f3j.

SPIRITUS ÆTHERIS AROMATICUS. L.

ÆTHER SULPHURICUS CUM ALCOHOLE ARO-MATICUS. E.

Elixir Vitrioli dulce. P.L. 1745.

This preparation, which was excluded from the London Pharmacopœia of 1787, is now restored. It consists of Sulphuric Ether, *one part*, rectified spirit *two parts*, impregnated with aromatics; the presence of spirit is necessary in this preparation, since the volatile oils would be insoluble in the ether, without it. MED. USES. A grateful stimulant.

SPIRITUS ÆTHERIS NITRICI. L.

SPIRITUS ÆTHERIS NITROSI. E.

SPIRITUS ÆTHEREUS NITROSUS. D.

Spiritus Nitri dulcis. P.L. 1745.

QUALITIES. A colourless fluid of the *specific gravity* ·850. *Odour*, extremely fragrant; *Taste*, pungent and acidulous; it is very volatile and inflammable. CHEMICAL COMPOSITION. A portion of nitric ether, and nitric acid, combined with alcohol. SOLUBILITY. It is soluble both in water and alcohol. INCOMPATIBLE SUBSTANCES. With a solution of *green sulphate of iron* it strikes a deep olive colour, owing probably to its holding a portion of nitrous gas in solution; with the *tinctures of guaiacum* it produces a green, or blue coagulum. MED. USES. When properly diluted, it is refrigerant, and diuretic; and has been long employed as a grateful draught in febrile affections; as a diuretic, it frequently proves a valuable auxiliary in dropsy, (see *Form.* 41, 44.) DOSE, mx to xl, in any aqueous vehicle. By age and exposure to the air, it is gradually decomposed, and gives rise to the reproduction of nitrous acid. When added, in a small proportion, to malt spirits, it gives them a flavour resembling that of *French Brandy*. I apprehend that the peculiar flavour of *Cogniac* depends upon the presence of an æthereal spirit, formed by the action of Tartaric or perhaps, acetic acid, on alcohol.*

SPIRITUS ÆTHERIS SULPHURICI. L.

ÆTHER SULPHURICUS CUM ALCOHOLE. E.
LIQUOR ÆTHEREUS SULPHURICUS. D.
Spiritus Ætheris vitriolici. P. L. 1787.
Spirit: Vitrioli dulcis. 1745.

QUALITIES. A fluid of the *specific gravity* ·816, consisting of *two parts* (by measure) of rectified spirit, and *one part* of sulphuric æther. MED. USES. It has all the properties of æther, but in an inferior degree. DOSE, fʒj to fʒiij.

SPIRITUS ÆTHERIS SULPHURICI COM-POSITUS. L.

This is intended as a substitute for the *Liquor Anodynus* of Hoffmann, although its composition was never revealed by him. In addition to its stimulating properties, it is supposed to add those of an anodyne nature. DOSE, fʒss to fʒij.

SPIRITUS RECTIFICATUS. L.

ALCOHOL FORTIUS. E. SPIRITUS VINOSUS RECTI-FICATUS. D.

In this preparation, alcohol is nearly in the highest state of concentration, in which it can be easily pre-

---

* In new brandy there also appears to be an uncombined acid, giving to it a peculiar taste and quality, which are lost by age. This explains the reason why the addition of five or six drops of " *liquor ammonia,*" to each bottle of *new* brandy, will impart to it the qualities of that of the oldest date.

pared, in the large way, for the purposes of trade; its specific gravity, however, varies in the different pharmacopœias, viz. the London and Edinburgh preparation is stated to have that of ·835, while the rectified spirit of Dublin is ordered to be only ·840. The former, at the temperature of 60° *Fah.* consists of 85 parts of pure alcohol, and 15 of water, the latter only of 83 per cent. of alcohol. It is a most powerful stimulant, but is rarely employed, except in combination; as a pharmaceutical agent, its use is highly valuable and extensive. (See *Tincturæ.*)

SPIRITUS TENUIOR. L.
ALCOHOL DILUTUM. E.
SPIRITUS VINOSUS TENUIOR. D.
Weaker, or *Proof Spirit.*

This is rectified spirit, diluted with a certain proportion of water, and it is to be regretted, that the quantity ordered for this purpose, should vary in the different Pharmacopœias; thus, according to the London and Dublin Colleges, its specific gravity is ·930, while the College of Edinburgh directs it to be of ·935. The former consists of 44 per cent of pure alcohol, and may be formed by mixing *four* parts, by measure, of rectified spirit, with *three* of water; the latter contains only 42 *per cent* of pure alcohol, and may be made by adding together *equal parts* of rectified spirit and distilled water. Alcohol in this state of dilution, is better adapted for taking up the principles of vegetables than rectified spirit; indeed, diluted alcohol acts upon bodies as a chemical compound, and will dissolve, what neither the same proportion of water, nor of alcohol would, if sepa-

2 B 2

rately applied ; we perceive therefore the importance
of ensuring uniformity of strength in our spirits.
(See *Tincturæ.*) It is necessary to remark, that
almost all the spirit sold under the name of " *Proof
Spirit,*" is contaminated with empyreumatic oil, and
is unfit for the purposes of pharmacy ; it ought therefore to be extemporaneously prepared by mixing
together rectified spirit and water, in the proportions
above stated. This however is rarely done, except
the liquors are intended for the toilette, and hence it
has been observed, that the cordials of the apothecary
are generally less grateful than those of the distiller,
the latter being extremely curious in rectifying and
purifying his spirit. If common water be employed
for the dilution of alcohol, the resulting spirit will be
turbid, owing principally to the precipitation of sulphuric salts ;. this circumstance lately occasioned
considerable embarrassment to the Curators of the
Hunterian Museum, at the College of Surgeons, who
were compelled to prepare their own spirit, in consequence of an excise regulation preventing the
distiller from sending out any spirit of that strength,
which is required for their anatomical purposes. A
curious fact has just been noticed in the Laboratory
of the Royal Institution, which is, that diluted spirit
becomes stronger by being kept in vessels that are
carefully closed by bladder ! whence it would seem,
that alcoholic vapour transpires through this animal
membrane less freely than aqueous vapour : we are
at present unable to offer a satisfactory explanation
of this anomalous case of distillation, bnt it is probably connected with the different solvent powers of
these two liquids, in relation to the animal membrane.
MED. USES. Alcohol, although diluted to the degree of proof spirit, is still too strong for internal

exhibition; indeed, where its use is indicated, it is more generally given in the form of wine, malt liquors, or ardent spirits, which must be regarded only as diluted alcohol, although each has a peculiarity of operation, owing to the modifying influence of the other elements of the liquid; thus *Brandy* is said to be simply cordial, and stomachic; *Rum*, heating and sudorific; *Gin* and *Whisky*, diuretic; and *Arrack*, styptic, heating, and narcotic; it seems also probable, that a modified effect is produced by the addition of various other substances, such as sugar and acids, which latter bodies, besides their antinarcotic powers, appear to act by favouring a more perfect combination, and mutual penetration of the particles of spirit and water. The effects also, which are produced by the habitual use of fermented liquors, differ essentially according to the kind that is drank; thus Ale and Porter, in consequence of the nutritive matter, and perhaps the invigorating bitter, with which they are charged, and the comparatively small proportion of alcohol which they contain, dispose to a plethora, which is not unfrequently terminated by apoplexy; Spirits, on the other hand, induce severe dyspepsia, obstructed, and hardened liver, dropsy, and more than half of all our chronical diseases; and Dr. Darwin remarks, that when they arise from this cause, they are liable to become hereditary, even to the third generation, gradually increasing, if the cause be continued, till the family becomes extinct : with regard to Wine, Rush has truly observed, that its effects, like those of tyranny in a well formed government, are first felt in the extremities, while spirits, like a bold invader, seize at once upon the vitals of the constitution; the different kinds of wine, however, produce very different and even opposite effects, as stated under the history of that article, (see *Vinum*.)

STANNI LIMATURA. L.E.D.

The Filings of Tin.

The anthelmintic properties of Tin have been explained by three different hypotheses, viz. 1. *That it acts mechanically by dislodging the mucus from the intestines ;* if this be true, it is difficult to explain the fact of its activity being increased by pulverization. 2. *That its efficacy depends upon the presence of arsenic* ; if so, why should the *purest* specimens act with equal efficacy? 3. *That it operates by generating hydrogen gas in the intestinal canal* : it has been observed that this opinion is rendered probable by the fact, that sulphur increases its powers. DOSE ʒj or ʒij, mixed with honey, treacle, or conserve, and exhibited for several successive mornings, a purgative medicine being occasionally interposed, (see *Form :* 122.) The use of this remedy however is entirely superseded by the more efficacous exhibition of oil of turpentine.

SULPHUR SUBLIMATUM, L.E.D.

Sublimed Sulphur. Flowers of Sulphur.

CHEMICAL COMPOSITION. It is, probably, a triple compound of oxygen, hydrogen, and some unknown base. SOLUBILITY. It is insoluble in water, and alcohol, but soluble in oils, especially in that of linseed, which is a powerful solvent of all sulphureous substances. MED : USES. It is laxative and diaphoretic ; it acts principally upon the large intestines, and very mildly, whence it proves useful in hemorrhoidal affections. (*Form:* 12) and in consequence of the diaphoresis which it also excites, it is useful in chronic rheumatisms, catarrhs, and in some cutaneous affections. To promote its purgative effects, *magnesia* will be found a serviceable adjunct in hemorrhoids; it may be given in the form of an electuary, or suspended in milk; its solution in oil, (*Oleum Sulphuratum*) is a most nauseous and acrid preparation. When sulphur is combined with metallic remedies, it generally lessens their activity. Its effects in curing psora are universally admitted, and the only objection to its use is the disgusting smell which accompanies its application, see *Unguent: Sulphuris*. Dr. Clarke of Dublin, recommends a lotion, which he says contains a sufficient impregnation of sulphur for the cure of psora in children, to be made, by adding an ounce of broken sulphur to a quart of boiling water, and allowing it to infuse for twelve hours. In this process, the water probably takes up a small portion of sulphureous acid; it is difficult to explain the efficacy of the lotion in any other manner. When sulphur is internally administered, it transpires through the skin, in the state of sulphuretted hydrogen, and blackens the silver in the pockets of those who take it. Dose ʒj to ʒiij. Officinal Prep : *Sulphur Lotum. L.E.D. Sulphur Præcipitatum. L. Unguent: Sulph: L.E.D. Unguent: Sulphur: comp: L.**

Sulphur Lotum. When sulphur is kept in loosely covered drawers, its surface is soon acidified, when it is said to operate with griping, hence the common *flowers* are directed to be washed with water to get rid of any sulphureous acid; it is however rarely performed, and would seem to be a useless subtlety.

Sulphur Præcipitatum. L. *Lac Sulphuris, P.L.* 1720. This, when pure, differs in no other respect from sublimed sulphur, than in its superior

---

* Sulphur Lozenges. Sublimed Sulphur *one part*, sugar *eight parts*, Tragacanth mucilage q. s. used in Asthma, and in Hæmorrhoids.

whiteness, which it owes to the presence of a small
proportion of water ; in consequence however of its
mode of preparation, it always contains a small
quantity of sulphate of lime, and, not unfrequently,
other impurities ; it may be assayed by pouring upon
a suspected sample a sufficient quantity of *liquor potassæ* to cover it, and setting it aside, in a warm place,
to digest, when the sulphur will be dissolved, and the
impurities remain ; or it might be at once subjected
to the operation of heat, which would volatilize the
sulphur, and thus separate it from its contaminations,

SYRUPI. L.E.D. *Syrups.*

These are solutions of sugar in water, watery infusions, or in vegetable juices ; the proportion of sugar
is generally *two parts* to one of the fluids ; if it exceeds this, the solution will crystallize, if it be less,
ferment, and become acescent.* The most certain
test of the proper consistence of a syrup is its specific
gravity, a bottle that holds three ounces of water at
55 *Fah:* ought to hold four ounces of syrup. Syrups
are introduced into medicinal formulæ, for several
purposes, viz.

* Sugar perfectly free from the extractive matter, with which it
exists in combination in nature, and which constitutes that compound
to which the name of *Sweet Principle* has been given, will not, however
diluted, undergo any kind of fermentation ; for it is the presence of
this peculiar extractive matter, the natural leaven of fruits, that enables it to undergo that process ; since, however, all clayed sugars, or
modifications of sugar which are short of perfect purity, still contain
a small proportion of this extractive, they are capable of fermenting,
when sufficiently dilute ; Dr. Macculloch, in his admirable essay on the
art of making wine, observes, that by the addition of a very small
quantity of the *Sulphite of Potass* the fermentation of syrups and preserves, may be effectually prevented ; he states also, that the same object may generally be attained by the use of *Oxy-muriate of potass*, a salt
absolutely tasteless, and easily procured.

1. *To correct, or disguise the flavour of disagreeable remedies.* Syrup: Aurantiorum. L.D. (*Form*, 35, 88, 102.)—Limonum. L.E.D.—Simplex (60, 85.)—Zingiberis (25, 33, 68). Bitter Infusions, and saline solutions are rendered more nauseous by the addition of syrups.

II. *To produce Medicinal Effects.* Syrup: Allii. D.—Altheæ. L.E. (49)—*Acidi Acetosi* E—Colchici. E.—Sennæ. E.D. (9)—Scillæ Maritimæ. E—Rhamni. L. *Papaveris.* L.E.D. (13, 117, 119)—Rosæ (12)—Zingiberis (82, 103.)

III. *To communicate peculiar forms.* Every syrup answers this purpose; for the necessary proportions, see *Electuaria.*

IV. *To communicate an agreeable colour.* Syrup: Croci. L.—Rhæados. L.D. (73, 75)—Caryophylli. Rubri. D.—Violæ. E. Except that of Saffron, these syrups are rendered green by alkalies, and red by acids.

GENERAL REMARKS. The practitioner should never introduce syrups into those medicines which are liable to be injured by the generation of acids: I have frequently seen the *cretaceous mixture,* when charged with syrup, increase, instead of check a diarrhœa ; and the syrup of poppies, from its disposition to become acescent, will often aggravate, rather than allay, the cholic of infants. The syrup of Senna furnishes the practitioner with a convenient purgative for children ; that of buckthorn is more violent, and is on that account but rarely used, besides which, in preparing it, the chemist not unfrequently substitutes the berries of the *Cornus Sanguinea,* the Dogberry-tree, or, those of the *Rhamnus Frangula,* the Alder-Buckthorn, for the Rhamnus Catharticus, a circumstance which necessarily renders the efficacy of this syrup variable and uncertain, The syrup of the rose,

when made with the leaves of the *Damask* rose, is
gently laxative, and is well adapted for weak children; it is however not unusual, *Coloris gratia*, to
substitute the leaves of the *red* rose, in which case
the syrup will possess astringent instead of laxative
properties. In the preparation of the syrup of poppies, the directions of the College are frequently not
obeyed; it is sometimes made by dissolving the extract in syrup, formed with coarse sugar, or even with
treacle; at others, by adding tincture of opium to a
coarse syrup, in the proportion of *mx* to every f℥j.
In the preparation of the syrup of violets, the juice
of red cabbage is generally substituted; this is at
least a harmless fraud. NOTE. The syrups which are
printed in *Italics*, are very susceptible of decomposition, and should be kept in cool places.

TABACI FOLIA. L.E. $\left(\begin{array}{l}\text{Nicotiana Tabacum.}\\\text{FoliaSiccata.}(\textit{Virginianæ})\end{array}\right)$
NICOTIANÆ FOLIA. D.
Tobacco.

QUALITIES. *Odour*, strong, narcotic, and fœtid;
Taste, bitter, and extremely acrid; *Colour*, yellowish
green, (its brown appearance is artificial, being produced by the action of *sulphate of iron*.). CHEMICAL
COMPOSITION. Mucilage, albumen, or gluten, extractive, a bitter principle, an essential oil, nitrate of
potass, which occasions its deflagration, muriate of
potass, and a peculiar proximate principle upon which
the properties of the plant are supposed to depend,
and which has therefore been named *Nicotin*. Vauquelin considers it as approaching the volatile oils,
in its properties; it is colourless, has an acrid taste,
and the peculiar smell of tobacco, and occasions violent sneezing; with alcohol, and water, it produces

TAB 387

colourless solutions, from which it is thrown down by
tincture of galls. SOLUBILITY. Tobacco yields its
active matter both to water, and spirit, but more perfectly to the latter ; long coction weakens its powers.
An oil of tobacco, of a most powerful nature, may be
obtained by distilling the leaves, and separating it
from the water, on the top of which it will be found
to float. MEDICINAL PROPERTIES. Tobacco is endued
with energetic poisonous properties, which appear to
depend on an especial action upon the nervous system, producing generally a universal tremor, which
is rarely the result of other poisons ; the experiments
of M. Orfila moreover demonstrate, that the action of
Tobacco is much more energetic when the soluble
portion is injected into the anus, than when it is
applied to the cellular texture, and for a still stronger
reason, than when introduced into the stomach. Mr.
Brodie, from the result of a well devised experiment,
has deduced the conclusion, that the infusion of Tobacco acts upon the heart, through the medium of
the nervous system. USES. As a powerful sedative,
it is sometimes valuable in medical practice ; the
leaves, when applied in the form of a cataplasm to
the pit of the stomach, produce an emetic operation;
(*Form*: 5.) In cases of obstinate constipation, depending upon violent spasmodic constriction, as in
ileus, or *incarcerated hernia*, clysters of the smoke of
Tobacco, or of an infusion, made according to the
London College, produce almost immediate relief;
(*Form*: 113.) the practice is not unfrequently attended with severe vomiting, extreme debility, and cold
sweats, circumstances which render its administration
highly dangerous in cases wherein the patient has
been already exhausted by previous suffering. I remember witnessing a lamentable instance of this

truth, some years ago : a medical practitioner, after repeated trials to reduce a strangulated hernia, injected an infusion of Tobacco, and shortly afterwards sent the patient in a carriage to the Westminster Hospital, for the purpose of undergoing the operation; but the unfortunate man arrived only a few minutes before he expired. Otherwise, the production of such a state of system appears essential to the successful operation of the remedy, Smoking, or chewing Tobacco, has been also advised in cases of spasmodic asthma, and as a general sedative to relieve suffering; in the process of *smoking*, the oil is separated, and being rendered empyreumatic by heat, it is thus applied to the fauces in its most active state. As a diuretic, it was successfully exhibited by Dr. Fowler, but as its operation is uncertain and violent, and appears to be very analagous to that of Digitalis, which is far more safe, and manageable, it has been very judiciously discarded from practice. The external application of Tobacco, in the form of cataplasm, or infusion, has been applied to several species of cutaneous disease, but even in this state it is liable to exert its virulent effects. A woman applied to the heads of three children afflicted with *tinea capitis*, a liniment consisting of powdered tobacco and butter, soon after which they experienced vertigo, violent vomiting, and fainting. (*Ephemerides des Curieux de la Nature*, Dec : ii, An : l, p. 46.) It is a curious fact, that the juice of the green leaves instantly cures the stinging of nettles.

ADULTERATIONS. When it exhales a fetid odour, we may infer that it has been badly prepared, and not deprived of all its mucus; when pungent, the presence of some deleterious drug is indicated : Cascarilla is very usually added to impart a peculiar flavour ; Nitre

TAB 389

is also employed for the sake of making it kindle
more rapidly, and to impress a lively sensation on the
tongue; its vapour is of course very injurious to the
lungs : its presence may be detected by treating a
suspected sample with hot water, and, after filtering
the solution through charcoal, setting it aside, in
order that it may yield its crystals by evaporation.
Traces of *Lead*, *Copper*, or *Antimony* may be discovered by boiling the Tobacco in strong vinegar,
and after filtering it, as before, by assaying it with appropriate tests. *Black Hellebore*, *Alum*, *Sugar*, and
Corrosive sublimate are amongst the more usual so-
phistications. *Dried Dock* leaves are also sometimes
substituted. OFFICINAL PREP: *Infus: Tabacci.* L.
Vinum Nicotian: Tabac : E.

SNUFF. This well known errhine is prepared from
the dried leaves of Tobacco ; in its manufacture, however, numerous additions are made, which are kept
secret; *Salt* is added for the purpose of increasing its
weight; *Urine*, Muriate of ammonia, and powdered
Glass, to heighten its acrimony. The varied flavour
of different *Snuffs* is owing to the leaf being in greater
or less perfection; or to its having undergone some
degree of fermentation; thus, for instance, the *Ma-
couba Snuff* of Martinique is principally indebted for
its acknowledged superiority to the fermentation which
the Tobacco undergoes, from being moistened with
the best cane juice ; other kinds are excited into fermentation by moistening them with melasses and
water.

Snuff possesses all the powers of Tobacco ; the celebrated Santeuil experienced vomiting and horrible
pains, amidst which he expired, in consequence of

having drank a glass of wine, into which had been put some Spanish snuff.*

TAMARINDI PULPA. L. Tamarindi Indicæ Fructus Conditus. E. Tamarindus: Fructus. D.

The Pulp, or preserved Fruit, of the Tamarind, vulgo *Tamarinds.*

Qualities. *Taste,* sweetish acid; *Odour,* none. Chemical Composition. ℥j of Tamarinds is composed of Citric acid grs. 45, Malic acid grs. 2, Supertartrate of potass grs. 15, together with sugar, gum, jelly, fecula, and woody fibre. Uses. A pleasant febrifuge may be formed by infusing Tamarinds in water, or milk; they improve the taste of the more nauseous cathartics. Officinal Prep: *Confectio Cassiæ.* L. E. D. *Infus: Tamarind: cum Senna.* E. D. Caution. Copper vessels should never be employed for the preparation of any compound which contains *Tamarinds.*

TARAXACI RADIX. L.E. (Leontodon Taraxacum) *Dandelion.*

Qualities. *Odour,* none; *Taste,* bitter,and somewhat sweet, and acidulous. Chemical Composition. The active principles appear to consist of extractive, gluten, a bitter principle *(not resinous),* and tartaric acid. Solubility. Water extracts its virtues much better than spirit. Incompatible Substances.

* Cephalic Snuff. The basis of this errhine, is powdered *Asarum,* diluted with some vegetable powder.

Infusion of Galls, Nitrate of Silver, Oxy-muriate of Mercury, Superacetate of Lead, and *Sulphate of Iron* occasion precipitates in its solutions. MED. USES. It has long enjoyed the reputation of proving beneficial in obstructions of the liver, and in visceral diseases; Bergius extolls its use in these complaints, and recommends the recent root to he boiled in whey or broth. Dr. Pemberton has more recently added his testimony to its value; he observes that he has seen great advantage result from using the extract in chronic inflammation, and incipient schirrus of the liver, and in chronic derangement of the stomach. FORMS OF EXHIBITION. In that of extract, or in decoction, made by boiling ℥j of the sliced root in ℥j of water, down to oss, adding to the strained liquid ℥j of Cream of tartar : the recent full grown root only should be used. DOSE f℥iij, twice or thrice a day. OFFICINAL PREP : *Extract* : *Taraxaci.* The roots are roasted, and used at Gottingen, by the poorer people, for coffee, from which, a decoction of them properly prepared can hardly be distinguished. The leaves of this plant are blanched, and very commonly used on the continent as a sallad.

TEREBINTHINA. *Turpentine.*

QUALITIES. *Consistence,* semi-fluid, and tenacious; *Odour,* aromatic; *Taste,* pungent. It is inflammable. SOLUBILITY. It is entirely soluble in rectified spirit, but not at all in water, and is capable of entering into combination with fixed oils. CHEMICAL COMPOSITION. Resin, and an essential oil, the proportions of which vary according to the species of pine from which it is obtained; they all

however possess the same general chemical, as well
as medicinal properties, viz. 1. TEREBINTHINA CA-
NADENSIS, Canada Turpentine, or Canada *Balsam*,
as it is sometimes improperly called, for it contains
no benzoic acid, is obtained from the *Pinus Bal-
samea.* 2. TEREBINTHINA CHIA, Chian, or Cyprus
Turpentine, from the *Pistachia Terebinthinus.* 3.
TEREBINTHINA VULGARIS, Common Turpentine,
Horse Turpentine, from the *Pinus Sylvestris* (the
Scotch Fir). 4. TEREBINTHINA VENETA, Venice
Turpentine, from the *Pinus Larix.* * MED USES.
All the Turpentines are stimulant, diuretic, and in
large doses cathartic, and, externally, rubefacient.
They may be either made into pills with liquorice
root, or suspended in water, by the intervention of
egg, or mucilage, for which purpose, 3j requires the
yelk of one egg, or 3iss of gum arabic. DOSE. gr. x.
to 3j. They have been principally recommended in
protracted gleets, and lucorrhæa, in mucous obstructions of the urinary passages, and in calculous affections.

TEREBINTHINÆ OLEUM. L. E. D.
Oil of Turpentine.

QUALITIES. *Form,* a limpid and colourless liquid,
whose *Specific gravity* is only 792. *Odour,* strong,
penetrating, and peculiar. *Taste,* hot, bitter, and
pungent. CHEMICAL COMPOSITION. It is an essential volatile oil, possessing however peculiar ha-

---

* A fluid extract prepared by decoction, from the twigs of this species of fir, is the well known *Essence of Spruce,* which, when fermented
with melasses, forms the popular beverage, called " *Spruce Beer*," (Cere
visia Pini Laricis.)
    TRUE RIGA BALSAM, *Baume de Carpathes.* From the shoots of the
Pinus Combra, previously bruised, and macerated for a month in water.
This same fir affords also *Briançon Turpentine.*

bitudes with respect to alcohol, it is readily dissolved by *hot* alcohol, but as the spirit cools it again separates in drops; in the cold, it is very sparingly soluble in the strongest alcohol, but it dissolves completely in six parts of sulphuric ether. MED. USES. It acts according to the dose, either on the primæ viæ, producing catharsis, or on the kidneys, exciting diuresis: thus its operation offers another illustration of the views which I have so anxiously pressed upon the attention of the practitioner, under the article *Potassæ Acetas*, furnishing a striking instance of the important influence of quantity or *dose*, in determining the specific operation of a remedy; in the present instance, 3ij of oil of turpentine may so excite the urinary organs, as to produce even bloody urine, whereas 3vj, or f℥j, will stimulate the bowels, and scarcely produce any apparent effect upon the urinary secretion. As a medicine acting powerfully on the first passages, its value seems only to have been lately appreciated; in Tænia, it may be said to act almost as a specific remedy, discharging it, in all cases, *dead*. In obstinate constipation, depending on affections of the brain, I have lately had several opportunities of witnessing its beneficial effects; in an unfortunate instance of *Hydrocephalus acutus*, in a boy of thirteen years of age,* it brought away an accumulation of feculent matter, almost incredible as to quantity, after the total failure of the strongest doses of ordinary purgatives; and I believe, if its dose be sufficiently large, that it may generally be administered with perfect safety and confidence. Dr. Latham has long

---

* This case, which I attended with Mr. Machell of Great Ryder Street, was occasioned by a violent whirling of the body in a frolic! the circumstances attending it are so interesting that I shall take an early opportunity of submitting the details to the profession.

regarded it as a valuable medicine in Epilepsy, in
which cases, it may in the first instance prove beneficial by unloading the bowels, and, subsequently, in
producing an affection of the head peculiar to its use,
and which generally succeeds a large dose, it is an
approach to intoxication, but is unaccompanied with
that hilarity and elevation of thought that so usually
follow the potation of spirituous liquors. In small
doses it produces diuresis, and is used with much advantage in sciatica and lumbago. *Form* : 107. This
oil has the effect of communicating the odour of
violets to the urine of those who take it, and what is
still more extraordinary, to those, even, who merely
expose themselves, for a short time, to its effluvia :
a mixture of mx of this oil with f℥j of almond oil,
introduced upon cotton into the ears, is serviceable
in cases of deafness, resulting from a diseased action
of the ceruminiferous glands ; it is also employed as
a local stimulant in a variety of cases : and in colic,
and obstinate constipation, it is sometimes exhibited
in the form of an enema. Dose as an anthelmintic,
f℥ss to f℥ij, repeated every eight honrs until the
worm is ejected ; in these large quantities it is more
convenient as well as more efficacious to administer
it like castor oil, floating upon some liquid vehicle :
as a diuretic or stimulant it may be given in the form
of an electuary, in doses of from mx to f℥j. Officinal Prep. *Liniment. Terebinth.* L. The Pharmacopœias direct the rectification of the oil by redistillation,* when it is commonly called *Spirit* of
turpentine, but it appears to be an unnecessary refinement.

* Scouring Drops. The peculiar odour which distinguishes oil of
turpentine, may be destroyed by the addition of a few drops of some
fragrant volatile oil, as that of lemons : a combination of this kind is
commonly sold under the name of Scouring Drops, for the purpose of
removing paint, oil, or grease, from cloth.

TINCTURÆ. L. E. D. *Tinctures.*

These consist of alcohol, or proof spirit, holding in solution one or more of those proximate principles of vegetable or animal matter, which are soluble in that menstruum, viz. *Sugar, resin, extractive, tannin, cinchonin, camphor, volatile oils, morphia, emetin, conein, elatin,* and *several acids.* The proper solvent of those bodies, termed *gum-resins,* appears to be proof spirit. The compilers of the *Codex Medicamentarius* of Paris, have defined the different degrees of spirituous strength, requisite for the full and perfect extraction of the active elements of different bodies, with great truth and nicety; thus they direct for these purposes a spirit of three different standards, viz. 36 *(Sp. gr.* ·8 37,) 32 (·856) 22, (·915) of Beaume's hydrometer; with the first are prepared the *resinous* tinctures; with the second those wherein the *resinous, extractive,* or *gummy* elements, hold nearly an equal place; and with the third those in which the latter predominate. We are moreover indebted to this committee for having set at rest a question which has been long doubtful, whether the addition of alkaline agents increase the extracting powers of the spirit ? They have, indeed, ascertained by experiment, that the reverse not frequently obtains; for instance, they found that a smaller proportion of *guaiacum* was dissolved by spirit of ammonia, than by alcohol of the same strength, and that the quantity of matter dissolved from the *root of Valerian* was the

* DUTCH, or HAERLEM DROPS. The basis of this nostrum consists of the residue of this redistillation, which is a thick, red, resinous matter, to which the name of *Balsam of Turpentine* has been given ; a preparation, however, is frequently vended as " *Dutch Drops,*" which is a mixture of oil of turpentine, tincture of guaiaeum, spirit of nitric ether, with small portions of the oils of amber, and cloves.

same in both cases. Very active substances, soluble in alcohol, are those which are more particularly adapted for tinctures, since they furnish preparations which are efficient in small doses, and very manage- able in extemporaneous prescription, such are the tinctures of *Opium, Digitalis, Hyoscyamus, Squill,* &c. and from the chemical analysis of *Elaterium,* there can be no doubt, but that a very active and useful tincture of that substance might be introduced into practice; on the contrary, substances of little activity, except in large doses, are the least adapted for this form of exhibition, as in such cases the solvent will act more powerfully on the living system, than the principles which it may hold in solution, and when continued for any length of time, will lay the founda- tion of the pernicious custom of dram drinking; such tinctures, however, are not without their value in combination; they sometimes increase the efficacy, and often corrrct the operation, or disguise the flavour of the medicines with which they may be united; for example, the cathartic tinctures, in *Formula* 9, aug- ment the purgative powers of the combination, at the same time that they correct its unpleasant operation; many other illustrations are presented in the different formulæ, for the explanation of which I must refer the student to the *Key Letters.* The addition of a tincture has likewise the effect of preserving decoc- tions and infusions from spontaneous decomposition, the *compound tincture of Cardamoms* answers such an object in the *compound decoction of Aloes.* Tinctures are sometimes made with ether, but they are generally more strongly characterised by the nature of the menstruum than by that of the substances dissolved in it, indeed ether is used in these cases, not to dissolve substances which would resist the action of

alcohol and water, but for the sake of its own direct
action on the body; thus the Edinburgh pharmacopœia
directs an *Ethereal Tincture of Aloes*, which is more
penetrating and stimulant than the alcoholic tinctures;
the London College, with the exception of the *Aromatic Spirit of Æther*, does not recognise any preparation of this nature : I have already alluded to the
Ethereal Tincture of Digitalis, of the French Codex,
than which, nothing can be more injudicious, for the
digitalis does not amount to more than 1-70th part of
the tincture, and must therefore be entirely counteracted by the stimulant effects of the menstruum.
The same objection cannot be urged against the
ethereal tinctures of *Castor*, *Musk*, and *Amber*, since
in these cases, the subject and the menstruum concur
in their mode of operation.

Tinctures derive their names from the substances
which impart activity to them, and, as the medicinal
history of each substance is detailed uuder its proper
head, it will be unnecessary to dwell at any length
upon the individual virtues of these tinctures.

1. *Prepared with Rectified Spirit.*

Tinctura Assafœtidæ. L. E. *Dose*, f3ss to f3j.
———— Benzoes Comp. L. E. D. *Balsamum
Traumaticum*, P. L. 1745. This is a combination of
Benzoin, Storax, and Tolu, with aloes; it is regarded
as a stimulating expectorant, but it is now very rarely
used, except as an application to wounds, and languid
ulcers. It is sold under the name of *Friar's Balsam*.

Tinctura Castorei. L. E. *Dose*, m xx to f3ij.
See Form. 14, 50, 70, 108, 111, 112.

Tinctura Castorei Composita. E. This is
much more active than the preceding tincture, as it
contains assafœtida, and its menstruum is ammoniated
alcohol.

TINCTURA GUAIACI. L. E. D. A simple solution
of the guaiac.

TINCTURA GUAIACI AMMONIATA. This is a solution of the guaiac in the aromatic spirit of ammonia,
and is consequently more stimulating than the preceding one, and more efficacious as a sudorific. *Dose*,
f3j to f3ij. It is worthy of remark, that nitrous acid
and the spirit of nitric ether occasion an extraordinary
decomposition in these tinctures, separating the guaiacum into coagulated masses, and imparting to the
whole an intense bluish green colour. I find that
chlorine has the same effect; but the sulphuric and
muriatic acids produce no disturbance. If equal
parts of quick-lime and powdered guaiacum be rubbed
together, and a quantity of water be poured over
them, and the mixture be allowed to stand until it
becomes fine, we shall obtain a solution of this
substance, which will mix, in any proportion, with
aqueous vehicles without decomposition, and to which
the aromatic spirit of ammonia may be subsequently
added with effect.

TINCTURA TOLUIFERÆ BALSAMI. E. D. This is
only useful as an adjunct, to impart agreeable flavour
and fragrance to other remedies.

The above tinctures, when added to water, are
instantly decomposed, the practitioner must therefore
remember, that when he prescribes them in aqueous
vehicles, it will be necessary to direct them to be
triturated with some viscid liquor, as mucilage,
previous to the addition of the water, in order to
suspend the resinous precipitate.

2. *Tinctures prepared with Spirit above Proof.*

TINCTURA ALOES COMPOSITA. L. D. *Elixir
Proprietatis.* P. L. 1720. Tincture of Myrrh is the

menstruum of the Aloes in this preparation, to which Saffron is added. *Dose*, f3j to f3ij. *Form.* 70.

Tinctura Myrrhæ. L. The strength of the spirituous solvent has been very judiciously increased in the *Editio altera* of the London Pharmacopœia, by which means a brighter tincture is obtained. It is rarely used except in astringent and detergent gargles, or as an external application to foul ulcers; diluted with water it presents us with an excellent lotion for spongy gums.*

3. *Tinctures prepared with Proof Spirit.*

Tinctura Angusturæ. D. See *Cuspariæ Cortex.*

Tinctura Aurantii. L. D. An agreeable adjunct to bitter infusions.

Tinctura Calumbæ. L. E. A valuable stomachic.

Tinctura Camphoræ Composita. *Tinctura Opii Camphorata.* P. L. 1787. *Elixir Paregoricum.* P. L. 1745. This preparation has undergone both change of name and composition in the present Pharmacopœia; its old name was thought improper from. its similarity to that of *tincture of opium,* and the *oil of aniseed* has been omitted on account of its disagreeable flavour; still, however, these perpetual changes are most distressing; the tincture, as it is now prepared,

---

* Hudson's Preservative for the Teeth and Gums. Equal parts of Tincture of Myrrh, Tincture of Bark, and Cinnamon water, to which are added Arquebusade and Gum Arabic.

Greenough's Tincture for the Teeth. The following receipt is given on the authority of Mr. Gray. Of *Bitter Almonds,* 2 oz. *Brazil Wood* and *Cassia Buds,* equal parts, half an ounce; root of the *Florentine Iris,* 2 dr.; of *Cochineal, Salt of Sorrel,* and *Alum,* equal parts, one drachm; *Rectified Spirit,* 2 pints; *Spirit of Horse Radish,* half an ounce.

Ruspini's Tincture for the Teeth. This consists of the root of the *Florentine Iris,* eight ounces.; *Cloves,* one ounce; *Rectified Spirit,* two pints; *Ambergris,* one scruple.

is very different from that which has been so long and
so generally sold under the name of *Paregoric Elixir*,
and the chemist is therefore obliged to keep both the
preparations, and to send the one, or the other, according as it may be required by the old, or new
name. One fluid ounce contains nearly two grains
of Opium, and of benzoic acid, and about one grain
and a quarter of camphor. In *doses* of fʒj to fʒiij, it
is anodyne.

TINCTURA CAPSICI. L.   It is an excellent stimulant. See *Capsici Baccæ.*

TINCTURA CARDAMOMI COMPOSITA. L. An agreeable cordial. See *Form.* 10, 88, 103.

TINCTURA CASCARILLÆ. L. D.   It is added with
much effect to different stomachic infusions. See
Form. 94, 96, 99.

TINCTURA CATECHU. L. E. D.   A warm and
grateful astringent; very useful as an adjunct to
cretaceous mixtures in diarrhœa, &c. See *Form.* 88.
90.

TINCTURA CINCHONÆ. L. E. D.   Used as an
adjunct to the decoction, or infusion of the bark.
See *Form.* 62, 63, 97.

TINCTURA CINCHONÆ COMPOSITA.   This resembles the celebrated tincture of Huxham, and although
it contains less cinchona than the simple tincture,
yet from the addition of aromatics it is more grateful
and stomachic.

TINCTURA CINNAMOMI. L. D.   See *Form.* 29.

TINCTURA CINNAMOMI COMPOSITA. L. E. D.
As this is a combination of aromatics with cinnamon,
it is more grateful and stomachic than the simple
tincture.

TINCTURA CONII MACULATI. E.   As *Conein* is
perfectly soluble in spirit, this tincture constitutes a

very elegant and efficient form for the exhibition of *Hemlock;* I have frequently experienced its effects, when added to febrifuge mixtures, with satisfaction. The London college has not hitherto admitted it into the list of tinctures, which is to be regretted.

Tinctura Croci. E. D. It has no medicinal use, independent of its colour.

Tinctura Digitalis. L. E. D. It is a very useful form for the exhibition of this valuable plant. *Dose, m* x, cautiously increased. See *Digitalis Folia,* and *Form.* 38.

Tinctura Gentianæ Composita. L. E. An elegant stomachic bitter, but less eligible as a remedy than the infusion.

Tinctura Hellebori Nigri. This preparation was strongly advised by Dr. Mead, in uterine obstructions. *Dose, m* xxx to f3j. See *Hellebori Radix.*

Tinctura Humili. L. E. It is supposed to possess the tonic and narcotic properties of the hop. *Dose,* f3ss to f3iij.

Tinctura Hyoscyami. L. This is a much more powerful narcotic than the preceding tincture; and it is not liable to affect the head, nor to produce that disturbance in the bilary secretions which so inevitably follows the use of opium. *Dose,* f3ss to f3ij.

Tinctura Jalapæ. L. E. As the activity of Jalap does not reside in any one principle, but depends upon the combination of its gum, extractive, and resin, *proof* spirit is, of course, its appropriate solvent: and the resulting tincture is therefore an active purgative, but it is rarely administered except as an *adjuvant,* to cathartic combinations. *Dose,* f3j to f3ss. See *Form.* 9, 14.

TINCTURA KINO. L. E. D. This is little else than a solution of *Tannin;* it is however less astringent than the tincture of Catechu. *Dose,* fʒi to fʒij.

TINCTURA LYTTÆ. L. *Tinct. Cantharides Vesicatoriæ.* E. *Tinct. Cantharides.* D. This tincture is highly stimulating, acting with great energy upon the urinary organs; it therefore offers a resource in gleets, fluor albus, incontinence of urine, &c. it has also proved serviceable as a highly stimulating diuretic, in cases of *Hydrops Ovarii.* See *Form.* 44. *Dose, m* x to fʒj, given in some demulcent infusion; it is likewise employed with advantage, as a stimulating embrocation, and rubefacient, in conjunction with *soap,* or camphor *liniment.*

TINCTURA OPII. L. E. D. This is at once a most convenient and elegant form for the exhibition of opium; *m* xix contain one grain of opium. See *Opium,* and *Form.* 13, 14, 35, 38, 50, 63, 79, 108, 117, 119, 120. As an external application, when rubbed upon the skin, it produces anodyne effects, and it is said that these effects are very much increased by combining it with acetic acid; an *acetate of morphia* is probably thus produced.

TINCTURA QUASSIÆ EXCELSÆ. E. D. The bitter principle of this root, *Quassin,* is completely extracted by proof spirit.

TINCTURA RHEI. L. E. D. Less purgative, but more astringent and aromatic than the infusion. That made with the *East Indian* variety, is of a deeper colour, with a tinge of brown.

TINCTURA RHEI COMPOSITA. L. A cordial, used principally as an adjunct to saline purgatives. *Dose,* fʒvj to fℨj; to produce purgative effects; from fʒj to fʒij, to act as a stomachic.

The Edinburgh Pharmacopœia directs two compound tinctures of Rhubarb for similar purposes, viz. *Tinct. Rhei et Aloes*, and *Tinct. Rhei et Gentiunœ*.

TINCTURA SCILLÆ. L. E. D. *Dose* mx to xxx. See *Form*: 3, 37.

TINCTURA SENNÆ. L. E. *Dose* fʒij to ʒj. See *Form*: 9.

TINCTURA SENNÆ COMPOSITA. E. In this tincture, the Senna is quickened by Jalap. *Dose* fʒij to fʒj.*

TINCTURA SERPENTARIÆ. L.E.D. *Dose* fʒi to fʒiij. It is principally employed as a stimulating adjunct to the infusion or decoction of Cinchona, in typhoid fevers.

TINCURA VALERIANÆ. L.D. It is only used as an adjunct to the infusion of Valerian.

TINCTURA VALERIANÆ AMMONIATA. L.D. This tincture is not more highly charged with the principles of the Valerian than the foregoing one, but as the ammonia corresponds with it in virtue, it is probably more powerful. *Dose* fʒi to fʒij. See *Form*: 111, 112.

TINCTURA ZINGIBERIS. L. D. A highly stimulating preparation. See *Form*: 99.

TINCTURA FERRI AMMONIATI. L.

As this is merely a spirituous solution of the *Ferrum Ammoniatum*, the title of tincture is improperly applied to it; it seems moreover to be a very superfluous preparation.

---

* DAFFY'S ELIXIR. This is the *Tinctura Sennæ Composita*, with the substitution of treacle for sugar candy, and the addition of anniseeds. Different kinds of this nostrum are sold, under the names of DICEY'S DAFFY, and SWINTON'S DAFFY; but they differ principally in some subordinate minutiæ, or unimportant additions.

TINCTURA FERRI MURIATIS. L. E. D.

QUALITIES. *Colour*, brownish yellow; *Taste*, styptic; *Odour*, very peculiar. CHEMICAL COMPOSITION. It is an alcoholic solution of muriate of iron; the iron being in the state of *per-oxide*. INCOMPATIBLE SUBSTANCES. *Alkalies* and their *carbonates ; the infusions of astringent vegetables*; *mucilage of gum arabic* : by this latter substance it is precipitated in gelatinous flakes. MED. USES. It is one of the most active preparations of iron which we possess, and it moreover appears to exert a specific influence upon the urinary organs. Mr. Cline informs us that mx, given every ten minutes, until some sensible effect is produced, afford, in dysuria, speedy relief; in hemorrhage from the bladder, kidneys, or uterus, it acts as a powerful styptic. See *Form*: 42, 70. Externally, it is very efficacious in destroying venereal warts, either used alone, or diluted with a small portion of water. *Dose* mx to fʒss, or fʒj.

TORMENTILLÆ RADIX. L.E.D. (Tormentilla Officinalis.)
Tormentil Root.

QUALITIES. This root is knotty, externally blackish, internally reddish ; *Odour*, slightly aromatic; *Taste*, austere and styptic. CHEMICAL COMPOSITION. Its active matter is chiefly *Tannin*, and, except galls, and catechu, it appears to contain a larger proportion than any other vegetable astringent. SOLUBILITY. Boiling water extracts all its virtues, as also does spirit. INCOMPATIBLE' SUBSTANCES. *olutions of Isinglass, the Salts of Iron ; Alkalies* and *Alkaline Earths*. MED. USES. It has been chiefly used in diarrhœa, and it is very efficacious in that, which is so frequently attendant on pthisis. Dr. Fordyce recommends its union with Ipecacuan, by which combination, he observes, we shall astringe the vessels of the intestines, and, at the same time, relax those of the skin. See *Introductory Essay*, p. 13. Forms of Exhibition. In substance, or in decoction, made by boiling ℥j of the root in oiss of water until reduced to oj. Dose of the substance in powder, ℈ss to ℈j : of the above decoction f℥j thrice a day. Officinal Prep. *Pulv : cret : comp :* L.

TOXICODENDRI FOLIA. L.E.
(Rhus Toxicodendron) *Sumach.*
Leaves, or *Poison Oak.*

Qualities. The leaves are inodorous, but have a sub-acrid taste. Chemical Composition. Gallic acid, tannin, and a certain acrimonious matter, upon which the virtues of the plant depend, and which, according to Van Mons, is disengaged from the leaves in the state of gas, during the night, or whilst they do not receive the direct rays of the sun. Med. Uses. Dr. Alderson of Hull introduced the leaves of this plant to notice, in whose hands they proved successful in several cases of paralysis; the same results however have not been obtained by other physicians; the plant has therefore fallen into disuse, and ought, in deference to public opinion, to be removed from the materia medica.

TROCHISCI. E. *Troches,* or *Lozenges.*

As these are regarded as objects rather of confectionary than of pharmacy, the London and Dublin colleges have not condescended to notice them; the Edinburgh pharmacopœia, however, contains several

formulæ for their preparation, and as the form of
lozenge offers a very commodious and efficacious
method of administering certain remedies, the theory
of its operation deserves some notice in the present
work. It is principally useful in cases where it is an
object that the remedy should pass *gradually* into the
stomach, in order to act as powerfully as possible
upon the pharynx and top of the trachea, as in certain demulcents, or astringents; for instance, *Nitre*,
when intended to operate in relaxed or inflamed states
of the tonsils, is best applied in this manner; so is
Sulphate of Zinc, in chronic coughs, attended with
inordinate secretion. In order to retard as long as
possible the solution of the lozenge in the mouth, it
ought to be composed of *several* demulcent substances,
such as farinaceous matter, sugar, gum, and isinglass;
for such a mixture will be found to answer the purpose better than any *one* of these articles taken by
itself; (see *Introductory Essay*, p. 4.;) thus the farinaceous matter will prevent the sugar and the gum
from being so soon dissolved; the viscidity of the
sugar and gum will prevent the farinaceous matter
from being swallowed so soon as it would otherwise
be; and the isinglass will give a softness to the whole,
and thus prevent any sharp points from stimulating
the membrane.

TUSSILAGO.   (Tussilago Farfara) *Coltsfoot.**
                     (*Folia, Flores.*)

This plant has been regarded as a powerful expectorant, from the earliest ages; it is, at present, only

* BRITISH HERB TOBACCO. The basis of which is *Coltsfoot*; this appears to have had a very ancient origin, for the same plant was
smoked through a reed in the days of Dioscorides, for the purpose of
promoting expectoration, and was called by him βηγίον from βηξ,
tussis, whence *Tussilago*.

valued for the mucilage which it affords; a handful
of the leaves boiled in oij of water, until reduced to
oj, will furnish, by the addition of a little sugar candy,
a very grateful demulcent.

VALERIANÆ RADIX. L.E.D.

(Valeriana Officinalis) *Valerian Root.*
     Sylvestris.

QUALITIES. *Odour,* strong, peculiar, and unpleasant; *Taste,* warm, bitter, and sub-acrid. CHE-
MICAL COMPOSITION. Extractive, gum, resin, fecula,
tannin, and a peculiar essential oil, which seems to
contain camphor, and on which its virtues probably
depend. SOLUBILITY. Its active matter is extracted
by boiling water, alcohol, and the solutions of the
pure alkalies. INCOMPATIBLE SUBSTANCES. *The
salts of iron.* MED. USES. It is antispasmodic, tonic,
and emmenagogue; and it is highly beneficial in
those diseases which appear to be connected with a
morbid susceptibility of the nervous system, as in
hysteria, hemicrania, and in some species of epilepsy;
and it would appear that its virtues, in such complaints, may be frequently increased by combining
it with cinchona. FORMS OF EXHIBITION. The
form of powder is the most effectual, and next to this,
a strong tincture made with proof spirit; by decoction
its powers are considerably impaired; and, consequently, the extract is an inefficient preparation.
DOSE of the powder Ɵj to ʒj; when the flavour dis-
gusts, the addition of a small portion of *mace* or *cinnamon,* will be found to disguise it. See *Form:* 93,
112. OFFICINAL PREP: *Infus: Valerian:* D. *Tinct:
Valerian:* L.D. *Tinct: Valerian: ammoniat:* L.D.
ADULTERATIONS. The roots of a species of *crowfoot*

are sometimes mixed with those of valerian; they
may be distinguished by a caustic taste on chewing
them; the roots have also often a disagreeable smell,
from the urine of cats, who are allured and delighted
by their odour; and they are sometimes inert, from
not having been taken up at a proper season, or from
not having been carefully preserved.

VERATRI RADIX. L. E. (Veratrum Album)
HELLEBORUS ALBUS. D.
White Hellebore Root.

QUALITIES. *Odour*, strong, and disagreeable;
Taste, bitter, and very acrid; by drying, the odour is
dissipated, and in this state it is found in the shops.
SOLUBILITY. Its active principles are soluble in
water, alcohol, and the alkalies. MED. USES. The
effects of this root are extremely violent and poisonous; the ancients employed it in various obstinate
cases, but they generally regarded it as their last resource; it acts as a violent emetic, and cathartic,
producing bloody stools, great anxiety, tremors, and
convulsions. Etmuller says, that the external application of the root to the abdomen, will produce vomiting; and Schroeder observed the same phenomenon
to take place in a case where it was used as a suppo-
sitory; notwithstanding these effects however the
veratrum has been very safely and successfully administered in cases of mania, epilepsy, lepra, and
gout: * but the most ordinary use of white hellebore

* In the former editions of this work, I stated the probability of the
veratrum being the active ingredient of the EAU MEDICINALE, and,
upon the authority of Mr. James Moore, I inserted a formula for its
preparation; subsequent enquiry however, has shewn the fallacy of

is as a local stimulant, as an adjunct to errhine powders, or in the form of decoction, as a lotion; or
mixed with lard, as an ointment in scabies,* and herpetic eruptions : great caution however is required
in its application, for several authors affirm, that as
an errhine, it has caused abortions, floodings which
could not be restrained, and fatal hemorrhages from
the nose. Dose, gr.iij to v, obtunded by the addition
of twelve times its weight of starch, a pinch of which
may be taken for several successive evenings ; for internal administration it ought not to exceed gr. ij.
OFFICINAL PREP : *Decoct: Veratri.* L. *Tinct: Veratri albi.* E. *Unguent: Veratri :* * L. *Unguent: Sulphur : comp:* L.

VINUM. *Wine.*

The term wine is more strictly, and especially,
applied to express the fermented juice of the *Grape,*
although it is generally used to denote that of *any*
sub-acid fruit. The presence of *Tartar* is, perhaps,
the circumstance by which the grape is most strongly
distinguished from all the other sub-acid fruits that
have been applied to the purpose of wine making ;
the juice of the grape, moreover, contains within
itself, all the principles essential to vinification, in
such a proportion, and state of balance, as to enable
it, at once, to undergo a regular and complete fermentation, whereas the juices of other fruits require

---

this opinion; but the fact of the medicinal efficacy of the *veratrum*,
when combined with opium, in the cure of gout, remains incontro-
vertible.

* EDINBURGH OINTMENT. The principal ingredients of which are
the *White Hellebore* and *Muriate of Ammonia.*

artificial additions for this purpose ; and the scientific
application, and due adjustment of these means, constitute the art of making wines.* It has been remarked, that all those wines that contain an excess
of malic acid, are of a bad quality, hence the grand
defect that is necessarily inherent in the wines of this
country, and which leads them to partake of the properties of cider, for in the place of the *tartaric* the
malic acid always predominates in our native fruits.

The characteristic ingredient of all wines is *Alcohol,*
and the quantity of this, and the condition or state
of combination in which it exists, are the circumstances
that include all the interesting and disputed points of
medical enquiry. Daily experience convinces us that
the same quantity of alcohol, applied to the stomach,
under the form of natural wine, and in a state of
mixture with water, will produce very different effects
upon the body, and to an extent which it is difficult
to comprehend ; it has, for instance, been demonstrated, that Port, Madeira, and Sherry, contain from
one-fourth to one-fifth their bulk of alcohol, so that
a person who takes a bottle of either of them, will
thus take nearly half a pint of alcohol, or, almost a
pint of pure brandy ! and, moreover, that different
wines, although of the same specific gravity, and
consequently containing the same absolute proportion
of spirit, will be found to vary, very considerably, in
their intoxicating powers ; no wonder then, that such
results should stagger the philosopher, who is naturally unwilling to accept any tests of difference from

* For an account of which the reader is referred to a most ingenious,
and interesting Essay, by Dr. Macculloch, entitled, " *Remarks on the Art
of making Wine, with suggestions for the application of its Principles to the improvement of Domestic Wines.*

the nervous system, which elude the ordinary resources of analytical chemistry; the conclusion was
therefore drawn, that alcohol must, necessarily, exist
in wine, in a far different condition from that in which
we know it in a separate state, or in other words, that
its elements only could exist in the vinous liquor, and
that their union was determined, and consequently
alcohol produced, by the action of distillation. That
it was the *product*, and not the *educt* of distillation,
was an opinion which originated with Rouelle, who
asserted that alcohol was not completely formed, until
the temperature was raised to the point of distillation;
more lately, the same doctrine was revived and pro-
mulgated by Fabbroni, in the memoirs of the Florentine Academy. Gay Lussac has, however, silenced
the clamorous partisans of this theory, by separating
the alcohol, by distillation at the temperature of 66°
Fah. and by the aid of a *vacuum*, it has since been
effected at 56°. besides, it has been shewn, that by
precipitating the colouring matter, and some of the
other elements of the wine, by *sub-acetate of lead*, and
then saturating the clear liquor with *sub-carbonate of
potass*, the alcohol may be completely separated without any elevation of temperature; and by this ingenious expedient Mr. Brande has been enabled to
construct a table, exhibiting the proportions of combined alcohol which exist in the several kinds of
wine: no doubt therefore can remain upon this subject, and the fact of the difference of effect, produced
by the same bulk of alcohol, when presented to the
stomach in different states of combination, adds another striking and instructive illustration to those
already enumerated in the course of this work, of the
extraordinary powers of chemical combination, in
modifying the activity of substances upon the living

2 D 2

system. In the present instance, the alcohol is so combined with the extractive matter of the wine, that it is probably incapable of exerting its full specific effects upon the stomach, before it becomes altered in its properties, or, in other words, *digested:* and this view of the subject may be fairly urged in explanation of the reason, why the intoxicating effects of the same wine are so liable to vary, in degree, in the same individual, from the peculiar state of his digestive organs at the time of its potation. Hitherto we have only spoken of *pure* wine, but it is essential to state, that the stronger wines of Spain, Portugal, and Sicily, are rendered marketable in this country by the addition of *Brandy,* and must consequently contain *uncombined* alcohol, the proportion of which, however, will not necessarily bear a ratio to the quantity added, because, at the period of its admixture, a renewed fermentation is produced by the scientific Vintner, which will assimilate and combine a certain portion of the foreign spirit with the wine: this manipulation, in technical language, is called *fretting-in.* The free alcohol may, according to the experiments of Fabbroni, be immediately separated by saturating the vinous fluid with *sub-carbonate of potass,* while the combined portion will remain undisturbed : in ascertaining the fabrication and salubrity of a wine, this circumstance ought always to constitute a leading feature in the enquiry ; and the tables of Mr. Brande would have been greatly enhanced in practical value, had the relative proportions of *uncombined* spirit been appreciated in his experiments, since it to *this,* and not to the *combined* alcohol, that the injurious effects of wine are to be attributed. " It is well known," observes Dr. Macculloch, " that diseases of the liver are the most common, and the most formidable of

those produced by the use of *ardent* spirits; it is
equally certain, that no such disorders follow the
intemperate use of *pure* wine, however long indulged
in : to the concealed, and unwitting consumption of
spirit, therefore, as contained in the wines commonly
drank in this country, are to be attributed the excessive prevalence of those hepatic affections which are,
comparatively, little known to our continental neighbours." Thus much is certain, that their ordinary
wines contain no',alcohol, but that which is disarmed
of its virulence, by the prophylactic energies of combination.

The odour, or *bouquet*, and flavour, which distinguish one wine from another, evidently depend upon
some volatile and fugacious principle, soluble in
alcohol; this in sweet and half fermented wines, is
immediately derived from the fruit, as in those from
the *Frontignan* and *Muscat* grapes; but in the more
perfect wines, as in *Claret, Hermitage, Rivesaltes*, and
Burgundy, it bears no resemblance to the natural
flavour of the fruit, but is, altogether, the product of
the vinous process; and in some wines it arises from
the introduction of flavouring ingredients, as from
almonds in Madeira wines, as well as in those of
Xeres, and Saint Lucar, and hence their well known
nutty flavour: among the ancients it was formerly,
and in modern Greece it is to this day, the fashion to
give a resinous flavour, by the introduction of Turpentine into the casks.

Wines admit of being arranged into four classes.

1. SWEET WINES. Which contain the greatest
proportion of extractive and saccharine matter, and
generally the least ardent spirit, though this is often
rather disguised than absent: as in these wines, a

proportion of sugar has remained unchanged during
the process of vinification, they must be considered as
the results of an imperfect fermentation, and are, in
fact, mixtures of wine and sugar; accordingly, whatever arrests the progress of fermentation, must have a
tendency to produce a sweet wine; thus, boiling the
must, or drying the fruit, will by partially separating
the natural leaven, and dissipating the water, occasion such a result, as is exemplified by the manufacture of the wines of Cyprus, the *vino cotto* of the
Italians, and the *vinum coctum* of the ancients, by
that of *Frontignac*, the rich and luscious wines of
Canary, the celebrated *Tokay*, *Vino Tinto* (Tent of
Hungary,) the Italian *Montefiascone*, the Persian
Schiras, the *Malmsey wines of Candia, Chio, Lesbos*, and
Tenedos, and those of the other islands of the Archipela-
go. The wines of the ancients, as Chaptal observes, were
so concentrated by boiling, that they rather deserve
the name of extracts, or syrups, than that of wines;
they must have been very sweet, and but little fermented; apparently, to remedy this, they were kept
for a great length of time; according to Aristotle and
Galen, seven years was the shortest period necessary
for keeping wine before it was fit to drink, but wines
of a century old were not uncommon at the tables of
the luxurious citizens of ancient Rome, and Horace
boasts of his drinking *Falernian*, born, as it were, with
him, or which reckoned its age from the same consuls.

2. SPARKLING OR EFFERVESCING WINES, as
Champagne, are indebted for their characteristic properties to the presence of carbonic acid; they rapidly
intoxicate, in consequence of the alcohol, which is
suspended in, or combined with this gas, being thus
applied in a sudden and very divided state to a large

extent of nervous surface; for the same reason, their effects are as transitory as they are sudden.

3. D R Y A N D L I G H T. These are exemplified by the more esteemed German wines, as *Hock, Rhenish, Mayne, Moselle, Necker,* and *Elsass,* and those highly flavoured wines, *Burgundy, Claret, Hermitage,* &c. They contain a very inconsiderable degree of ardent spirit, and combine with it the effect of an acid.

4. D R Y A N D S T R O N G, as *Madeira, Port, Sherry,* &c. The name *Sec,* corruptly written Sack, signifies dry; the *Sec* wine prepared at Xeres,* in Spain, is called according to our orthography *Sherris,* or *Sherry.* In the manufacture of Sherry, *Lime†* is added to the grapes, a circumstance, observes Dr. Macculloch, apparently conducive to its well known dry quality, and which probably acts by neutralizing a portion of *malic,* or *tartaric* acid.

By the adulteration and medication of wines, three principal objects are attempted, viz. 1. *To give them strength,* which is effected by adding any ardent spirit; but the wine is slowly decomposed by it. 2. *To perfect or change their colour.* It is very usual to change *white* wines, when they have grown brown or rough, into *red* wines, by means of sloes, or other colouring matter. 3. *To lessen, or remove their acidity.* It is well known that lead in different forms has frequently been employed for this purpose; the practice however is attended with most dangerous consequences; but which Dr. Macculloch is inclined to believe has been over-

---

* ξηρος signifies *dry.* This is a curious coincidence.

† The *Sack* of Shakespeare was probably *Sherry*; a conjecture which receives additional strength from the following passage.

Falstaff. — "You rogue, here's *lime* in this Sack too: There is nothing but roguery to be found in villainous man: yet a coward is worse than a cup of sack with *lime* in it; a villainous coward."

rated, since the compounds which this metal forms with the tartaric and malic acids are insoluble ; but against this argument, the decisive results of experience may be opposed, and Fourcroy conceived, that by the addition of lead, a soluble triple salt, an *aceto-tartrate of lead*, was produced. The fraud may be easily detected by the test * invented by Dr. Hahnemann. The ancients, it appears, were acquainted with this property in Lead, for according to Pliny, the Greeks and Romans improved the quality of their wines by immersing a plate of lead in them.‡ Wine, as a pharmaceutical agent, is employed to extract several of the principles of vegetables, and to dissolve certain mineral bodies : as a solvent, however, it is liable to many serious objections, as inequality of strength, and uncertainty of composition ; thus, sound, and perfectly fermented, dry wine as *Sherry*, is frequently unable to dissolve iron, while tartarized antimony is instantly decomposed by every other. As a menstruum, to obtain an extract, it is quite inadmissible, on account of the residuum which it leaves by evaporation.

VINUM ALOES. L. E. D. This solution contains all the virtues of the Aloes, and is more agreeable than the tincture. It is a warm stomachic in doses of

---

* Expose equal parts of sulphur and powdered oyster shells, to a white heat for fifteen minutes, and, when cold, add an equal quantity of cream of tartar : these are to be put into a strong bottle with common water to boil for an hour ; and the solution is afterwards to be decanted into ounce phials, adding 20 drops of muriatic acid to each. This liquor will precipitate the least quantity of Lead, from wines, in a very sensible black precipitate. As Iron might be accidentally contained in the wine, the muriatic acid is added to prevent its precipitation.

‡ Lead will not only correct the acidity of wines, but remove the rancidity of oils: a property which is well known to Painters, and which affords an expedient for making an inferior olive oil pass for good.

f℥j to f℥ij, and a stimulating purgative when given from f℥j to f℥ij.

VINUM FERRI. L. D. When prepared according to the London college, each pint is stated to contain 22 grains of the red Oxide of Iron ; the strength however must, in every case, depend upon the quantity of *tartar* contained in the wine. Very dry Sherry is frequently incapable of acting upon the iron, until a small proportion of Cream of Tartar be added to it; would it not therefore be adviseable to direct at once a given portion of *ferrum tartarizatum* to be dissolved in wine? The Dublin formula is more eligible than that of the London Pharmacopœia, since it directs the use of *Rhenish* wine, instead of Sherry, as a solvent; and iron *wire* in preference to iron *filings*; this last circumstance is important, for the purest iron can only be drawn, and this is most easily acted upon by the super-tartrate of potass. *Med. Uses.* It is the least unpleasant of all the preparations of iron, and its medicinal activity is supported by the testimony of ages, for it is one of the oldest preparations with which we are acquainted. *Dose* f℥j to f℥ss.

VINUM IPECACUANHÆ. L.E.D. The virtues of this root are completely extracted by Wine. *Dose* as an emetic from f℥ij to f℥ss : as a diaphoretic from mxx to xl. *See Form.* 1, 51.

VINUM OPII. L. E. This is a vinous solution of the *extract* of Opium, combined with various aromatics, which are supposed to modify the effects of the opium, while, by the substitution of the extract, for the crude of opium, it is considered as being less likely to disturb the nervous system. I submit, whether the views offered under the history of Wine respecting the relative effects of combined and uncombined Alcohol, might not lead us, by analogy, to prepare a more efficient *vinum opii*, and a preparation less likely to affect the stomach : by adding the opium to the wine during its state of fermentation, it would enter into intimate union with its elements, in the same way that brandy is incorporated, by the technical manipulation of *fretting in* : this suggestion is also sanctioned by the generally acknowledged superiority of the *Black Drop*, which I have little doubt is indebted for its peculiar efficacy to the state of combination in which the *acetate of morphia* exists in the vinous menstruum. See p. 313. The present preparation is nearly analogous to the celebrated *Liquid Laudanum* of Sydenham, and its degree of narcotic power is nearly the same as that of the ordinary tincture.

VINUM VERATRI. L. Since the discovery of the real nature of the *Eau Medicinale*, this preparation has fallen into disuse, and might be now removed, to make room for a *Vinum Colchici*.

ULMI CORTEX. L. E. D. (Ulmus Campestris).

Elm Bark.

QUALITIES. *Odour*, none ; *Taste*, slightly bitter, and mucilaginous. CHEMICAL COMPOSITION. Gum, extractive, gallic acid, and super-tartrate of potass. SOLUBILITY. Water is its appropriate solvent. MED. USES. It has been commended in hepetic eruptions, but in the hands of Dr. Willan and others, it has not proved successful ; it is one of those articles that might be discarded from our pharmacopœia with much propriety. OFFICINAL Prep : *Decoct: Ulmi.* L. D.

UNGUENTA. L. E. D. *Ointments.*

These are unctuous substances, analogous to *ce-rates*, except in consistence, which is much less firm, and scarcely exceeds that of butter : formerly, ointments were numerous, and complicated in their composition, and surgeons adapted, with much technical formality, different ointments to answer different indications : this practice however has undergone a very judicious reform, and it is now well understood, that *in general*, all that is required- in an ointment is a suitable tenacity and consistence, to keep the parts to which it may be applied soft and easy, and at the same time, to exclude from them the atmospheric air; in some cases, however, these simple compositions are made the *vehicles* for more active remedies, as in the following preparations, *viz.* UNGUENTUM ELEMI COMPOSITUM. L. The elemi and turpentine in this ointment, render it stimulant and digestive. UNGUENTUM HYDRARGYRI FORTIUS. L. The precise nature of this compound does not appear to have been known until the late researches * of Mr. Donovan (*Annals of Philosophy, November* 1819,) which pro-

---

* It is to be hoped that a quantity of the ointment will be prepared according to these views, and be submitted to a more extended series of experiments. The oxide may be procured by decomposing *Calomel* by a solution of pure potass, or, by pouring a solution of the nitrate of mercury into a caustic, alkaline solution; this oxide should be at first triturated with a little lard, in the cold, to make the penetration complete, taking care that the lard be quite free from common salt, or else, *Calomel* will be the ultimate result : the mixture is now to be submitted to the action of heat, and it is very important to attend to the necessary temperature, for at 212° the oxide and lard will not unite, at 600° the oxide will be decomposed, and the mercury volatilized, at 500°, and 400°, the oxide is partially decomposed, some red oxide being formed, and mercury reduced; the proper temperature is between 300° and 320°, at which it should be maintained for an hour, and the ointment should be stirred until cold.

mise to lead to a more uniform, efficacious, and economical mode of preparing it, for they * shew, that in the officinal ointment, the mercury exists in two different conditions, in the state of metal, *mechanically mixed*, and in that of an oxyd, *chemically combined* with the lard ; and, that the medicinal activity of the ointment exclusively resides in this latter portion, the presence of metallic mercury, not only being useless, but injurious, by obstructing the absorption of the ective compound of the oxide. Mr. Donovan accordingly formed a direct chemical combination, by continually agitating together lard and black oxide of mercury at the temperature of 350° *Fah.* for two hours. At the end of the process it appeared, that every ounce of lard had dissolved, and combined with, 21 grains of oxide ; and, from the trials which have been made respecting its activity, it would seem to be as efficient as the officinal ointment, and, moreover, that it may be introduced by inunction in one third of the time. The investigation is highly important, for it not only offers the means of preparing a mercurial ointment more economically, but one more active and manageable, and less liable to that want of uniformity in strength, which must always attend a preparation in which so much labour is required for its completion, for independent of that variation in strength which will arise from imperfect triture, it is by no means an uncommon practice to use chemical means, which are not admissible, to facilitate the process,

* Four ounces, *troy*, of mercurial ointment, prepared six months before, were kept at 212°, when it separated into two distinct strata, viz. the *upper* one which was light grey. and extremely active as a medicine, and the *under* one, which upon being triturated with magnesia, yielded a large proportion of metallic mercury, and which was not found to possess any activity.

such as the addition of *Sulphur*, which is found to abridge very considerably the labour requisite for the extinction of the mercury, but it converts a portion of the metal into a *Sulphuret*, and diminishes the power of the unguent. There is however a method of facilitating the process, which is not liable to any apparent objection, but the theory of its operation is obscure; it consists in adding to the half prepared ointment a portion of that which has been long kept; which appears to act as a *leaven* to the whole mass.

The following table exhibits the relative quantity of mercury contained in each of the different ointments directed by the British Pharmacopœiæ, and in that prepared according to the process of Donovan.

One Drachm { *stronger ointment* contains of Merc : 30 grs.
of the Lond : { *weaker ointment* .... 10·—
of the Edinb : *common ointment* .... 12 —
of the Dub : { *stronger ointment* .... 30 —
{ *weaker ointment* .... 20 —
of that prepared according to Donovan .... 2½ —

Mercurial ointment furnishes the most prompt, and least exceptionable mode of impregnating the system. The external method of administering mercury, says Mr. John Hunter, is always preferable to the internal, because the skin is not nearly so essential to life as the stomach, and therefore is capable in itself of bearing much more than the stomach. The inunction is generally performed by rubbing ʒss to ʒj, on some part of the body, where the cuticle is thin, generally on the inside of the thigh, except perhaps in cases of chronic hepatitis, when it is more usually applied to the region of the liver, care being taken that the friction is continued until every particle of the ointment

disappears, and, for obvious reasons, the operation
ought, if practicable, to be performed by the patient
himself: where it has been an object to saturate the
system with mercury, as quickly as possible, I have
witnessed the advantage of confining, by means of
slips of bladder, a drachm of mercurial ointment in
each axilla, in addition to mercurial friction : camphor, turpentine, and other stimulants have been
sometimes added to the ointment, with a view of promoting its absorption ; this however is an erroneous
practice, since these acrid ingredients soon produce
pustules on the skin, which prevent the continuance
of the friction ; the warm bath is a more certain, and
less objectionable *adjuvant*, many practitioners therefore advise the body to be immersed in a warm bath,
once, and again, before the course is commenced, and
to repeat it once or twice a week, during its continuance : the length of time to be employed in a course
of mercury, and the quantity to be given, are circumstances that must, in every case, be left to the discretion of the practitioner. Mercury, when introduced
into the body, acts as a powerful stimulant, and per-
vades every part of the system, hence it is the most
powerful evacuant belonging to the Materia Medica,
and, from its stimulant operation, exerted directly or
indirectly, we are able to explain its utility in the
cure of disease, and it may be made to act according
to management and circumstances, as a tonic, antispasmodic, diuretic, cathartic, sialogogue, emmenagogue, or alterative ; but its most important operation
is that displayed in removing the diseases induced by
the syphilitic poison, although its *modus operandi* is
still buried amongst the many other arcana of physic.
The mode of directing and controlling the influence
of mercury, in the cure of the venereal disease, is

now very generally understood, and it is to be hoped
that a full confidence in its anti-syphilitic powers is as
universally maintained, in spite of the late opinions
which tend to depreciate its value, and to question its
necessity; there is however no advantage to be
gained, as was once imagined, by exciting profuse
salivation. In its next important application, that of
curing chronic affections of the liver, and dropsy, a
remark which has been suggested to me by the results
of practice, may not be unacceptable. I think I have
generally observed, that when the remedy has been
pushed to such an extent as to excite the salivary
glands to excessive secretion, the urinary organs
cease to participate in its stimulating action ; and
vice versa, for the mouth is rarely affected, when the
mercury runs off by the kidneys ; this may suggest a
precaution of some practical moment, in the treatment of dropsy, and it will be generally judicious to
accompany the administration of this metal with certain diuretics, in order to direct its operation to the
kidneys ; and it would seem, that for such an object,
those diuretic medicines should be preferred, that act
primarily on the organs, as alkalies and their combinations, squill, &c : the success of such a plan of
treatment will also depend greatly upon the exact
period at which these remedies are administered ; it
will, for instance, be right to wait until the system is,
to a certein degree, under mercurial influence. It is
hardly necessary to observe, that if the mercury runs
off by the bowel, we shall be deprived of all, or of a
great share, of the benefit to be expected. In certain
cases, the lymphatic vessels seem to resist the ad-
mittance of mercury, and to refuse the conveyance of
it to the general circultion : I have already thrown
out some vague hints upon this subject, in my Intro-

ductory Essay (p. 8), and I must refer the reader to some farther remarks, which I apprehend bear upon this question under the following article.

UNGUENTUM OXIDI HYDRARGYRI CINEREI. E. This consists of a mixture of *one part* of grey oxide of mercury, and *three parts* of axunge : it was reasonable to suppose, *a priori*, that as the whole of the mercury is, in this ointment, oxidized, its adoption would supersede the necessity of the labour required for the preparation of the common mercurial ointment, and, at the same time, afford a combination of equal, if not of superior efficacy ; but experience has not justified the conclusion, for it has been found to possess little, or no activity ; the consideration of it is therefore introduced into this work, not on account of its utility, but as an object upon which I may pause with advantage, to offer those observations which its history is so well calculated to call forth and illustrate : the circumstance which renders this preparation inert, will now receive a satisfactory explanation from the experiments of Mr. Donovan, as related in the preceding article ; in short, it is a *mechanical mixture*, instead of a *chemical combination ;* and I beg again to urge the importance of this distinction, and to offer the present example as a farther illustration in support of my opinion, respecting the preparation of certain extracts, (*see page* 217). By subjecting this ointment for some hours to a heat of 300°, it would, without doubt, become an active preparation. It is probable that the lymphatics offer less resistance to the ingress of a mineral body into the system, when it is presented to them in combination with some animal substance, which must alone be regarded as their peculiar stimulus, and the only matter which they are destined perpetually to receive and convey ;

for the same physiological reason, the lacteals may
probably take up iron with greater readiness, when
in combination with vegetable matter, than when introduced into the stomach in a more purely mineral
form ; (*see page* 228.)

UNGUENTUM HYDRARGYRI MITIUS. L. This
weaker preparation is sometimes preferred, as it irritates the skin less ; it is, however, principally used
as a topical dressing to venereal sores, and as an application to kill vermin on the body.

UNGUENTUM HYDRARGYRI NITRATIS. L.E.D.
vulgo *Citrine Ointment.* It is stimulant, detergent,
and alterative ; when diluted with an equal quantity
of simple ointment, or almond oil, it may be almost
regarded as a specific in opthalmia tarsi, smeared
upon the cilia every night at bed time.

UNGUENTUM HYDRARGYRI NITRICO-OXYDI. L.
An- excellent stimulant application, well adapted
for giving energy to indolent ulcers. If mixed with
any ointment containing resin, it loses its red colour,
passing through olive green, to black, which depends
upon the conversion of the *red*, into the *black* oxide
of mercury.

UNGUENTUM HYDRARGYRI PRÆCIPITATI ALBI.
L. Stimulant, and detergent.

UNGUENTUM LYTTÆ. L. As the active ingredient in this ointment is derived from an infusion of
the Lyttæ, it is extremely mild, and frequently inefficacious ; the *ceratum lyttæ* furnishes a more certain
application.

UNGUENTUM PICIS LIQUIDÆ. L.E.D. *Tar Ointment.* This ointment has been much extolled for the
removal of tetter, and for the cure of tinea capitis.

UNGUENTUM RESINÆ NIGRÆ. L. olim, *Ung :
Basilicum nigrum.* Digestive and stimulant.

2 E

UNGUENTUM SAMBUCI. L.D. It possesses no advantage over the simple ointment.

UNGUENTUM SULPHURIS. L. E. D. A specific in the itch. Dr. Bateman proposes a combination, equally efficacious, but which has not the same disagreeable smell; *viz.* " Take of sub-carbonate of potass, *half an ounce*; rose water, *one ounce*; red sulphuret of mercury, *one drachm*; essential oil of Bergamot, *half a fluid-drachm;* sublimed sulphur, hog's lard, of each *eleven ounces.* Mix them."

UNGUENTUM SULPHURIS COMPOSITUM. L. More stimulating than the simple ointment, from the addition of white hellebore; it is frequently found to excite too much irritation.

UNGUENTUM VERATRI. L.D. It is used for the cure of scabies, but is less certain than the ointment of sulphur.

UNGUENTUM ZINCI. L. E. D. Astringent and stimulant ; very beneficial in some species of ophthalmia, smeared upon the tarsi, every night.

UVÆ URSI FOLIA. L.E.D. (Arbutus Uva Ursi.)
Uva Ursi, Bear-berry, or *Trailing Arbutus.*

QUALITIES. *Odour,* slight, resembling that of hyson tea ; *Taste,* bitterish, and sub-astringent. CHEMICAL COMPOSITION. Tannin, mucilage, gallic acid, extractive, resin, and traces of lime. SOLUBILITY. Both water and alcohol extract its virtues. MED. USES. The ancients employed it on account of its astringency, the moderns, however, have exhibited it for various diseases, and, it would seem, without any theory respecting its *modus operandi* ; but it has at length fallen into disrepute, and, probably, with justice; when it is administered, the form of powder is preferred, and in doses from ℈j to ℨj.

ZINCI OXYDUM. L.E.D.

Oxide of Zinc.

This is occasionally used internally, as a tonic, and may be exhibited in the form of pill. It is however principally employed externally, as a mild, but efficient astringent; viz. *Ung: Zinci.* ADULTERA-TION. Dr. Roloff, of Magdeburgh, has lately discovered the casual presence of *Arsenic* in this oxide; by boiling the substance in distilled water, and assaying the solution with the ammoniaco-nitrate of silver, its presence may be instantly recognised ; *Chalk* may be detected by sulphuric acid, exciting an effervescence; and *White Lead,* by its forming an insoluble sulphate of lead. It ought to be volatile.

ZINCI SULPHAS. L.E.D.

Sulphate of Zine, olim, *White Vitriol.*

QUALITIES. *Form,* crystals, which are four-sided prisms, terminated by four-sided pyramids; they are slightly efflorescent ; *Taste,* styptic, metallic, and slightly acidulous. CHEMICAL COMPOSITION. One proportional of oxide, and one proportional of acid ; its crystals contain seven· proportionals of water. SOLUBILITY. It is soluble in 2·5 times its weight of water at 60°, and in less than its own weight of boiling water, but is quite insoluble in alcohol. IN-COMPATIBLE SUBSTANCES. *Alkalies ; earths ; hydro-sulphurets ; astringent vegetable infusions ; Milk.* MED. USES. Tonic, astringent, and, in large doses emetic, (Form. 4.) As an emetic it operates directly, and offers therefore a prompt resource in cases of poison, or where an immediate discharge from the stomach is required ; it appears to differ from most remedies of this nature, in not proving diaphoretic in smaller doses : in spasmodic* coughs it is administered with the best effects, especially when combined with camphor, or myrrh, (Form. 105) in affections of the chest, attended with inordinate secretion, I have witnessed much benefit from its exhibition, particularly when presented in the form of lozenge; and, when dissolved in water, in the proportion of grs. ij to f℥j, it forms a useful injection in fluor albus, &c. Dose, as an emetic from grs. x to ʒss—as a tonic, and astringent, from grs. j to ij. Officinal Prep. Liquor : Alum : comp : (a,) L. Solutio Sulphatis Zinci. E. Solutio Acetatis Zinci, (f.) E. Tinctura Acetatis Zinci. (f.) D. Adulterations. The white vitriol of commerce ought never to be used in medicine, without previous purification, since it generally contains the sulphates of copper and iron.

ZINGIBERIS RADIX. L.E.D. (Zinziber Officinalis.) *Ginger Root.*

Chemical Composition. Volatile oil, fecula, and resino-extractive matter ; on the first of these principles its well known flavour and odour depend ; but its pungency resides in the last. Solubility. Water, alcohol, and ether, extract its virtues. Med. Uses. It is highly stimulant, and is therefore frequently beneficial in flatulent cholic, dyspepsia, and

---

* The various quack remedies advertised for the cure of the *hooping cough* are either *Opiates*, or medicines composed of *sulphate of zinc*.

gout; it is however more generally employed as an adjunct to other remedies to promote their efficacy, or to correct their operation, (see *Form.* 40, 67,) and it is found, that it does not produce the ill effects of those species, whose virtues reside in an acrid oil. Dose, of the powder grs. x to ʒj. Officinal Prep. *Syrup: Zingib:* L. E. D. *Syrup: Rhamni: (c.)* L. *Tinct: Zingib:* L.D.* *Tinct: Cinnamom: comp: (a.)* L. *Acid: Sulphuric: aromat:* E. *Confectio Opii.* L. *Confectio Scammon: (c.)* L. D. *Infus: Sennæ. (c.)* L. *Pulvis Cinnamom: comp: (a.)* L. E. D. *Pulv: Scammon: comp: (c.)* L. D. *Pulv: Sennæ comp: (c.)* L. *Pil: Aloes.* D. *Pil: Scillæ comp:* L. D. *Vinum Aloes.* L. E. D. Adulterations. The powder is rarely met with in any tolerable degree of purity: there are two varieties of ginger in the market, viz. the *Black*, produced by scalding the root, and afterwards hastily drying it in the sun; and the *White*, being that which has been carefully washed, scraped, and gradually dried.

* Oxley's Concentrated Essence of Jamaica Ginger.—A mere solution of Ginger in rectified spirit.

Ginger Beer Powders.—White sugar ʒj ʒij, ginger grs. v, sub-carbonate of soda grs. xxvj, in each *blue paper.* Tartaric acid grs. xxx, in each *white paper.* These proportions are directed for half a pint of water.

Preserved Ginger. That from India is almost transparent, while that manufactured in Europe is always opaque, and fibrous.

FINIS.

INDEX

TO THE PATENT MEDICINES, and NOSTRUMS,

DESCRIBED IN THIS WORK.

" Arcana revelata fœtent." —BOERH.

INDEX.

London : Printed by William Phillips,
George Yard, Lombard Street.